The
ALPHA BOOK
on Cancer and Living

For Patients, Family,
and Friends

$20⁰⁰

1/96

The
ALPHA BOOK
on Cancer and Living

*For Patients, Family,
and Friends*

Published by:
The Alpha Institute
PO Box 2463
Alameda, CA 94501

1-800-866-4111

Printed in the
United States of America
98 97 96 95 94 93   5 4 3 2

Library of Congress
Catalog Card Number 93-71332

ISBN 0-9632360-0-8

ISBN 0-9632360-1-6 pbk.

The Alpha Institute Ideal

The Alpha Institute is a group of individuals united by a commitment to an ideal. That ideal is to gather and present research that will help people to deal with personal crises involving their health and their well-being. The Institute is dedicated to making available a broad spectrum of information, undistorted by personal bias, and to communicating this information in everyday language, making even the most technical concepts accessible to lay people.

We recognize that everyone is different, that there is rarely a single solution to any problem. Our ideal, then, is to provide information in a way that presents alternatives and options—in a way that promotes an attitude of discovery, a way that leads to effective solutions.

Each member of the Institute helps to make our ideal a reality. Some members are specialists, chosen for their professional expertise. Others are lay people, chosen for their direct experience of the topic under investigation. Still others are people who, because they are unfamiliar with that topic, are able to see it in a fresh light. The Alpha process, then, is a collective effort. It integrates many separate perspectives into a unified whole.

In modern society it is easy to be overwhelmed by the excess of information available to us. This excess makes it difficult for the individual to find the information that would most benefit him personally. The Alpha Institute is committed to helping to solve this problem. The Alpha Institute ideal is to present solid, impartial facts, valuable insights, and helpful concepts in a way that makes them accessible to everyone.

Director
Brent G. Ryder

Editor
Brent G. Ryder

Associate Editor
Irene Elmer

Advisory Board
Hal Zina Bennett, PhD
Vincent P. Bynack, PhD
Paula Carroll
William Collins, CPA
James W. Davis, MD
Irene Elmer
Robert Fuhr, PhD
Jane Hebler, EdD
Nancy Heck, RPT
Theresa Koetters, RN, MS
Andrew Kneier, PhD
Carol Landt, MA
Lawrence A. Lippman, MD
Pat Markley
Andrew W. Moyce, MD
Janet S. Ranney, PhD
Anne M. Rogel, PhD
Lois Ryder
Michael Samuels, MD
Robert J. Sinaiko, MD
George Somogyi, MA
Samuel D. Spivack, MD
John Toth, MS, MBA
Phillip C. Zinni III,
   DO, MS, ATC

Head Writers
Mason Drukman, PhD
Irene Elmer

Writing Team
Stephen Altschuler
Pat Farewell
Vicki Nelson
Tom Riley
Brent G. Ryder
Gloria St. John

Head Researcher
Robert Fuhr, PhD

Research Team
Monica Downer
Patricia Fitzpatrick, MS
Reina M. Galanes, PhD
Kimberly J. Jinnett, MSPH
Jean C. Mitchell
Janet S. Ranney, PhD
Julie Wellik

Head of Photography
Al Wright

Art Director
Suzanne Anderson-Carey

Elfriede Adams
A.H. Alexander, MD
Katie Allen, RN
Stephen Altschuler
Dennis Aman
Ann Anderson
Cherie Anderson
Kare Anderson
Michael Ashburne
Beth Ashley
Ruth Ayer
Carly Ayres
Mark J. Azevedo
Rev. Darrold Barber
Mary Barnett
Gayle Bartolomei
Chick Bataille
Julie Benbow
Nancy A. Bennett, MS, RD
William L. Berg
Rick Bernardo
Paul Brenner, MD
W. Douglas Brodie, MD
Dennis Brown
Marie Butler
Grant Butterfield
Vincent P. Bynack, PhD
Linda Campbell
Paula Carroll
James P. Carse, PhD
Alice Challen, MD
John Chapman
Linda Cohn
William Collins, CPA
Carol Costello
Myrna Cozen
Kelly F. Crane, MBA, CFP
Laurie Cross
Sharlynn Crutcher
Barney Currer
James W. Davis, MD
Martha M. Davis
Michelle DeMarta
Ellen L. Denebeim
Grayce DeWeese

Ralph J. DiClemente, PhD
Ricki Dienst, PhD
Robin K. Dorn
Monica Downer
La Vera Crawley Draisin, MD
Mason Drukman, PhD
Kay Dyer
Dick Elliot
Donna Epstein
Pat Farewell
Sheva Feld, PhD
Patricia Fitzpatrick
Betsy Ford
James W. Forsythe, MD
Carol Freed
Jay and Barbara Fritz
Robert Fuhr, PhD
Charles Fuhrman
Reina M. Galanes, PhD
Yvette Gan
Johana Garrison
Paul Geffner
Eric Gilsenan
Pat Gisonno
Lisa Goldoftas
Norman N. Goldstein, EdD
Kristen Gomez
Julien M. Goodman, MD
Melissa Gosland, MD
Kathy E. Goss
David Grassetti, PhD
Marge Gray
Diane Greenleaf
Morris Grossman, PhD
Melissa Gullion
Sandy Hackman
Leslie Haines
Maire Hanley
Fran Hargraves
Nan Harvey
Peter Hass
Donna Hawley
Jane A. Hebler, EdD
Nancy Heck, RPT
June Heitz
Nancy Heitz

Sheri Henderson
Joyce Herron
Kay Hickox
Lee Hilborne, MD
Chris Hill, LTC, CANG
Jerry Hill, PhD
Jeri Hobramson
Jerry Hutton, PhD
Karen Hutton
Kathryn Jackson
Ken Jacopetti
Alan Jas
Tracy Jesson
Kimberly J. Jinnett, MSPH
Barbara Johns
Barbara Johnson
Ashley O. Jones, MA
Kathryn H. Jones
Teri Kanefield
Andrew Kanka
Katherine Keiffer
Joe King
Andrew Kneier, PhD
Theresa Koetters, RN, MS
Lily Kravcisin, MA, LMFCC
Samantha Lachapelle
Judy Lakotas
Carol Landt, MA
Ann E. Lawrence
Thomas V. Leavitt, MD
Erika Leder
Lois A. Leveen
Valentina Lewis
Rev. Greg Lindsay
Lawrence A. Lippmann, MD
Andrea Lockwood
Virginia Logan
Jeff and Diane Losea
Julie Lowe
Steve Lubar
Chris MacIlvaine
Ben Maggart
Chris Maggart
Denise Manning
Richard B. Marill, DDS

Dwight Markley
Pat Markley
Caroline Marringa
Patty McCann
Elizabeth A. McCarthy
Shannon Behrens McGowan,
 MFCC
Tegan M. McLane
Polly McMahon
Joellen A. Miller
Kristiina Miller, RN
Joan Minninger
Jean C. Mitchell
Michael Modzelewski
Linda Morganstein, MA
Chris Morrison
Sandy Moses
Andrew W. Moyce, MD
Latifu Munirah, PhD
Laura Nathan, PhD
Pat Nisson
Chris Ann Ohler, DVM
Arnold and Sue Olitt
David Oliver, MD
Elizabeth O'Neal
Andy O'Neill
Ginny Paolazzi
Val Paraschak
Carol Peters
Debra Phairas
Christine Picinich
Fred Plumer
Annette Pont-Gwire, PhD
Gail Raborn
Janet S. Ranney, PhD
Anne Reinke
Linda Reister, RN
Kris Richardson
Tom Riley
Russ Robertson, MS
Anne M. Rogel, PhD
Charles Rojer, MD
Leonard Roth, MD
Eric Roudabush
Beverly Rubik, PhD

Jean Ruxton
Lois Ryder
Juana Samayoa
Suzanne G. Schaff
E.F. Schmerl, MD
Arnold Schraer
Mary Lou Schram
Karin Selbach, RN
Harry and Debra Shaich
Floyd Sharp
Kirsten Akash Simon
Robert J. Sinaiko, MD
Marilyn Smiler
Joyce J. Smith
George Somogyi, MS
Karin Somogyi
Vincent Spiaggia
Samuel D. Spivack, MD
Gloria St. John
Beth Stern
Frederick Stugard, PhD
Diane Summers
Linda Sumner
Fred and Ruth Swain
Martha Tonsing
John Toth, MS, MBA
Ursula Unger, RN
Sonja Von Kampermann
John Wadsworth
Aaron Waldier
Rev. Brian Waldier
Vickie Waldier
Dorothy Wall, MA
Debra L. Waterhouse,
 MPH, RD
Barbara M. Waxer
Paul D. Wcislo
John Wienecke
Evangeline Welch
Julie Wellik
Lari B. Wenzel, PhD
Dick Williams
John Wong, EdD
Roxann Wurst
Barbara Yoder

Gary York
Claudia T. Zdral, DC
Brad Zebrack
Joanna Zinni
Phillip C. Zinni III, DO,
 MS, ATC

ACKNOWLEDGEMENTS

Book Design
Anderson-Carey Design
Suzanne Anderson-Carey
Leslie Dickersin

Cover Design
Suzanne Anderson-Carey
Melissa Jacoby
Brent G. Ryder

Illustrator
Leslie Laurien

Production Consultants
Zipporah W. Collins
Candice Fuhrman
Michael Samuels, MD

Transcriber
Joanna Zinni

Proofreader
Catherine Cambron

Indexer
Elinor Lindheimer

Special Consultants
Debra Atlas
Stevanne Auerbach, PhD
Hal Zinna Bennett, PhD
Eileen Duhné
Karen Hutton
Bill Lekas
Jan Lekas
Floyd Sharp
Traudl Stangl
Bonnie Weiss

Table of Contents

Chapter 6: Coping: Meeting the Challenges

About This Book

In 1979 my father, Paul Ryder, was diagnosed with cancer. I found myself facing the same ordeal that you may be facing now. I needed to learn all I could about the disease, about the available treatment options. I needed to learn to deal with the emotional challenges that my father and our family faced. That is how the *Alpha Book* came to be written. It has taken the Alpha team eight years to collect this material and to present it in a way that is easy to read and reassuring to those who need it most—to you, the cancer patient, and you, the patient's family and friends.

The Alpha team includes physicians, nurses, psychologists, and other health care professionals. Above all, it includes people who have had cancer and their loved ones. In the stories these people shared with us, you will find not only practical advice but also courage, inspiration, and hope. It is with heartfelt gratitude that I thank the many people who have helped to create the *Alpha Book on Cancer and Living*.

You can use this book in two ways. You can pick it up and read it from cover to cover, going back later to reread the parts that you found especially helpful. Or you may prefer simply to thumb through the *Alpha Book* for answers to the questions that concern you the most.

The patients we interviewed helped us to develop the five concepts on which this book is based. The first concept we call the *step process*. In this process, you focus on one step—one aspect of the cancer experience—at a time. Throughout this book we show you how to use the step process to find out exactly what you are facing, to deal with the stresses that go with having cancer, to discover ways to improve your quality of life. The step process increases efficiency and

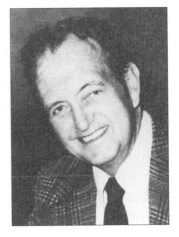

Paul Ryder

reduces anxiety. It is an invaluable problem-solving tool.

The second concept we call the *individual approach.* The people who shared their stories with us led us to realize that everyone is different. This means that no one answer is always right, that no one approach—no matter how good it is—will work for everyone. You need to find the approach, the treatment, the coping program that is right for *you.* We believe that the greatest shortcoming of most self-help books, even books that are otherwise excellent, is that they give the reader too few options—the ones that the authors found worked best for *them.* The *Alpha Book on Cancer and Living* offers you many different options. Our goal is not to provide you with "the answer" but to promote an attitude of discovery.

The third concept we call *patient responsibility.* We believe that most people do best when they participate as fully as possible in the decisions that concern their treatment and their recovery program. But since everyone is different, there are exceptions to this rule. You may choose to delegate some, or even all, of the decision making to others, if you feel that this is more appropriate for you. Our point is simply that the choice—and the responsibility—are yours.

If you are reading this book, you already appreciate the advantages of *becoming informed.* We believe that knowledge reduces fear. Knowing what you face can give you more confidence in your decisions and help to increase your sense of control. These are ways of getting in touch with hope.

This brings us to the fifth and last concept, the one we call *thinking positive.* If there is one thing we want you to learn from reading our book, it is this: you don't have to be a victim. You can assert at least some control over cancer, and over the effect that cancer has on your life. We are not saying that positive thinking cures cancer. We are saying— and we firmly believe—that a positive attitude can make a difference, and that you can even benefit from the cancer experience. As you use this book, as you listen to some of the many patients we have interviewed, we hope that you will come to share this belief.

—Brent G. Ryder
Publisher
Founder of the Alpha Institute

The Verdict Is Cancer

The Verdict
Is Cancer

Julie Benbow hadn't been feeling well. Her head ached; she couldn't sleep; she was edgy and restless. Finally the young graphic artist went to the hospital. The doctor checked her over, administered some tests, and gave his verdict: Julie had cancer of the thyroid gland.

Stunned by the news, Julie cried all the way home. "I had gone to the hospital feeling distressed in a sick, headachy way, and I came out having the world blown from underneath me."

Charles Fuhrman, a book designer, was constantly tired; he had vaguely defined pains all over his body. One day he discovered a golf ball-sized lump in his neck. His doctor told him that the lump was a cancer known as Hodgkin's disease, and that he would be under treatment "for a long, long time."

"My world dropped out," Charles told us. "You know, 'cancer,' it's a death word–the worst thing you can hear."

Paula Carroll learned that she had breast cancer at the age of forty-four, when she and her husband were busy managing a successful business. She said that getting the news was like stepping on a rake. "The handle comes up and hits you in the face. You think you're going to die. It's right here, and it's frightening."

If you have been diagnosed with cancer, or if your cancer has recurred, you know how Charles and Julie and Paula felt. You too may have been terrified. You too may have thought, *"Can this be happening to me? Why me? Maybe they made a mistake. How do I tell my family and friends? Why do I feel so guilty? How much pain will there be? I'm going to die. What about my children? What*

"My world dropped out. You know, 'cancer,' it's a death word–the worst thing you can hear."

–Charles Fuhrman

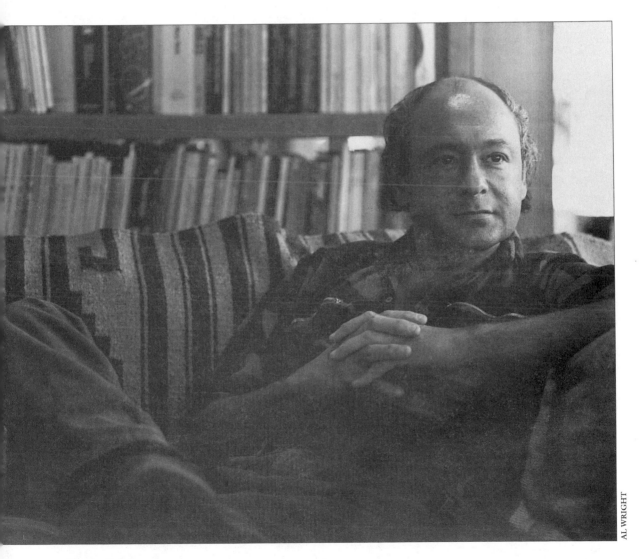

Charles Fuhrman

AL WRIGHT

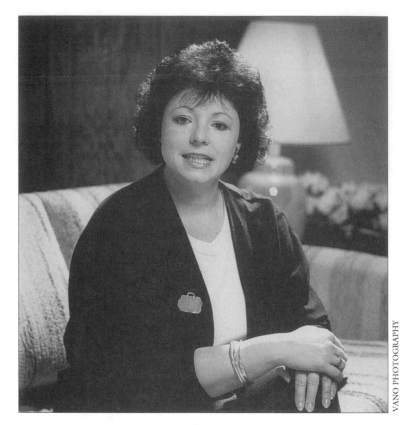

VANO PHOTOGRAPHY

Julie Benbow

> *"I had gone to the hospital feeling distressed in a sick, headachy way, and I came out having the world blown from underneath me."*
>
> **–Julie Benbow**

about all the things I wanted to do? I'm all alone. No one can help me. No one can ever know how I feel."

These thoughts are entirely natural. It would be surprising if you didn't have them. Cancer evokes a wide range of reactions–fear, anger, guilt, denial, depression, grief. And as anyone who has ever had to deal with it can tell you, cancer continually tests your courage and your strength.

The act of confronting cancer honestly and directly can help you to deal with this emotional stress. As Julie, Charles, and Paula went on to discover, their individual worlds did not dissolve overnight. They managed, slowly and painfully, to get through their initial despair. They learned to understand their condition and to make informed decisions about the future. Not only did they learn to deal with their situation, but they actually used their experience to improve the quality of their lives.

Julie Benbow, Charles Fuhrman, and Paula Carroll are three of the hundreds of cancer patients whom we interviewed for this book. With their help and that of others like them, we will try in this chapter to give you an overview of the cancer experience. This will help you to make positive decisions during the anxious period following your diagnosis. If you have already passed through this difficult period, you may still want to learn how others handled it. In this chapter we shall also introduce briefly some of the subjects that we discuss later in the book.

Making positive decisions means taking control of your illness *insofar as you are able*. It means asking the right questions. It means learning to communicate with doctors, family, and friends. It means finding the best medical care available; it means finding ongoing sources of emotional support. Above all, it means knowing that you are doing everything you can to make yourself as healthy as you can possibly be.

How Do They Know You Have Cancer? Waiting for the Results

Diagnosing cancer may be a relatively simple process. Or it may be a complicated one, involving intricate lab tests, X rays, and examinations by a whole range of specialists. Doctors usually look at the most obvious symptoms first and then decide whether further investigation is needed.

A test was performed on the lump in Charles Fuhrman's neck. A tiny bit of it was removed and sent to a *pathologist,* a physician who specializes in studying the effects of disease on body tissue. It was the pathologist who concluded that the lump was cancer.

The scientific name for such a lump is a *tumor.* Tumors may or may not be cancerous, and this can often be determined almost immediately. But not always. Pathologists may have to consult other specialists for help in confirming their findings, and in difficult cases tissue samples may be sent to a national referral center for verification.

The time you spend waiting for the test results is a time, in Charles's words, "full of horrible anxiety." Most of the cancer patients we interviewed felt that their tests should have been done faster, in a way that took their emotional needs into account. Paula Carroll, a cancer survivor who became a counselor to other cancer patients, agrees. "Doctors, hospitals, and technicians must realize," she says, that "when cancer patients are dealing with something as frightening as the possibility of death, they can't be kept waiting an indefinite period for their test results."

Paula encourages fellow patients to speak up rather than to suffer in silence. "Ask the doctor, 'When is this test going to be back? I want to know immediately. I don't want to have to wait. I need to have those results.'"

Charles Fuhrman got similar advice from a physician friend. Charles had been told that, due to scheduling problems, no date could be set for his biopsy. "I'm just sitting there," he told us, "every moment thinking the cancer is spreading." Acting on his friend's advice, he insisted on having the biopsy done at once. He got immediate results. The biopsy was done the following day, and Charles had his answer within twenty-four hours.

Do you suspect that the lab is giving you this kind of bureaucratic runaround? Some delays are unavoidable; in the most difficult cases, doctors and technicians may have to check and recheck the evidence to arrive at an accurate diagnosis. But if you think you have been waiting too long, and you don't know what is happening or why, we urge you to speak up as Paula suggests and to do it as assertively as Charles did.

You and Your Doctor: Questions, Questions, Questions

Most doctors don't go into great detail during that first discussion. Newly diagnosed cancer patients are often in a state of shock (Paula Carroll described herself as "terrified"). They may have trouble hearing what the doctor says, let alone understanding it. If you have this experience–or even if you don't–you may want to set another meeting at a later date, after you have had time to digest the news and talk things over with your family and friends.

Be Prepared

Come to this second meeting prepared to learn. Bring with you a list of written questions, a tape recorder, and, if possible, a friend or relative. This person will provide emotional support and will help you to remember what the doctor said. He or she can be, as Dr. Samuel Spivack puts it, your "reality person"–someone who can communicate regularly with your medical team and be there when you make the tough decisions.

Dr. Spivack, a highly respected West Coast oncologist, says that most doctors won't object if you use a tape recorder. "I'm always glad," he says, "when someone wants to tape my words. I never view it as a threat."[1]

The written list of questions is especially important. People under stress, Dr. Spivack says, "frequently lose their heads in a doctor's office." He feels that coming armed with a shopping list of questions is a good way to keep your wits about you. Looking back, Julie Benbow recalls that she suffered unnecessarily at the outset because "I didn't ask the right questions."

Never be embarrassed to ask questions. No question is unimportant, if it's important to you. And questioning doctors closely doesn't mean that you have to give them the third degree. Most doctors know that they will perform better, and that you will do better too, once a good dialogue has been established. Asking questions does more than satisfy your need to know. It also tells your doctor that you want to be an informed patient, an active partner in the decision-making process. As one doctor remarked to Paula Carroll, "It's so wonderful to

> *"I'm always glad when someone wants to tape my words. I never view it as a threat."*
>
> – Dr. Samuel Spivack

work with informed consumers." Dr. Spivack carries the process one step further: he asks patients to keep a diary so that they can write down their questions as they think of them. That way they won't forget what it was they wanted to ask.

What to Ask

You should raise the following questions at the first meeting after your diagnosis is made. Copy the list and take it with you, along with any other questions you may think of. Before you run through your list, however, listen carefully to what your doctor has to say. You may find that at least some of your questions will be answered even before you ask them.

The answers to these questions will give you any basic information you didn't already have. This will reduce the fear that comes from not knowing.

- What kind of cancer do I have?
- Has it spread to other parts of my body?
- What are these tests we are doing?
- How accurate are the tests?
- How soon will the results be back, and how will I be notified?
- Will more tests be required?
- Did the pathologist check his (her) findings with others?
- Is there any doubt about my diagnosis?
- How many cancers of my type do you see in a year?
- Did you consult with your colleagues before you made the diagnosis?

Next, it is best to get a general idea of the issues surrounding treatment. This subject is discussed at length in Chapter 4 and Chapter 5. Later you can make a special appointment with your doctor to decide which treatment program is right for you. For now, you should simply raise the following questions:

- What procedure (or procedures) do you recommend?
- What are my chances with this treatment?
- What are the potential risks and benefits? What are the side effects?
- Are there alternative ways to proceed?
- How much will the treatment cost?
- Can I resume my normal life after treatment?
- What might happen if I decide not to undergo treatment?

The question about resuming your normal life is directly related to the treatment you and your doctors choose. This is an important issue. A radical treatment may increase your chance of survival, but the cost to your life-style may be more than you are willing to pay. Dr. Andrew Moyce, a practicing surgeon in Oakland, California, told us how an elderly attorney with cancer of the larynx solved this problem. Surgery offered this man the best chance of a cure, but if he had surgery, he would lose his voice. After weighing the pros and cons, the attorney chose radiation therapy instead. "There are certain things I have left to do in this life," he said, "things I can't do without my voice. I'll take my chances with radiation." He lived the life he wanted for a few more years, knowing that he might have lived longer had he chosen surgery.[2]

Many of the patients we interviewed saw things differently. Some were ready to try almost anything in the hope of effecting a lasting cure. They were willing to endure being seriously disabled in order to get in as many more years as they could.

Two Points That Make a Big Difference

We conclude this section with two critical points. First, think seriously about getting a second opinion. Most doctors are more than willing to cooperate–some even find it a relief–and getting a second opinion is no longer unusual. Indeed, says Dr. Spivack, it is "always advisable"

For more on these two points, see Chapter 3.

in dealing with matters as serious as cancer. Even the very best doctor is sometimes wrong. Getting a second opinion ensures the best possible health care for you.

Second, your doctor should be someone you are comfortable with—somebody you can trust. He or she is a vital member of your health care team. Your faith in your doctor will give you confidence, and a feeling of comfort and security in the challenging days that lie ahead.

Deciphering the Terminology

See the Glossary for a list of technical terms used in this book.

Dealing with cancer means dealing with a world where everyone seems to be speaking a foreign language. The jargon comes at you thick and fast, and at times you may feel like shouting, "Why can't you say it in simple English?" But like it or not, the terminology is going to be important to you, so it's a good idea to learn some of the basics. This will help you to understand what the medical professionals are talking about.

The term *cancer* has traditionally been used to describe more than 100 different diseases located in various parts of the body. However, some researchers see cancer as a single disease with many subcategories. All researchers agree that every type of cancer involves the uncontrolled increase of abnormal new cells. These cells can destroy surrounding tissue, and they can spread throughout the body.

Carcinomas are cancers that originate in epithelial tissue, that is, in the glands, the skin, and the lining of the internal organs. Since 80 percent to 90 percent of all cancers are carcinomas, doctors sometime use the terms "cancer" and "carcinoma" interchangeably.

Sarcomas are cancers that originate in nonepithelial tissues, that is, in bone, cartilage, muscle, or fat.

A *tumor* (fig. 1) is a mass of tissue formed either by excessive cell division or by some other cause. It may or may not be cancerous. When it involves new and abnormal growth, a tumor is also called a *neoplasm*.

When doctors speak of a *primary* or *parent* tumor, they are referring to the site where the tumor first appeared,

Fig. 1. Tumors

Benign Tumor
Abnormal growth of cells (shown here surrounded by healthy cells) produces a self-contained mass with normal-looking cells.

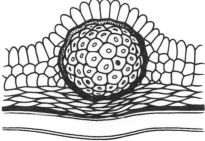

Malignant Tumor
Uncontrolled growth of cells produces a mass with mutated cells, which can break away and travel to other parts of the body.

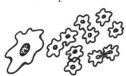

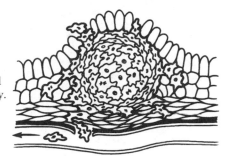

before it spread to other parts of the body. When they speak of a *secondary* tumor, they are referring to a tumor that has spread from the primary tumor to another part of the body. And an *occult* tumor is a primary tumor that cannot be found but that is known to exist because its secondary tumors have been discovered.

A *benign* tumor is an abnormal growth, but its cells—unlike cancer cells—are not reproducing rampantly or uncontrollably. Nor are they spreading into other parts of the body. However, a benign tumor may have to be removed anyway. This may be because it is damaging one or more organs as it grows, because it detracts from your appearance, or because it could become malignant later.

Being told that a tumor is *malignant* is the same as being told that you have cancer. Indeed, "malignancy" is another term for cancer.

A *biopsy* is performed to determine whether a tumor is malignant or benign. This is done by removing a bit of tumor tissue and looking at its cells under a microscope.

Fig. 2. Tumors and Metastasis

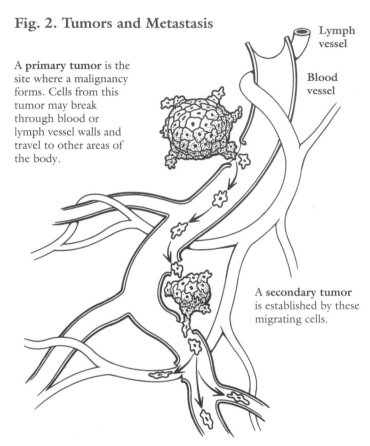

A **primary tumor** is the site where a malignancy forms. Cells from this tumor may break through blood or lymph vessel walls and travel to other areas of the body.

Lymph vessel

Blood vessel

A **secondary tumor** is established by these migrating cells.

Taking a tissue sample can mean something as simple as doing a blood test or as complicated as doing major surgery. Modern technology—CAT scans, ultrasound, and MRI (magnetic resonance imaging)—has reduced the need for diagnostic surgery, however.

You may have heard that, in the course of doing a biopsy, cancer cells are sometimes spread from the parent tumor. This is not impossible, and you may want to ask about it. But under normal conditions, the risk is exceedingly low, certainly far lower than the risk of *not* doing a biopsy when one is called for.

When cancer travels from its point of origin to other parts of the body, it is said to have *metastasized* (fig. 2). Cancer cells spread by moving through the bloodstream or the lymph system. Your treatment—and your chance of recovery—will greatly depend on whether and how much metastasis has taken place.

The *lymphatic system* (fig. 3) is separate from the bloodstream. It is made up of a series of vessels similar to blood vessels, through which an infection-fighting, plasmalike substance called *lymph* is carried. At various intervals along the channels are *lymph nodes*–usually called "glands"–where white blood cells are produced and where harmful agents such as bacteria, viruses, and even cancer cells are destroyed. You can sometimes feel the lymph nodes under your jaw, or in your armpits, abdomen, or groin. Because they act as filter stations, cancer often spreads to the lymph nodes first.

The standard treatments for cancer are surgery, radiation, chemotherapy, and hormonal therapy. *Radiation therapy* uses high-energy X rays in four ways: to effect a cure by destroying all the cancer cells, to reduce the size of the tumor before surgery, to destroy cancer cells that might remain after surgery, and to shrink certain cancers to relieve symptoms. *Chemotherapy* simply means the treatment of cancer (or any disease, for that matter) through the use of drugs. In the case of cancer, the drugs are intended–just as radiation is intended–to kill malignant cells while destroying as few healthy cells as possible. *Hormonal therapy* is often used to treat breast cancer in women and prostate cancer in men. Hormones are complex chemicals secreted by various glands. Each hormone regulates the function of certain groups of cells. The standard treatments for cancer are discussed at length in Chapter 4.

One of the newest treatments for cancer involves the *immune system,* one of the body's vital defenses against infection and disease. The pus that you see in a sore is composed partly of white blood cells fighting infection– an example of the immune system at work. *Immunotherapy* attempts to stimulate the immune system to kill or control cancerous cells.

Two more terms you may expect to encounter are *remission* and *recurrence*. Remission occupies a gray area somewhere between survival and cure. You are said to be

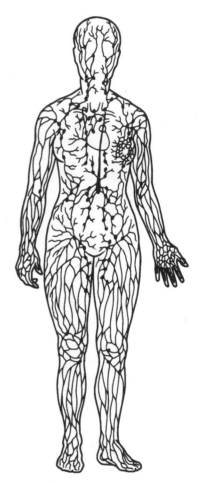

Fig. 3. Lymph Nodes and Vessels

Lymph nodes are indicated here by dark spots in the head, arm, and torso areas.

in remission if your cancer has remained inactive for any period up to five years. If it remains inactive for five years, you are said to be cured.

Sometimes the cancer reappears after a period of remission. It may reappear at its original site, or it may metastasize to a new site. In either case, you are said to have a recurrence.

Can You Be Cured?

"Doctor, what are my chances?" This was probably the first question you asked when you were told you had cancer. To answer it, your doctor relied heavily on statistics. But there are problems with using even the best statistical information, and especially with trying to apply it to a specific person. In this section we shall discuss some of those problems. But first, let's define two important terms.

Survival Rates and Cure Rates

The terms *survival* and *cure* are sometimes used interchangeably, but strictly speaking they do not mean the same thing. In discussions of cancer, the term "survival" refers to a period covering five years from the end of treatment. That is, if you are alive during any part of this period, you are said to have survived up to that point.

What is the *survival rate?* It is the percentage of people who have survived a given cancer up to a given time. It is found by dividing the number of these survivors by the total number of people who were originally diagnosed with that particular cancer.

To illustrate: suppose that 100 people have a particular cancer. If, after three years, 85 of those people are still alive, the three-year survival rate for that cancer is 85 divided by 100, or 85 percent. This statistic can be further refined by comparing only tumors of a specific size, tumors that have spread only a specific distance, tumors that have been treated with a specific therapy, and so on.

For most cancers, once five years have elapsed, the

term "cured" replaces the term "survived." Thus if you are alive five years after your cancer treatment ends, and there is no sign that your cancer has reappeared, you are said to be cured. So if 70 out of 100 people are alive and free of symptoms after five years, the *cure rate* for their type of cancer is 70 percent.

We should point out that the distinction between cure and survival is by no means universally accepted. Because cancer can recur many years after all of the symptoms have disappeared, some doctors don't *ever* like to use the term "cured." They prefer to describe *any* patient without symptoms as being in remission.

Although we speak often of cure rates and of being cured, we agree that "cure" is not an absolute concept. Some cancers do return after five years, as we have just explained. And the term doesn't indicate anything about the patient's quality of life. A cured patient may be totally disabled or playing six sets of tennis every day. Remember too that most cure rates are based on patients who have received only standard treatment. They do not include those who have received alternative treatment, or those who have received no treatment at all.

Nevertheless, statistics indicate that, in most cases, once you reach the five-year point, the odds of recurrence diminish greatly with each passing year. This is what we mean, then, when we refer to cure rates for particular cancers.

However, cure rate statistics tell only part of the story. Your actual chances depend on a host of other factors: your age, your sex, your previous medical history, your overall health and attitude, the extent to which your cancer has progressed, and your ability to undergo certain kinds of treatment. Take two people with virtually identical cancers. One is forty and can endure a long and intensive treatment program; the other is eighty, with a bad heart and weak lungs, and cannot tolerate aggressive treatment. The odds are that the first person will have a better chance of recovering than the second person.

Ask your doctor whether the statistics being cited take

all of these various factors into account. You might have, say, a 75 percent chance of being cured, even though the cure rate for your kind of cancer may be only 45 percent.

Interpreting the Numbers

"One of the worst things that we can do as cancer patients is to say, 'All right; here's my life, doctor or clinic or whatever— you take care of it.'"

—Paula Carroll

Progress in science could not take place without the use of numbers. It must be said, however, that statistics do not parade automatically in the direction of truth. They march to the beat of the person who recorded them, and sometimes they are used as a drunk uses a lamppost—more for support than for illumination.

We know, for example, of one researcher whose statistics "prove" that he has by far the best acute-leukemia cure rates in the country. Looking closely at his numbers, however, we find that his category of cured patients includes only those who have survived the first, and most dangerous, phase of treatment. Why doesn't it include the patients who didn't make it through the first phase? Because if it did, this researcher's cure rates might look like everyone else's—or maybe even worse.

We don't mean to imply that this leukemia study is typical of the profession. Most widely published cancer statistics are basically reliable, since, like most of the statistics cited in this book, they are taken from long-term national averages. Nonetheless, it is always wise to be wary. This is especially true in the area of alternative treatment, where impressive claims are often made without any evidence to back them up.

And remember that doctors cannot predict the future. When they make a *prognosis*—that is, when they try to anticipate how your cancer will progress—the best they can do is to give a rough estimate. This estimate is based on ever-changing statistics gathered from research on other patients. A degree of doubt, sometimes a lot of doubt, is inevitable when it comes to interpreting the numbers.

The fact that there *is* doubt, however, can be seen as cause for hope. The bleakest prognosis can sometimes be wrong. "Miracle" cures do happen, even when the cure rate for a given cancer is close to zero. "I have seen patients who defied the statistics," Dr. Spivack tells us. In dire cases, he says, "you should be prepared for the worst. But you should keep on hoping for the best."[3]

We agree. There are always grounds for hope. If the odds for survival are one in ten, why shouldn't you be that one? Paula Carroll suggests that if the cure rate for your type of cancer is under 50 percent, you say to yourself, "Hey...I'm going to be a winner." And Dennis Brown, a middle-aged executive whose cancer of the kidney spread to the bone, put it like this:

"I feel that I'm enough of an individual that statistics really don't apply to me. It isn't just a matter of chance. The survivors are going to survive because of factors other than just luck. They aren't going to survive because they were that one out of a hundred. They're going to survive because of the way they approach their course of treatment. Because of their attitude and strength. More than anything else, the will to be that survivor."

In medical literature, patients like Paula Carroll and Dennis Brown are referred to as *fighters*–people who are determined (sometimes belligerently determined) to beat the odds. An impressive body of research suggests that fighters do in fact tend to do better–to recover more quickly, to survive longer–than patients who passively accept their fate. And even when they don't live longer, fighters seem to improve the quality of their lives simply by engaging in the battle.

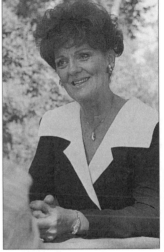

Paula Carroll

JEFFREY STEPHENS

For more on fighters, see Chapter 6 and Chapter 8.

Making Choices

Working with doctors, getting a second opinion, understanding the terminology, interpreting statistics–not an easy set of tasks, especially when you are feeling ill, uncertain, and afraid. If you feel better not dealing with these issues, if you'd rather have a friend or an advocate or your doctor make the big decisions for you, then that is what you should do. Don't feel guilty. You have the right to do whatever you decide is best for you.

You are, however, apt to feel more in control if you know what is happening to you—why certain things are being done, why other things aren't, how best to proceed under your special sct of circumstances.

Learning to Take Control

Depressed by her condition and reacting to her chemotherapy, at first Julie Benbow just wanted someone to make all her decisions for her. "I felt that I didn't have control over anything," she told us. "And I wanted somebody else to take it."

Had Paula Carroll been there, having fought through her own indecision and depression, she might have tried to persuade Julie to take control herself. "One of the worst things that we can do as cancer patients is to say, 'All right; here's my life, doctor or clinic or whatever—you take care of it,' says Paula. "We have to take an active responsibility for our health care." She believes that patients who relinquish control tend to become the victims of their own illness—and current research bears her out. Dr. Spivack feels that patients are most in control when they are part of the decision-making process. And he adds: "Anything the patient can do to improve his or her feeling of control and state of positive thinking is beneficial."[4]

Learning to take control is not always easy. For Julie, one of the biggest obstacles was depression. Part of this depression stemmed from guilt, from the idea, common to many patients, that she had somehow deserved to get cancer, that she was a "bad person." Part of it stemmed from the results of her chemotherapy. Her hair and eyelashes fell out, her skin became mottled, and her fingernails stopped growing. "Cancer is traumatic," she told us, partly because "your body is not under your control anymore." And this loss of control made her feel even more depressed.

It took six months for Julie to hit bottom. "I was so disgusted with myself," she recalled. "I was so unlike me." But the despair of hitting bottom changed Julie's thinking, led her to view her experience in a new light. She began to see that she had no reason to feel guilty, that she *could* learn to take control. She began to see that "for every cancer patient, there is hope at the end of the tunnel." And this discovery carried over into other parts of Julie's life. "You know," she told us a year later, "I *do* have some control over how I cope with the things in my life that are negative. Cancer taught me that."

For more on cancer as teacher, see Chapter 8.

Using What You Know

The best way to take control of your situation is to arm yourself with knowledge and then use it. As Dr. Spivack says, you are most in control when you have all of the facts that you need and can participate in the decision-making process.

You can begin to take control of your own situation by finding out, for example, what your rights as a patient are, and by learning how to stand up for them. You can also learn as much as possible about your condition. Here your doctor is your most important source of information. Other sources include your local library, the nearest branch of the American Cancer Society (ACS), and the National Cancer Institute (NCI) Cancer Information Service (1-800-4-CANCER). You will also find suggestions for further reading at the end of every chapter in this book.

On patients' rights, see Appendix 2.

When it comes to informing yourself about cancer, we can think of no better example than that of John Chapman, who developed bone cancer at the age of twenty-eight. When asked if he had done any research into his condition, John replied:

"I just had to know what I had. How do they treat my type of cancer? What is the prognosis? What is the likelihood of my surviving? What can I expect in my future life? Am I going to be able to have children? Will my hair grow back? Will it grow back a different color? So, yes, I did a lot of outside research."

You may not want to seek information as vigorously as John did, or feel up to doing so. Just do the best you can, remembering that your best may change from day to day, even from hour to hour, depending on how you are feeling. At the same time, you may find that merely starting to look for answers gives you new energy and improves your morale.

Finally, when it comes to using what you know, don't forget what you know about yourself. Even if you don't want to learn more about cancer, you may find it useful to examine your own reactions as you move through the course of your illness. How are you reacting to your health care team? How are you reacting to your situation? Can you let go of things that are unimportant and devote yourself to the things that matter most? Are you being realistic, yet hopeful? Concentrating on questions like these, and finding satisfactory answers, are also ways of taking control.

Using what you know, being, in John Chapman's words, "a positive force in the treatment program," can help you to feel better not only psychologically but also physically. Participating in treatment decisions can give you a sense of control over your cancer. Mounting scientific evidence indicates that this can actually affect the course of the disease. In Chapter 2 and Chapter 6 we discuss the connection between attitudes and illness, and especially the role played by mental stress.

Beyond Survival

In the course of your illness, you may find, as so many of our cancer patients did, that the question of survival – at first the crucial issue – tends to diminish in importance, while questions about the quality and meaning of life become more significant. Questions like these:

- Is there anything about my life – diet, exercise, work, stress, relationships – that I need to think about changing?
- What can I do to feel the best I possibly can today?
- What can I do to help others in my situation?

- What or who is most important to me and why?
- What are my goals in life, and how can I achieve them?
- How can I help my friends and family to deal with my situation?

There are no statistics on how patients respond to these questions, and they are not normally addressed as part of a medical treatment plan, but we believe that they are important, and we discuss them at length in Chapter 6 and Chapter 8. Meanwhile, here are a few ideas for you to think about.

Setting goals is an excellent way to improve the quality of your life. You can set long-term goals, things that you want to accomplish in your lifetime, or short-term goals, things you can do to improve your life right now. Paula Carroll says that she's happiest when she has a major goal to strive for. But she also finds great satisfaction in achieving short-term goals. "Today I'm going to dress up and I'm going to go downtown," she might tell herself, "and I'm going to have lunch with a friend. That's a goal."

It's important to learn to live in the present too. Having faced the possibility of death, Charles Fuhrman began to see his life in a new light, and to live accordingly. "I started to really nourish myself, give myself terrific things. I'd go to bed if I was tired during the day. I'd read. You know, I don't do those things ordinarily. I'm too busy."

Paula, who had to battle a new cancer ten years after her first diagnosis, feels that much may be lost by concentrating too heavily on five-year survival periods. "Because we're thinking about a distant number, we're not living life to the fullest in the present." Her advice? Don't give up trying to survive. But in the meantime, live your life to its absolute maximum. If you want to carve or sketch or travel, do it now, she told us. "If there's something in your life that you have always wanted to do, do it."

Behind such advice, of course, lurks the very real possibility of having to face death—imminent death or death in the not-too-distant future. In Appendix 1 we treat this issue at length. For now it is worth noting that, for many

> *"If there's something in your life that you have always wanted to do, do it."*
>
> —Paula Carroll

of the people we talked to, looking squarely at death proved to be a liberating experience, one that allowed them to take stock of where they had been and what they could most productively do with the days they had left. At the very least, thinking about death made them more acutely aware of all that life has to offer. As Charles Fuhrman put it, "I literally stopped, and started smelling the roses."

Having had cancer himself, and having therefore been on both sides of the examining table, noted oncologist Dr. John Laszlo also found that facing death can make one more sensitive to life. In *Understanding Cancer* he writes about the "courage and determination" of people with cancer "who lived and experienced life to the fullest after they decided to get on with it and did. To sit around and grieve our fate is also a kind of death. I often wish the well could learn from our patients who better appreciate the beauty of life *after* learning that it is in serious danger."[5]

We encountered patients who displayed yet another kind of courage in the face of death. At age fifty-nine, restaurateur Paul Ryder was diagnosed with prostate cancer that had spread to other parts of his body. His doctors told him he would die within a matter of months. Paul's way of responding was not that of Paula Carroll and Charles Fuhrman. His way was to carry on as he always had, only more so, striving with all he had in him to keep cancer from interfering with his normal routine. Although he carefully followed medical instructions, he assigned his wife the task of acquiring information and communicating with his doctors.

While Paul did not take control in the way we have recommended, it would be wrong to think that he lacked either courage or determination. We advise you to become an active partner in the task of dealing with cancer because, like most of the people we interviewed, we believe that this approach is the best one for most patients. But not everybody is alike, and there is no universally correct way to cope with cancer, no one way that is perfect for everybody. In Chapter 6 we will have more to say about the various approaches to coping.

Though he always remained hopeful and in no way denied the existence of his illness, Paul preferred to discuss it and think about it as little as possible. Patients who take this approach may give up the chance to reexamine their long-term goals and to reassess the quality and meaning of their lives. But in so doing, they undoubtedly remain true to their characters—confronting cancer in the way that best fits their personalities. As for Paul, his own way seemed to serve him well: choosing to work a full and strenuous schedule much of the time, while continuing to enjoy many of the things he most loved to do, he lived more than six years from the day his doctors told him that his case was hopeless.

Getting Support

Everyone needs support. People who have cancer need it more than most; cancer support groups and your own support team can play a vital role in your recovery. In Chapter 6 we suggest ways to gather support, to build a network of people who can help you, so that you need not face your illness alone. For now, it is our hope that this chapter, that all of our chapters, will reach out to provide you with some measure of support and guidance. Every word has been written with that purpose in mind, and we would like nothing better than to have you finish this book feeling as confident as Julie Benbow ultimately came to feel. After a year in remission, Julie was eager to think of herself as being cured. "But," she immediately added, "whether or not I am cured, if it comes around the next time, I'm going to beat this. Because I am armed now. Spiritually, psychologically, and emotionally, I'm armed for it."

In order of their first appearance, the patients who contributed to this chapter are: Julie Benbow, Charles Fuhrman, Paula Carroll, Dennis Brown, John Chapman, and Paul Ryder.

"If it comes around the next time, I'm going to beat this. Because I am armed now. Spiritually, psychologically, and emotionally, I'm armed for it."

–Julie Benbow

Recommended Reading

Dollinger, Malin, Ernest H. Rosenbaum, and Greg Cable, eds. *Everyone's Guide to Cancer Therapy.* **Kansas City, MO: Andrews & McMeel, 1991.**

A collection of articles by oncologists and other specialists, written for the general reader. Part 1 covers diagnosis and treatment; Part 2 covers supportive care; Part 3 covers risk factors, genetics, and the Physicians Data Query (PDQ); and Part 4 discusses in detail the causes, diagnosis, and treatment of four dozen common cancers. This book is well designed, easy to use, and very clearly written, with excellent illustrations. The discussion of emotional issues and coping is useful but brief; the discussion of the disease itself and of the various forms of treatment is extremely thorough. In this respect it complements the *Alpha Book*. For this reason, and because it is an excellent resource, we recommend *Everyone's Guide* very highly. If you read only one other book besides ours, let it be this one.

Holleb, Arthur I., ed. *The American Cancer Society Cancer Book.* **Garden City, NY: Doubleday & Co., 1986.**

A collection of articles by noted specialists. Part 1 covers various forms of therapy, pain, genetics, prevention, and questionable remedies. Part 2 covers specific cancers and their treatment. The emotional aspects of living with cancer are discussed only briefly. The writing is on the technical side.

Larschan, Edward J., with Richard J. Larschan. *...The Diagnosis Is Cancer....* **Palo Alto, CA: Bull Publishing Co., 1986.**

This short, readable book treats subjects that are not discussed at length in most other books. The author is an attorney, a clinical psychologist, and a cancer patient; his book covers emotional, legal, and financial issues.

Laszlo, John. *Understanding Cancer.* **New York: Harper & Row Publishers, 1987.**

This book focuses on learning about, rather than on dealing with, cancer. It discusses causes, prevention, and treatment; the mind–body connection; current research; and alternative treatments. There is a helpful chapter on reducing costs and a short but useful appendix on legal issues. The author, an oncologist and himself a cancer survivor, is vice president for research at the American Cancer Society.

Morra, Marion, and Eve Potts. *Choices: Realistic Alternatives in Cancer Treatment.* **New York: Avon Books, 1987.**

This useful reference book focuses on diagnosis and treatment and provides detailed information about common types of cancer. There is a helpful section on diagnostic tests and an excellent chapter on where to get help. The question-and-answer format is reader friendly.

Understanding Cancer

Understanding Cancer

In the last chapter you heard mainly from patients who overcame the first shock of their diagnosis by learning more about cancer and by learning to take control. Not everyone we interviewed took this approach. As you know, Paul Ryder asked his wife to get the facts and to communicate with his doctors. A few of the patients we talked to were even less interested in learning about cancer than was Paul. These people cared nothing for the facts behind their condition. They only wanted to get well as quickly as possible.

A veteran railroad worker, Joe Dodig developed throat cancer at age fifty-five. From the beginning, and consistently thereafter, Joe regarded his cancer solely as an annoyance, as something not to be thought about but to be eliminated. "It was an inconvenience to me," Joe told us. "Something bugging me. The sooner we get it over with, the better off I'll be."

Joe stands in marked contrast to Charles Fuhrman, Paula Carroll, and most of the other cancer patients we interviewed. As Charles said, "The more you know the better. You're more in control." Paula—a patient advocate who wrote a book about her cancer experience[1]—agrees; the more you know, she adds, the less likely you are to be paralyzed by fear. Cancer patients, she says, "fear the unknown more than the known. If you don't know the facts, you fabricate all sorts of fears and build them up out of proportion."

We lean heavily toward Charles's and Paula's way of thinking. Almost all of the patients we interviewed told us that they were stunned by their diagnosis, and that

*"If you don't know the facts, you
fabricate all sorts of fears and build
them up out of proportion."*

–Paula Carroll

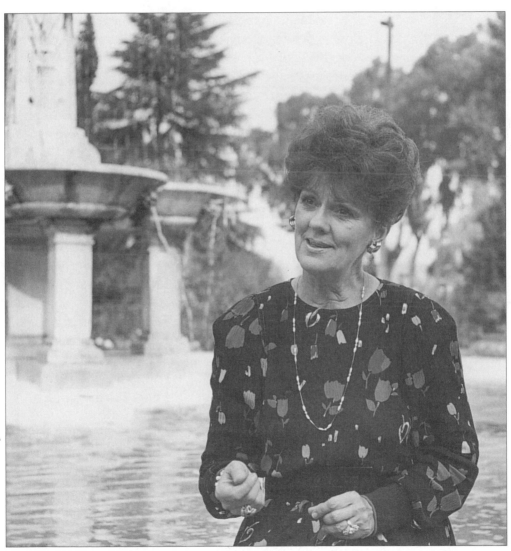

Paula Carroll

"In my mind, the only way to cure it was to cut it out."

–Joe Dodig

learning the facts helped them to overcome their fears and to deal with the enormous changes that they suddenly had to face. This, however, is not to belittle Joe Dodig, whose approach seems perfectly suited to his personality. And apparently it paid off–Joe had been without symptoms for four years when he died in an accident. Whether his approach would benefit most cancer patients, however, is highly questionable.

For one thing, Joe's refusal to find out more about his disease left him with some of the same misconceptions he'd had before he developed cancer. He saw his tumor as consisting of strange little creatures "creeping in every-where, just chewing away, getting bigger and bigger, a parasite eating me up. Like when you're a kid and you go to school and you catch lice." As we shall see, likening cancer to an onslaught of body lice is far from realistic. And unrealistic conclusions can lead to hasty decisions, decisions that you may later come to regret.

In Joe's case, the idea that his cancer was a parasite led him to reject every treatment except surgery. The "parasite" must be exterminated immediately. "I automatically kicked out radiation," Joe told us. "In my mind, the only way to cure it was to cut it out." He told his doctor, who had asked him to think about radiation, to "fix this up with an operation."

Joe had his operation. But he was later surprised to meet people with cancers like his who had been successfully treated with radiation alone. Had he learned more about cancer in the first place, he might have chosen this alternative himself. He might have discovered that when two therapies look equally promising, the less aggressive one, hence the one that entails less risk, is often the better choice.

Apart from its implications for treatment, not knowing the facts can make you feel worried, helpless, and depressed. Our assumption throughout this book is that, for *most* patients, knowledge is power, and that, like the majority of those we interviewed, you will draw strength and perhaps some comfort from learning as

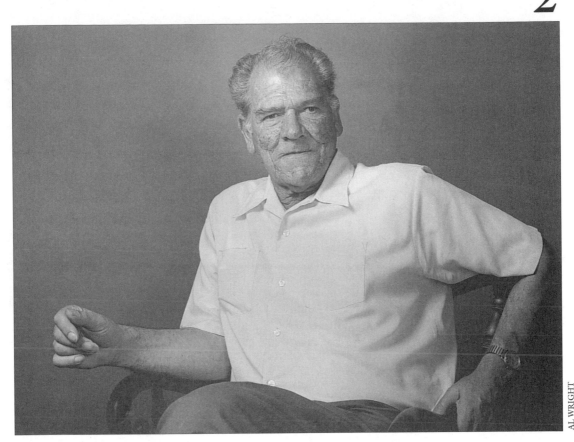

Joe Dodig

AL WRIGHT

much as you can about your illness.

In this chapter we present a very brief overview of the facts about cancer—what it is and why some people get it. If you want to learn more, see the Recommended Reading. If you plan to do real, in-depth research, see the notes to this chapter. There we cite scientific sources for the various points that we touch on—briefly—in the discussion that follows.

What Is Cancer?

You learned in Chapter 1 that cancer develops when abnormal new cells in your body grow out of control. But where do those abnormal new cells come from?

49

The human body contains up to a trillion cells. Each cell is a living organism; it takes in food, grows, reproduces, and eventually dies. Indeed, millions of cells die every second, while millions more are created. In this ongoing process the number of dead cells is balanced by an equal number of replacements.

The core of the cell is called the *nucleus*. The nucleus is a small balloon-shaped control center containing a miniature master plan or blueprint of the body, in a substance known as *deoxyribonucleic acid,* or *DNA*. Within the DNA reside approximately 100,000 *genes,* which interpret the blueprint and direct the cells to behave in designated ways. One gene, for example, determines eye color; another hair color. Still others tell cells whether they are to be blood cells, liver cells, skin cells, and so forth. And—the point that concerns us here—genes also tell cells when they should reproduce and when they should not. This is the mechanism that makes it possible for cancer to develop.

Cells reproduce by dividing. When they do, they pass their exact genetic blueprints on to the cells that descend from them. Consequently, if a particular cell goes wrong—that is, if it has its blueprint altered in such a way that it becomes cancerous—so too will every cell that descends from it.

A cell begins to go wrong when it has been structurally changed, or *mutated*. But not all mutated cells grow into cancer cells. Most researchers today believe that for a cell to become cancerous the mutation must involve a particular kind of gene—known as an *oncogene*—which disrupts the nucleus and causes a breakdown in the normal controls over cell division. When this happens, the mutated cell continues to reproduce. In time its millions of offspring form into an ever-growing tumor. They may also disperse into the lymphatic system, the bone marrow, or the other blood-forming organs.

It is generally accepted that oncogenes do not become active on their own. They are apparently activated when they are bombarded, probably many times over, by carcinogens—external forces that promote the development of cancer—such as solar radiation, harmful chemicals, or viruses. Once activated, an oncogene may alter the cell's structure so badly that it cannot be repaired.[2]

As they multiply, these cancer cells become dangerous. They begin to take nutrition meant for healthy cells. If they grow into tumors, they can get in the way of vital organs, sometimes causing pain and often making it impossible for these organs to function. If left unchecked, they may destroy the organs, and in some cases the patient as well.

Cancer can also prove fatal in other ways. It can obstruct air passages or major blood vessels. It can destroy blood coagulants, so that hemorrhaging from an injury cannot be stopped. It can block the immune system so that other deadly diseases cannot be suppressed. And it can generally weaken the body so that it cannot sustain itself—a condition known as *cachexia*.[3]

The fact that your body produces cancer cells does not necessarily mean that you will develop cancer. One theory even suggests that everyone, even the healthiest among us, produces a few cancer cells every now and then.[4] Almost always, however, the body's natural defenses attack and kill these cells before they can divide and multiply. It is believed that when a cancer does form, and when it spreads throughout the body, it is because the natural defenses, including the immune system, fail to do their job. We shall have more to say about this presently.

Talking about Tumors

In order to treat your cancer, your doctors must first know what kind of cancer it is. This means classifying it and charting its development.

How Cancers Are Classified

Although there are thought to be more than a hundred varieties of cancer, most of them fall into one of eight

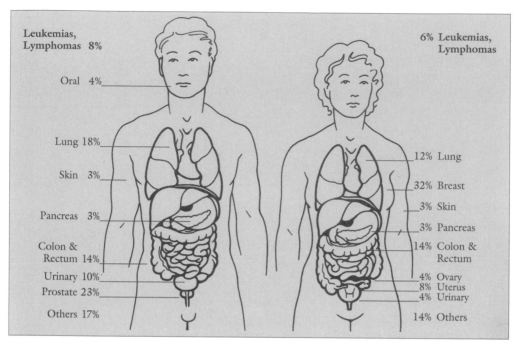

Fig. 4. Commonest Cancers, 1992 Estimate   (ACS data)

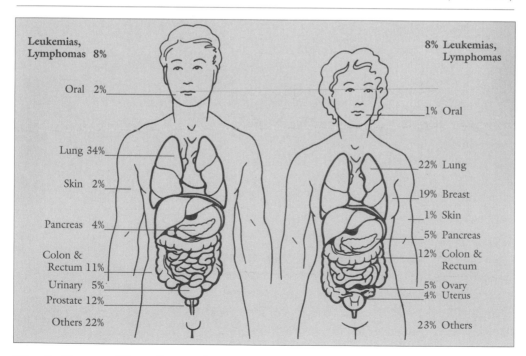

Fig. 5. Cancers That Cause the Most Deaths, 1992 Estimate   (ACS data)

classifications, according to the type of body tissue in which they first appear.

In Chapter 1, we mentioned *carcinomas.* These represent 80 percent to 90 percent of all cancers.[5] They originate in epithelial tissue–in the glands, the skin, and the lining of the internal organs. We also mentioned *sarcomas,* which originate in nonepithelial tissue–bone, cartilage, muscle, blood vessels, lymph vessels, and fat. Much rarer are *mixed tumors,* which originate in both kinds of tissue. The other common classifications are listed below.

Leukemias are cancers of the blood-forming tissues, primarily of the bone marrow. These cancers produce an overabundance of white blood cells. They spread through the body without forming secondary tumors.

Lymphomas resemble leukemias in cell type. They originate in the lymph glands, which are located in the neck, groin, abdomen, and armpit, and like leukemias they produce an oversupply of white blood cells. Unlike leukemias, they form a mass, or tumor, and frequently give rise to secondary tumors. One of the more common lymphomas is *Hodgkin's disease.*

Myelomas are like some leukemias in that they usually originate in bone marrow. Typically they involve a malignant growth in the plasma cells of the blood.

Melanomas arise in the cells that give color to the skin. Unlike most skin cancers, they spread easily to other parts of the body and are very virulent.

Gliomas are tumors that originate in the nervous system.

Cancers are also classified according to *site*–that is, according to the part of the body in which they first appear. Figure 4 shows the commonest cancers in the American population, classified by site. Figure 5 shows the cancers that cause the most deaths. The percentages in these two figures are current as of this writing. However, such percentages can change, sometimes dramatically, over a few years. The incidence of breast cancer, for example, has increased about 3 percent a year since 1980–or a total of 29 percent between 1980 and 1988, the most recent year for which figures are available.[6]

Charting Your Tumor

If you have a cancerous tumor, your doctors will want to know three other things about it before they recommend treatment. They will want to know its stage, its grade, and its doubling rate.

The *stage* of a tumor is determined by establishing how far it has spread from its point of origin. Cancers range from stage one–a tumor that has not spread at all–to stage four–a tumor that has metastasized to distant parts of the body and has penetrated other organs.

The *grade* of a tumor describes the extent to which its cells resemble ordinary cells. Tumors are usually graded on a scale of one to four. Grades one and two have cells that more closely resemble the normal cells of the organ in which they originated. Such tumors tend to act in a predictable manner, are usually slow growing, and are relatively easy to destroy. Grades three and four only slightly resemble their cells of origin, often behave errati-cally, and can be extremely difficult to destroy.

The *doubling rate* is the time it takes a tumor to double in size. Some tumors double in a few days; some can take months or years. Most tumors cannot be detected until they have reached the size of a small pea. But a fast-doubling tumor that is already as big as a pea will grow very much larger in a very short time. For example, a tumor with a ten-day doubling rate that has taken a year to grow to the size of a pea will grow to the size of a tennis ball in the next six weeks. Obviously, the fastest-doubling tumors require the most immediate attention–to destroy them while they are small enough to be destroyed, or, failing that, to slow down their growth if possible.

If a patient has a stage one, grade one cancer with a slow doubling rate, that patient's chances of being cured are usually excellent. Patients with stage four, grade four, fast-doubling cancers face much worse odds. Ask your doctors how your tumor is charted. (And just to be certain, ask if they are following the staging and grading systems outlined above. Some systems use scales with

Fig. 6. Causes of Cancer   (NCI data)

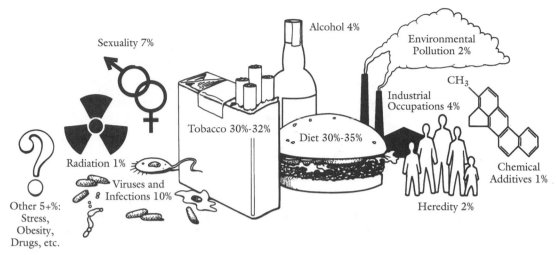

Sexuality 7%

Alcohol 4%

Environmental Pollution 2%

CH_3

Industrial Occupations 4%

Tobacco 30%-32%

Radiation 1%

Diet 30%-35%

Chemical Additives 1%

Viruses and Infections 10%

Heredity 2%

Other 5+%: Stress, Obesity, Drugs, etc.

numbers higher than four and lower than one, or with smaller increments between the numbers.)

One reason why you might want this information is that your treatment could be based on it. For example, other things—such as age and overall health—being equal, patients with stage one, grade one, slow-doubling cancers might be given the least intensive therapy, while those at the other extreme might be given much more aggressive treatment. Ask how these factors relate to the treatment that is being prescribed for you. Merely having this kind of knowledge—knowing what is going on and why—can make you feel better and give you some sense of control.

Why Did You Get Cancer?

The honest answer to this question is that no one knows for sure. You can sometimes form an educated guess as to how you might have developed cancer, or even why you were at a high risk of developing it. But why *you* did, while others with similar medical histories did not, cannot be determined with certainty. It is possible, however, to list the factors that cause cancer in the population as a whole (fig. 6).

Exposure to carcinogens is probably the most important of these factors. Cigarette smoke is one of the most dangerous of the common carcinogens. It is a *cancer initiator,* an agent that, by itself, can cause cells to mutate. Cigarette smoke can induce lung cancer, a major killer with an overall cure rate of only 13 percent. Smoking accounts for 30 percent of all cancer deaths.[7]

Carcinogens are discussed in Chapter 8.

Alcohol is a factor in the development of many cancers. It is a *cancer promoter,* an agent that weakens the body's resistance to carcinogens. Together, alcohol and tobacco make a particularly lethal combination. People who smoke and drink heavily are in one of the highest-risk categories. They are particularly vulnerable to cancers of the mouth and throat.

On the risks of smoking and drinking, see page 328 and page 336.

There are other well-known carcinogens—asbestos, arsenic, certain kinds of pesticides, and formaldehyde, to name a few. There are also what might be called natural carcinogens—sunlight, for instance, and atmospheric radiation, both of which can cause skin cancer; and even sawdust, which, if inhaled in large enough quantities, can lead to cancer of the nasal sinuses. Some carcinogens are initiators; others are promoters. Some carcinogens may be both.[8]

To repeat, according to one theory, everyone produces *some* cancer cells in the course of a lifetime. Thus it may be that you developed cancer, while others much like you did not, not because your cells mutated and theirs didn't— but because their immune systems killed off their cancer cells while, for whatever reasons, yours did not. For regardless of *why* cancer cells are produced, it is the immune system's job to destroy them.

The Immune System

The ever-vigilant immune system is the body's front-line defense against disease. Employing a vast army of killer cells, antibodies, and chemical messengers, it wages unrelenting biological warfare against a teeming array of

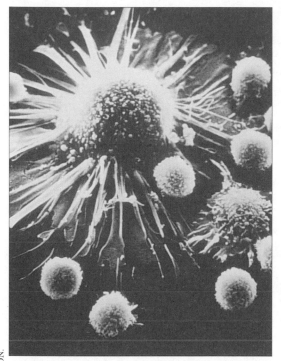

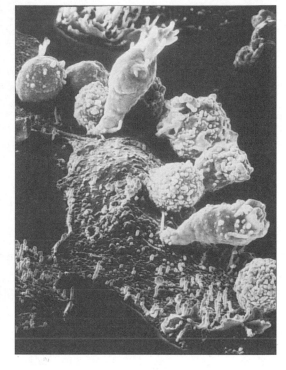

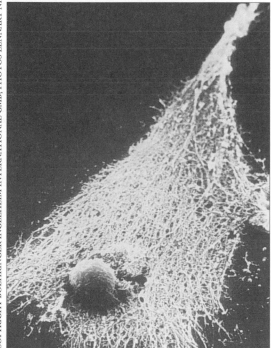

Death of a Cancer Cell

Magnified thousands of times, these microscopic photographs by Lennart Nilsson show killer T-cells in action.

Upper left: attracted to the abnormal cell by surface antigens, the T-cells begin to take action.

Above: normally round in appearance, the killer cells change shape as they work to break down the membrane of the cancer cell.

Left: the cancer cell ruptures and dies, leaving only its cellular skeleton behind.

viruses, bacteria, pollutants, and other foreign invaders. It uncovers foreign cells by "reading" the *antigens,* or markers, on their outer surfaces and then attacks these cells in an effort to neutralize them or destroy them. As soon as the foreign cells have been destroyed or disarmed, scavenger cells called *macrophages* clear away the debris, allowing the body to return to normal.

The immune system goes quietly about its business keeping most people healthy most of the time. And yet people sometimes do get sick–because the immune system doesn't work perfectly. In roughly 1 out of every 400 people, at least one component of the immune system malfunctions or is missing altogether. And even in a normal immune system, things can go wrong.

Exactly what goes wrong in cancer cases is a matter of speculation. There are several widely accepted theories. One is that some immune systems are simply overwhelmed by the sheer number of cancer cells developing at a given moment. Another is that some immune systems are themselves altered by the impact of cancer cells so that they cannot operate normally. A third is that some immune systems lose their ability to distinguish cancer cells from normal cells. Why they do so nobody knows for sure.[9]

When the Immune System Breaks Down

Furthermore, the immune system itself can break down. Some researchers believe that this breakdown is part of the aging process, that as one grows older, the immune system grows weaker, less able to fend off disease. If this is true, it is probably no accident that a higher percentage of the elderly are stricken with cancer than any other age group.[10]

Other studies, however, suggest that old people are more likely to develop cancer simply because, over the course of their long lives, they have been exposed to more carcinogens. And the longer one is exposed to carcinogens, the greater one's chance of developing cancer *regardless* of the condition of one's immune system.[11]

In any event, it is generally accepted that anything that

damages the immune system can lower resistance to cancer. This includes certain contagious viruses. AIDS is the most notorious of the conditions that are caused by a contagious virus—its very name, *acquired immune deficiency syndrome,* describes its destructive effect on the immune system. When a person has AIDS, invading viruses damage or destroy the *lymphocytes*—the disease-fighting white blood cells. This leaves the body susceptible to innumerable diseases, including lymphomas and a once-rare malignancy known as *Kaposi's sarcoma,* a cancer of the blood vessels.

Other viruses (apparently only a few) are also associated with particular cancers—for example, hepatitis B virus with liver cancer and certain wart-forming viruses with cervical cancer. In such cases, again, it is believed that you contract the virus, not the cancer, but that the immune system damage caused by the virus increases the odds of developing cancer later on.[12]

Much attention has been given lately to *cancer immunotherapy,* the attempt to strengthen the immune system to make it more cancer resistant. This subject is discussed in Chapter 4.

What Makes You Vulnerable to Cancer?

The answer is: Several factors. Diet is one. Being malnourished can leave the body unable to fight back when cancer strikes. And research shows that even if you have enough to eat, *what* you eat can be a factor too. For example, most nutritionists and many cancer researchers believe that if you eat a lot of high-fat, low-fiber foods, you will increase your chance of developing gastrointestinal, breast, colon, or prostate cancer, and that if you reverse this diet, you will reduce your risk accordingly.

If poor nutrition must be guarded against, so must obesity, which is linked to cancers of the uterus, gallbladder, prostate, ovary, colon, and breast. The ancient prophecy "In old age they shall be fat and flourishing" misses the mark as far as cancer is concerned. Evidence

For more on diet and cancer, see Chapter 8.

To learn how to control your weight, see Chapter 8.

We discuss stress and immune response in Chapter 6.

indicates that old age and obesity can be a deadly combination, and that you are more likely to reach old age, and flourish when you get there, by keeping your weight within accepted standards. In fact, controlling your weight at any age can shift the odds in your favor.

Controlling the amount of stress in your life may be as critical as controlling your weight. While research on stress-associated illness does not prove a cause-and-effect relationship, it does suggest a strong connection between emotional stress and cancer. Though it is a controversial point in medical research, many studies have demonstrated that stress, prolonged stress in particular, can lower immune system response. This leaves the body either unable to kill off the earliest cancer cells or unable to keep them from spreading once they are established.

Can cancer be inherited? The tendency to develop specific types of cancer seems to be. Defects in certain genes, susceptibility to various illnesses, an impaired immune system—all are occasionally known to run in families. When they do, they may increase the family members' risk of developing cancer. Note, however, that this increased risk can only be identified after a long-term pattern has become clear. Usually a significant number of family members must have had a specific cancer over at least two generations before it can be determined that the risk of developing that cancer is hereditary. Hereditary cancers commonly involve the large intestine, stomach, lungs, prostate, breast, endometrium, and ovaries.

Although they comprise only a very small percentage of all reported cases,[13] hereditary cancers are especially important for research purposes. By studying the history of cancer-prone families, scientists can make an educated guess about the risk to descendants of those families. It is known, for example, that a woman whose female relatives had breast cancer *prior* to menopause and in *both* breasts is at higher risk than a woman whose relatives had breast cancer *after* menopause and in only *one* breast.[14] And members of families that are at very high risk for one of the common cancers can have as much as a 50 percent chance of developing that cancer at some time in their lives.[15]

If you have any doubt about your own family's odds, and if your doctor isn't entirely certain, ask for a referral to a *genetic counselor,* someone who specializes in this field and can help you to understand your particular situation.[16]

Reasons for Hope

Will science ever find a cure for cancer? Can a disease that has plagued humanity since prehistoric times be overcome? We believe that the answer is yes–but first let us raise a more basic question. What real progress has been made to date? The answer to this question depends a lot on who is being asked.

Cancer counselor, author, and patient Paula Carroll remembers appearing on national television with a noted St. Louis oncologist who had been part of the government-sponsored "war on cancer" in the late 1960s. The doctor had been an eager researcher during those optimistic days when it was thought that unconditional victory was nearly at hand. Twenty years later, when Paula met him, he no longer believed that the war on cancer could be won.

Though she personally has never lost hope, Paula is nonetheless skeptical of those who claim stupendous advances in the treatment of cancer. She believes that alternative treatments (which she chose not to explore) owe much of their appeal to the fact that standard treatments have had limited success.

Dr. Vincent T. DaVita, past director of the National Cancer Institute (NCI), would disagree. In 1987 Dr. DaVita was quoted in the *New York Times* as saying, "There are literally hundreds of thousands of people alive today who wouldn't be here if new treatments introduced over the past fifteen to twenty years were not available."[17]

Estimates compiled by the American Cancer Society (ACS) support this optimistic point of view. In 1992 40 percent of cancer patients were expected to be alive five years after diagnosis. "In the early 1900s," the ACS observes, "few cancer patients had any hope of long-term survival." In the 1930s, less than 20 percent of patients survived five years. In the 1940s it was 25 percent; in the 1960s 33 percent. The difference between the survival rates for the 1960s and for today represented 79,000 persons in 1992. That is, 79,000 cancer patients who will survive today would not have survived if they had got cancer in the 1960s.

Furthermore, the 40 percent figure represents what is called the "observed" survival rate. Allowing for normal life expectancy (that is, not counting the deaths of cancer patients who would have died of old age, heart disease, and so forth if they hadn't died of cancer), the five-year survival rate in 1992 was actually 51 percent—or about 576,300 Americans. This so-called "relative" survival rate indicates the percentage of cancer patients who are potentially curable today.[18]

Although the exact amount of progress may be controversial, everyone does agree that at least some genuine progress has been made. It is generally agreed, for example, that refinements in technique—in the more precise use of drugs and in the computerized application of radiation—have made traditional treatment for many cancers more effective and less debilitating than it was just a few years ago. And the recent explosion of knowledge in cancer research has resulted in many promising new therapies and other discoveries.

See Chapter 4 for new directions in research.

It is this area of biomedical research that appears the most promising. Dr. Lewis Thomas, past president of the Memorial Sloan-Kettering Cancer Center, took part in the national war on cancer in the 1970s. He too came to believe that a "silver bullet" cure would never be found. But by 1986, recent breakthroughs in biomedical research had given him a totally different perspective. "Now," he said, "it's hard to imagine...that cancer will not be overcome."[19]

Like Dr. Thomas, we think it makes sense to remain optimistic. Even if the great breakthroughs are slow in coming, we believe that there are always reasons to be hopeful. Here is our summary of a "cancer patient's

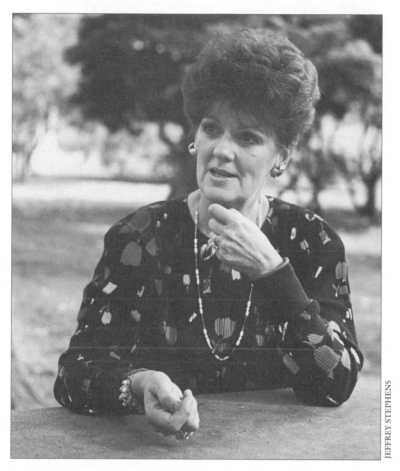

JEFFREY STEPHENS

Paula Carroll

Though she has never lost hope, Paula is skeptical of those who claim stupendous advances in the treatment of cancer.

hope list" put together by one noted specialist.[20]

> *The hope that your treatment will have the best possible outcome*
> *The hope for time to attain a cherished goal*
> *The hope for time to share what matters the most to you with family and friends*
> *The hope for freedom from pain and from the worst side effects of treatment*
> *The hope that you will have time for personal growth, time to reach an "awareness of the beauty of life not achieved before the prospect of dying came so near"*
> *The hope for a rare and extraordinary healing*

"There are literally hundreds of thousands of people alive today who wouldn't be here if new treatments introduced over the past fifteen to twenty years were not available."

–Dr. Vincent T.
DaVita

While this last hope may seem extravagant, we think it is entirely justifiable. Medical literature records hundreds of spontaneous remissions, even of advanced cancers. Who knows how many thousands may have gone unrecorded? It is always important to be realistic, to understand that cancer is a serious illness. But it is equally important to remain optimistic. We believe that in the vast majority of cases there is always reason to hope.

In this spirit we add the following more general hopes–hopes that are eminently reasonable, given what is already known about cancer and about the advances in treatment that are currently taking place:

The hope that science will learn to detect and treat premalignant conditions–that is, to treat people who are cancer prone but who have not yet developed cancer

The hope that science will learn to treat the cancers that are currently the hardest to treat

The hope that more and more carcinogens will be removed from the environment

The hope that the public can be educated to adopt a healthier life-style

These do not seem pie-in-the-sky hopes to us. We believe that they can be realized in our lifetime.

In order of their first appearance, the patients who contributed to this chapter are: Paul Ryder, Joe Dodig, Charles Fuhrman, and Paula Carroll.

Recommended Reading

Cox, Barbara G., David T. Carr, and Robert E. Lee. *Living with Lung Cancer.* **Gainesville, FL: Triad Publishing Co., 1987.**

Funded by the NCI and written by two oncologists and a specialist in patient education, this book explains how lung cancer begins, how it is diagnosed, and how it is treated. Nutrition, stress, and cancer quackery are also discussed. The writing is concise and readable.

Dollinger, Malin, Ernest H. Rosenbaum, and Greg Cable, eds. *Everyone's Guide to Cancer Therapy.* **Kansas City, MO: Andrews & McMeel, 1991.**

Part 4: "Treating the Common Cancers." Forty-six chapters, each covering one kind of cancer in detail. The authors explain how the cancer in question develops, list the known causes, and describe each stage.

Hirshaut, Yashar, and Peter Pressman. *Breast Cancer: The Complete Guide.* **New York: Bantam Books, 1992.**

The latest information on diagnosis, treatment, and life after breast cancer from two leading specialists in the field. Extremely well done; full of good advice.

Kelly, Patricia T. *Understanding Breast Cancer Risk.* **Philadelphia, PA: Temple University Press, 1991.**

This concise, clearly written book discusses the various risk factors associated with breast cancer and benign breast disease. It also offers guidelines on choosing the best treatment. Breast cancer risk analysis services and patient education resources are listed in the appendices. The author is a medical geneticist; she directs the cancer risk analysis service at Children's Hospital in San Francisco.

Laszlo, John. *Understanding Cancer.* **New York: Harper & Row Publishers, 1987.**

Chapter 5: "What Is Cancer and How Does It Kill?" This chapter clearly describes how tumors grow and metastasize.

Chapter 7: "The Causes and Prevention of Cancer." This chapter describes in detail the various nongenetic causes of cancer. It is full of interesting anecdotes and examples.

Potts, Eve, and Marion Morra. *Understanding Your Immune System.* **New York: Avon Books, 1986.**

A good overview of the immune system, written for the general reader. This book is well organized, credible, and comprehensive.

Getting the Best Care

Getting the Best Care

D o you want the best possible care? Of course you do. In this chapter we'll tell you how to get it.

To get the best possible care, you must know how to choose the best resources. You must also know how to make the best use of the resources you choose. This usually means maintaining some control over your treatment. Studies have shown that most patients do best when they have a sense of control–when they work in active partnership with their health care teams.[1] However, not all patients want to be, or can be, active partners. You need to know your own personal style and know how to make that style work best for you.

Your Doctor

Finding the right doctor is "crucial," says oncology nurse Theresa Koetters. "It's probably the most important relationship the patient has during the disease process." And, she adds, patients must be able to talk to their doctors. "They have to be able to cry with them, if that's what they need."[2]

The patients whom we interviewed would agree. Without exception, they said that trusting their doctor was the most important aspect of their treatment. As John Chapman said, "You have to believe in your doctors and the choices they make for you." Even the self-reliant Joe Dodig was glad to have a surgeon who was "a straight shooter"–someone whom he could trust:

"He's got a professional manner. He doesn't give

*"You have to believe
in your doctors and the choices
they make for you."*

–John Chapman

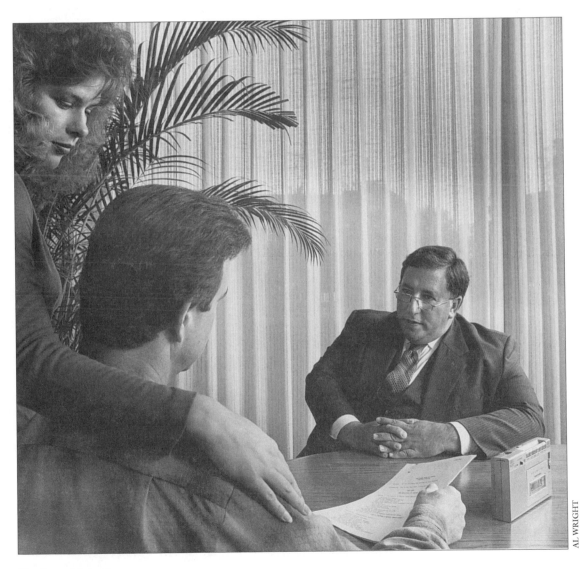

Dr. Samuel Spivack

AL WRIGHT

you the doom signal, you know. You can talk to him. He understands your problems."

So successful treatment depends on having a doctor you can trust. How do you go about finding such a doctor?

Choosing a Doctor

Start by asking yourself what you mean by "a doctor I can trust." Above all, you probably mean someone who is well qualified, someone whose medical skills you have confidence in. You probably also mean someone you can work with, someone you can understand and respect, someone who listens to what *you* have to say, someone who is willing to answer your questions. Someone, in short, whom you feel comfortable with.

It may take a little searching to find that someone. Charles Fuhrman was put off by the first doctor he saw:

"I felt insecure in his hands. He seemed very flip about a lot of things. I didn't trust the man. I couldn't wait to get out of the office. I didn't ever want to see him again."

He had the opposite reaction when he met his oncologist:

"I felt, 'Now there's a sane person, and I like him.' He had an intelligent look. He looked wholesome. I felt, 'Now here's a man I can trust.'"

"If you feel good about a doctor, stay," Charles says. "If you feel indifferent, get away."

Jeri Hobramson resorted to trial and error. It took her three tries before she found a doctor she could feel good about. Although it did work for Jeri eventually, we do not recommend the trial-and-error method. You can save time and get better results if you take a systematic approach, first to find the best-qualified candidates and then to identify the one you like best.

Pick someone who is well qualified

We put the following question to oncologist Dr. Samuel Spivack, of the University of California at San Francisco:

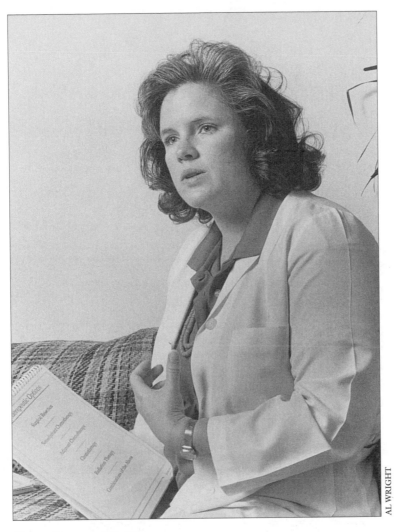

Theresa Koetters, RN, MS

Patients must be able to talk to their doctors. "They have to be able to cry with them, if that's what they need."

–Theresa Koetters

Alpha: Suppose you had a close relative in a faraway city who had developed a serious cancer. You yourself know nothing about this city and you know no one in the medical profession there. What would you tell your relative to do to find the right doctor?

Dr. Spivack: First I would tell the relative to ask his own physician–assuming he has a good relationship with that doctor–to provide the names of two or three specialists. The next thing to do is to assess whether or not any of

71

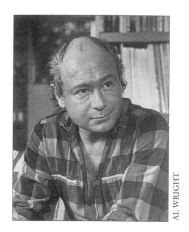

Charles Fuhrman

"I felt, 'Now there's a sane person, and I like him.' ...I felt, 'Now here's a man I can trust.'"

–Charles Fuhrman

them are board certified in oncology (or, in the case of a young doctor, eligible for board certification). Finally, seek a doctor who is on the staff of a teaching hospital. That will generally guarantee a certain excellence.[3]

Let's take a look at Dr. Spivack's suggestions. His first point assumes that the patient has a good, long-term relationship with a primary-care physician. The importance of such a relationship cannot be emphasized strongly enough. However, if you are uncomfortable with your current physician–or if you currently have no physician at all–there are other ways to get the names of specialists.

Start by calling the local hospitals and asking to be put in touch with the nearest cancer support group. (Usually you connect with these groups only after you have begun treatment, but you may do so at any time.) Ask the members of the group for their recommendations. These people are cancer patients like you, and they tend to know who the best doctors are.

If there are no cancer support groups in your area, ask a local hospital for its physician referral service. (You can even specify that you want the names of male–or female–physicians.) You could also check with your county medical association or with the state and local offices of the American Medical Association (AMA).

Dr. Spivack's second point is that you should go directly to an oncologist. We think this is good advice. We don't mean to imply that cancer patients can't be treated by primary-care physicians. Your own doctor will be a vital member of your health care team. But because they have three or four years of specialized training, and because they treat cancer patients exclusively, oncologists keep abreast of the latest developments in diagnosis and treatment. This is especially important in cases involving complicated or unusual cancers. It is also important in advanced cases, where the patient's symptoms require expert attention.

When Dr. Spivack speaks of a "board-certified" doctor, he means one who is certified by the American Board of Internal Medicine and who belongs to the American

Society of Clinical Oncology.* How do you find out whether a doctor is board certified? Simply telephone the doctor's office, or the American Board of Medical Specialties (1-800-776-2378). You can also look your doctor up in the *Compendium of Certified Specialists* or the *American Medical Dictionary,* available in many libraries. These reference books list physicians geographically and by specialty. They describe each doctor's training, certification, and practice; and indicate which doctors are affiliated with university hospitals.

Dr. Spivack's third point is that you should choose a doctor on the staff of a teaching hospital. This has two advantages. First, your case will be reviewed by several physicians. Second, you will be in the hands of someone who is familiar with the latest clinical research. (The advantages and disadvantages of the teaching hospital itself are discussed later in this chapter.)

When you have a list of well-qualified doctors, it's time to find out about each candidate's office policy. Call the doctor's office, or have someone else call, and ask the following questions:

- What are the doctor's office hours?
- Does he or she take Saturday or evening appointments?
- How soon can I make an appointment?
- Is the doctor normally on time for appointments?
- What is the doctor's fee schedule?
- Is the doctor available for telephone consultation after the first visit?
- What kind of medical insurance does the doctor accept?

If you don't like what you hear, cross that candidate off your list.

Pick someone who feels right to you

Once you have lined up two or three promising candidates, make an appointment with each one of them. Explain that you want to discuss your situation. At that

*Note that oncologists who have not been, or are not eligible to be, certified are not necessarily incompetent. For example, many highly skilled older physicians may have specialized in oncology before certification examinations were established. Certification is just one criterion for choosing a qualified oncologist.

Dr. Andrew Moyce points out that there are some doctors "who happen to be good salesmen but aren't very good physicians."

first meeting, try to get a sense of the doctor's approach to medicine, and to his or her patients. Do this with each candidate. Use your intuition to find the doctor who feels right to you.

Gut reaction may be your most reliable indicator here. Most of the patients we interviewed sensed, often very quickly, how they felt about a particular doctor. But if you have trouble deciding how you feel, take a minute to ask yourself the following questions:

● Does this doctor give me straight answers?
● Do I understand what he or she is saying?
● Does this doctor see me as an *individual* and not just another case?
● Does this doctor's treatment philosophy make sense to me? Is it consistent with my values? (For example, should I be treated by a doctor who recommends chemotherapy when I have never believed in taking drugs of any kind?)
● Will this doctor be available throughout my treatment?
● Does he or she return my phone calls?
● Does this doctor seem warm and personable or cold and remote?
● Have I been listening carefully to what the doctor is saying? Have I given him or her a chance to be helpful?

Thoughtful answers to these questions will help you to decide whether this doctor is right for you.

A word about reputation

Wherever you get recommendations—from your own physician, from friends, from a support group—you are likely to hear about the doctor's "reputation." Reputations are important, but it's often hard to tell what they are based on. You may hear that so-and-so is "a brilliant doctor," but you may have no idea what is meant by "brilliant." In any case, however glowing a doctor's reputation, you should still trust your own judgment.

A doctor with a deservedly good reputation for treating cancer may be far less skilled at interacting with patients. You may require both skills. Most patients do.

On the other hand, be wary of a reputation that is built solely on a good bedside manner. Dr. Andrew Moyce points out that there are some doctors "who happen to be good salesmen but aren't very good physicians." These doctors, he says, "have their patients' confidence because they are so good at interpersonal things." And he adds:

"The best surgeon I've ever seen operate had no interpersonal skills. His approach to a cancer patient was 'It's cancer; it's got to come out'—and that was it. I certainly didn't admire that approach, but I admired his surgical skills."[4]

Dr. Spivack believes that you should consider a doctor's reputation, but only up to a point, and only insofar as the source is reliable:

"I would rather talk to the families of previously treated patients than, say, the public at large, who think that Dr. X has a very busy practice—they always hear him being paged, or he dresses well, or something like that. The real criterion is: How available was the doctor when the family needed him, when the patient needed him? Talk to family members, to hospice workers, to oncology nurses. Those are the best sources of reputation."

If you aren't up to doing it yourself

It's all very well to say that you should choose your own doctor. But some people simply can't shop around. Maybe they don't have the time or the strength. Maybe they just don't have the emotional energy. If this sounds like you, what should you do?

Your best option is to delegate the job to someone else. Choose someone who has shown a genuine interest in your well-being, someone who you think would be willing to do you a favor. Choose someone who is *able* as well as willing. That means someone who has the time to do the job; someone whose judgment you instinctively trust; some-one who will understand what you are looking for in a

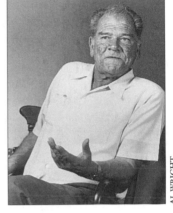

AL WRIGHT

Joe Dodig

"He's got a professional manner. He doesn't give you the doom signal, you know. You can talk to him."

–Joe Dodig

75

physician. Ideally this means someone who knows you well.

And if there is no such person? Don't give up. The important thing is to locate a competent doctor. So ask around until you find someone who is willing to take on the job—even if it's someone you hardly know.

You may find it very difficult to do this, and there's always the risk that the person you ask will say no. But the potential benefits far outweigh the risks. So reach out, even if you don't want to, even if it's painful. And remember: most people really do want to help.

Look for the best doctor you can find, but don't look forever, expecting to find perfection. Linda Sumner, who has been treated by many doctors, tells us that she has yet to find "that dream oncologist." But, she says, "some are much more helpful than others." She recommends working with a doctor whom *you* find helpful for as long as you feel comfortable doing so, remembering always that doctors "are human and have their own insecurities and their own problems."

Finally, if all else fails, remember that even an uncongenial doctor can provide you with excellent medical care. This is not the ideal situation by any means. But if it's your only option, don't be afraid to take it.

In short, a "dream" doctor may be beyond your reach. But with a little effort, you should be able to find a competent doctor, one whom you can trust.

Working with Your Doctor

What if you are basically satisfied with your doctor but are dissatisfied with one aspect of your treatment? Often it's a communication problem. If that is the case, here are a few things to try.

Ask questions and express concerns *each* time you see your doctor. This will show that you want to be involved in your treatment. It will also prevent you from building up a backlog of resentment. Use paper and pencil, a tape recorder, a supportive friend or relative—anything or anyone to help you to remember what to ask *and* what

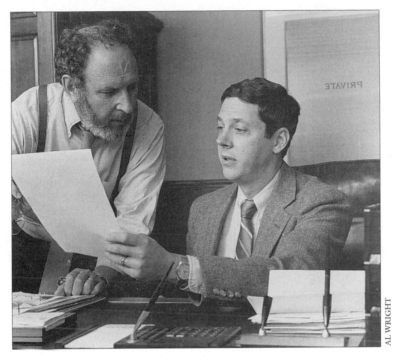

Dr. Andrew Moyce

the doctor answered.

Keep on asking questions until you get an answer that you can understand. If you feel intimidated by the scientific language, ask for an explanation in simple English. Better yet, ask for an illustration. For instance, have the doctor draw a picture of the organ or tumor under discussion.

Try to be firm but understanding in expressing your needs. If, for example, the doctor acts rushed (most doctors are extraordinarily busy), you might say, "Could you spare me an extra few minutes—if not now, then later when you aren't so busy? This is really bothering me." Or if the doctor hasn't explained something fully, try saying, for example, "I appreciate your explaining this to me. But I'm just not getting the picture. Could you tell me exactly *how long* the treatment will last?"

Give your doctor ongoing feedback. Tell him or her in your own words what you heard, to be sure that you have it right. For example, "As I understand it, with the chemotherapy you say I have a 70 percent chance of recovery." And remember that it never hurts to let the doctor know when you do in fact understand what was said.

Sometimes the problem involves your own emotions. Don't be surprised if you have mixed feelings about your doctor. After all, you are an adult; up until now you've managed your own affairs. Now, like it or not, you are heavily dependent on someone else, on an authority. It's natural to feel resentful sometimes, no matter how much you admire, trust, or like your doctor. As long as you are aware of this problem, it isn't likely to cause trouble – provided that you *talk it over with someone.* If you don't want to talk to the doctor personally, confide in a nurse, a friend, a counselor, your cancer support group, or your spouse. Talking it over does two things. First, it helps to keep the problem in perspective, by getting it out in the open, where people can give you feedback. Second, it keeps the problem from festering. Talking it over helps you to work through it and let it go.

Getting a Second Opinion

Never be afraid to get a second opinion. You owe it to yourself to do so if you have any doubt about your diagnosis, your doctor's competence, or your treatment program. And even if you don't have any doubts, a second opinion can add to your peace of mind.

Either you or your doctor may seek a second opinion. Usually this is done not to confirm that cancer is present but to decide on the best treatment in light of the diagnosis or to confirm the type of cancer involved – its stage, grade, and rate of growth. In our view, a second opinion should be routine in cases involving major surgery or involving one of the rarer forms of cancer. (Your health insurance company may insist on a second opinion before it approves payment for extended cancer treatments.)

How do you go about obtaining a second opinion?

Start with your doctor. If you feel shy about asking, take a friend or relative along for support. Ask for a referral to an oncologist, as described in the section on choosing a doctor. You want someone who has had experience with your kind of cancer. Get a couple of names and check the doctors out, using the methods outlined above.

You can assume that your doctor will refer you to the best-qualified person. But it never hurts to make sure. Paula Carroll recommends asking, "Would you send your wife to this doctor that you're referring me to?" Or, "If I were your father, where would you send me?" This allows you to benefit from your doctor's personal, as well as his or her professional, perspective.

If you don't want to get a referral from your doctor, you can obtain a second opinion through the National Cancer Institute (NCI) Hotline (1-800-4-CANCER). An Institute representative will give you the names of doctors in your area who specialize in treating your type of cancer. These physicians are accustomed to being asked for second opinions; they will usually see you and report back to your doctor promptly. In many cases, especially those involving surgery, health insurance will cover the cost of a second opinion.

Once again, local cancer support groups are an excellent source of information. Talk to as many members as you can, particularly those with cancers similar to yours, and find out whom they asked for a second opinion before they started treatment.

For the diagnosis itself, you can, if you wish, act on your own behalf. If a biopsy was taken, your slides can be sent at your request to the Armed Forces Institute of Pathology, which reviews cases from all over the country and is generally regarded as being a very reliable second-opinion center (phone 1-202-576-2800). If X rays were taken, they can be examined by another radiologist, preferably one who works at a major cancer center in your area. We know of one patient who took the unusual step of talking directly to the pathologist who analyzed his tissue. He asked his doctor for the pathologist's name, made

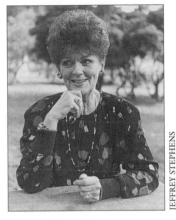

JEFFREY STEPHENS

Paula Carroll

> *"Would you send your wife to this doctor that you're referring me to?"*
>
> **–Paula Carroll**

79

an appointment to see him, and got a first-hand description of the findings.

You might also want to seek a second opinion in order to learn about all of the treatment options. One of the partners in H&R Block, Inc. reports that he was successfully treated for lung cancer only after he learned of standard treatments that his original physician had not considered useful.[5] Often you will find that there is a standard treatment for cases like yours, an approach that, under similar circumstances, has produced the best results for the most patients. There may, however, be innovative methods and research programs that offer wholly new therapies or that apply old therapies in new ways. Seeking a second opinion is one way to find out. This is particularly important if your case is complicated or unusual, or if the cure rate for your kind of cancer is not very promising.

If you are especially motivated to research potential treatments on your own, you may wish to look into the Physician Data Query (PDQ) service. PDQ is an up-to-date, computerized data bank on treatments—standard and investigational—for all types of cancer. To consult PDQ, call the NCI Hotline or ask your doctor's office to secure a printout from a medical library. PDQ information is presented in everyday language that the lay reader can understand. You may wish to do this even before you get a second opinion, so that you will be well informed when you talk to the doctor.

With or without PDQ data, it is always preferable to obtain a *multidisciplinary* second opinion—that is, one that comes from a variety of specialists. To do this, you can consult a second-opinion clinic, or your doctor can consult a tumor board.

A *second-opinion clinic* is a group of specialists who collaborate to diagnose cancers and recommend treatment. Along with pathologists, any of the following might be members of a second-opinion clinic:

Oncologists, internists who have had additional training in the study and treatment of cancer

Surgeons, who perform biopsies and other diagnostic

procedures and who remove tumors

Radiation oncologists, who prescribe radiation therapy
to treat cancer

Diagnostic radiologists, who use X rays to perform
diagnostic tests for cancers involving bone or dense tissue
and to analyze soft tissue, such as the lungs or brain

Nuclear medicine physicians, who trace radioactive
material introduced into the bloodstream in order to
determine how soft tissue and other organs are functioning

Geneticists, who examine evidence of cancer in light of
the patient's long-term family history

One advantage of second-opinion clinics is that in them
your condition is discussed from many points of view by
people who are experts in their respective fields. Another
is that these clinics do not usually require a referral. Simply
ask your physician to supply the necessary records, X rays,
and slides. The clinic will take it from there.

Because second-opinion clinics are relatively new, you
may have to do some looking to find one in your area. But
wherever you live, you are probably within reach of either
a state medical school or a hospital designated by the NCI
as a Comprehensive Cancer Center. Most of these institutions will, upon request, review your pathology report,
your diagnosis, and your doctor's treatment plan and will
render a second opinion on each.

If you cannot get to one of these centers in person,
you can have your records sent through the mail, and a
second opinion will be mailed back to you. Paula Carroll
suggests that if you have an unusual cancer, you request a
second opinion from a clinic that specializes in treating
that cancer.

For a list of Comprehensive Cancer Centers, see Appendix 3.

Tumor boards, which are associated with many hospitals,
are made up of specialists who assist doctors in prescribing
treatment. As a rule, however, tumor boards look only at
unusual cases, cases that involve rare tumors or in which
there is some question regarding therapy. It is up to your
doctor to request a tumor board review, but you should
certainly feel free to ask whether such a review might be
worth having.

With tumor boards, the question arises as to whether you should be present when the specialists meet to discuss your case. Dr. Moyce says yes—as long as the tumor board is open to patient appearances (some are not). He believes that you *and* the specialists will benefit from an in-person exchange of ideas, that it's important for them to see you as a living, breathing man or woman, not merely as a set of X rays and slides. He feels that this is particularly important if, as sometimes happens, these specialists are going to participate in your treatment.

Other physicians disagree. Some of the ones we consulted said that your presence would inhibit the board from speaking freely. They added that most patients would be overwhelmed by a blunt, clinical discussion of their symptoms and of their chances of survival. You might want to compromise by asking to appear at the tumor board for a short question-and-answer session, leaving the rest of the meeting to the professionals.

What do you do if your first and second opinions conflict? If you are truly unsure, get a third opinion. And try to get all of your doctors to communicate with one another to discuss the points on which they disagree. Sometimes misunderstandings occur over minute differences in the way test results are interpreted.

Finally, remember that you have every right to obtain a second opinion. Most doctors understand this and are glad to cooperate. If yours resists, you should probably find another doctor. Linda Sumner wanted a second opinion, but she felt a little timid about asking; she was afraid that her doctor might be offended. She took herself off the spot by reporting that her mother was the one who was insisting. "You know how mothers are," she told her doctor.

But don't waste too much time getting second opinions. Cancer usually calls for a prompt response; the sooner you are treated, the better your chances are of being cured. And it doesn't make sense to keep looking in the hope of finding someone who will suddenly tell you that you don't have cancer after all. Once there is general agreement on your diagnosis, it's time for you and your doctors to map out a strategy to combat your illness.

Your Hospital

Nobody really looks forward to a stay in the hospital. But your hospital is a valuable part of your treatment program. That's where you'll get the concentrated care, the care that will give you your best chance of recovery. Try to see your stay in the hospital not as a problem to be endured but as part of the solution to your problem—as a chance to help yourself to get well.

Choosing a Hospital

Most people don't choose their own hospital. If hospitalization is called for, they are admitted to the hospital their doctor selects. Is there anything wrong with this? Generally speaking, no. Unless they practice in an isolated area, most doctors are affiliated with a number of hospitals and will know which one is best suited to your needs. (Doctors with *no* hospital affiliation—those, for example, who operate exclusively out of their own private clinics—might not be your best choice to begin with. Unaffiliated doctors may not be held to the standards imposed by most reputable hospitals and may not have access to the subspecialists and up-to-date equipment found in those hospitals.)

This is not to say that you have no role in the decision. You are always part of the decision-making process. Although the final decision is the doctor's, you can always ask the doctor to refer you to the hospital that you prefer.

Why might you ask to be referred to a particular hospital? Perhaps because it specializes in your type of cancer. You should be aware that certain hospitals do specialize. For example, "Stanford Hospital has a reputation and a special interest in lymphomas that is unmatched anywhere," says Dr. Spivack. "I would say that [in the San Francisco Bay Area] someone with lymphoma should go to Stanford."

Dr. Spivack refers lymphoma patients to Stanford even though he himself is affiliated with another of the top cancer centers in the United States.

You may want to ask your doctor whether there is a hospital in your area that specializes in your type of cancer and, if so, whether he or she will refer you to it. If you are treated in such a hospital, you will be assigned to a qualified staff physician, who will act as a specialist member of your team, working together with your own physician.

Or you might ask to be referred to a teaching hospital. Fifty-seven institutions, most of them teaching hospitals, have been designated as Cancer Centers by the NCI. They include *Laboratory Centers,* which do basic research; *Clinical Centers,* which do patient treatment research; and *Comprehensive Centers,* which do all kinds of research. Call the NCI Hotline (1-800-4-CANCER) to find out whether there is a center doing research in your type of cancer. If so, you can find out whom to contact for further information.

Being treated in a teaching hospital has both advantages and disadvantages. In teaching hospitals, students do their residence work under the supervision of senior physicians in a program that is affiliated with a university. Dr. Spivack and Dr. Moyce both told us that teaching hospitals have a higher level of medicine. If you choose a teaching hospital, you should find yourself in competent hands.

However, the sheer number of those hands could make you uneasy. In a teaching hospital, you are sometimes a case study for medical students as well as a patient being treated for cancer. Depending on how the hospital is administered, you may have little or no privacy; students may be examining you and asking you questions at any time. If you think this would bother you, a teaching hospital may not be the right place for you.

Finally, you may want to think twice about choosing a teaching hospital if you don't like being just another number in a big institution. "Teaching hospitals tend to be short on personal care," says Dr. Moyce.

Some patients felt that teaching hospitals were excellent

for inpatient treatment, but that their outpatient clinics were impersonal and bureaucratic. Others complained of a lack of continuity–they said that when one resident doctor's rotation ended, they had to start all over again with a new resident. However, some teaching hospitals have continuity clinics, where patients retain the same resident throughout their stay. Ask which practice your hospital follows.

In choosing a hospital, size is another important consideration. Large hospitals have very sophisticated equipment operated by highly trained technicians following the latest procedures–all of which can sometimes mean the difference between life and death. At the same time, because the equipment and personnel are so expensive, they are most cost effective when they are used on a regular basis. For this reason, and also just because the resources are there, doctors sometimes order tests and procedures that aren't strictly essential. This is a serious issue if your insurance coverage is limited, or if you are paying entirely out of pocket. In that case, ask your doctor whether each test and procedure is absolutely necessary. If you are told, "I just want to rule something out," find out what that something is and whether it is really at all likely. Keep in mind, however, that many doctors are afraid of being sued for malpractice. They often feel pressured to conduct the widest range of tests, so that if they are sued, they cannot be accused of ignoring any possibility, no matter how remote.

Many large hospitals have self-contained oncology units where only cancer patients are admitted and where multidisciplinary treatment is coordinated by oncologists, oncology nurses, social workers, and other specially trained personnel. Is it worthwhile to be admitted to such a unit? Dr. Moyce and Dr. Spivack both believe that being treated by specially trained staff is a definite plus if not an outright necessity. However, neither feels that it is essential for the patient to be placed in a separate unit.

Many of the patients and nurses we interviewed strongly support the use of oncology units. They like the emphasis on teamwork among health care professionals, patients, and patient families. They like the fact that the units often include such amenities as common kitchens, lounges, libraries, and even overnight accommodations for family members. John Chapman described his oncology unit in one word: "Superb." All things considered, oncology units seem to us to offer many benefits. You might want to find out whether your hospital has one.

Although small community hospitals (those under 300 beds) lack some of the facilities offered by large hospitals, they may have certain other advantages. These include a more relaxed atmosphere and more personalized care. If you have a fairly uncomplicated cancer for which the treatment is more or less routine, you may get adequate care from an attending physician in a community hospital. But "fairly uncomplicated" and "more or less routine" are terms that are subject to interpretation. Be quite sure about the nature of your cancer before you and your doctor choose a small community hospital. Of the patients we interviewed who had been treated in both, most preferred large hospitals, despite their bureaucratic tendencies.

Checking In

Your first stop upon entering the hospital will be the admitting office, where a staff person will discuss financial arrangements, insurance coverage, hospital procedures, and your room assignment. Some of these topics can be complicated and confusing; you may want to bring along a friend or family member to help you out. If you have a strong preference for a private room, a private bath, a window bed—now is the time to discuss it. It's not easy to change rooms once you have been admitted.

For more about your rights as a patient, see Appendix 2.

You may also be given literature dealing with hospital–patient relationships and obligations. Study it when you have the time and energy, or have someone study it for you. Finally, you will be issued a plastic bracelet with your name and ID number on it.

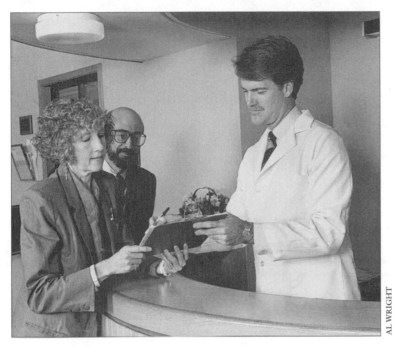

AL WRIGHT

Patient at hospital admittance

Your hospital room will be your home away from home for the length of your stay. Even if you will be there for only a few days, make it as pleasant as you can. Bring along some of your favorite things–lounging clothes, books, a tape player (battery operated, with a headset), your favorite photo. (Don't bring anything valuable, though; most hospitals do not guarantee the security of valuables.) We cannot prove that you will get well faster in pleasant surroundings, but we believe that you will, and in any case, it certainly can't hurt. You might as well be as comfortable as possible.

Many hospitals provide a list of things that you *should* bring with you–toothbrush, razor, and so forth. Have this list sent to you a few days before you check in.

Your Teammates: The Hospital Staff

You will be attended by a sizable staff. There will be nurses, nurse's aides, medical assistants, therapists, clinical

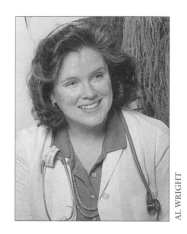

Theresa Koetters, RN, MS

"Nurses are the translators, the buffers, the map readers, the shoulders when people need them, the hand holders, the explainers..."

–Theresa Koetters

specialists, and volunteers. With three shifts a day plus weekend personnel, you may have trouble remembering who is who from one day to the next. Try to learn as many names as possible; it helps to write them down. And try to be friendly. You're likely to get better service – and to feel better yourself.

Being friendly, however, doesn't mean being passive or agreeing with everything that the staff does. If you aren't getting adequate attention, if you have a need that isn't being met, don't hesitate to make your feelings known. Assert yourself firmly but politely. (Be sure that the matter is important, though, to avoid being labeled a chronic complainer.) If you still don't receive satisfaction, ask to speak to the head nurse or the patient representative for your floor, or have a friend or family member do so. Next, complain to your doctor. One of our consulting nurses recommends that, if all else fails, you complain directly to the hospital administration.

Doctors' visits usually last only a few minutes, so make the most of them. Jot your questions down beforehand, or have someone do it for you, and have them ready when the doctor arrives.

Sometimes a *nurse practitioner* or a *physician's assistant* may visit you instead of your doctor. These professionals are qualified to do many of the things that doctors do, from interpreting lab reports to ordering tests and adjusting medication; however, your doctor must approve their decisions within a specified time. They can usually spend more time with you and your family than the doctor can, and they are often a valuable source of information.

Remember, however, that nurse practitioners and physician's assistants are *not* doctors. Always insist on speaking directly to your physician when important decisions must be made.

Your nurses are a vital link between you and the medical establishment – "in one word," says Theresa Koetters, your "advocates." "While the physician is the key player," she says, "the nurses are the translators, the buffers, the map readers, the shoulders when people need them, the

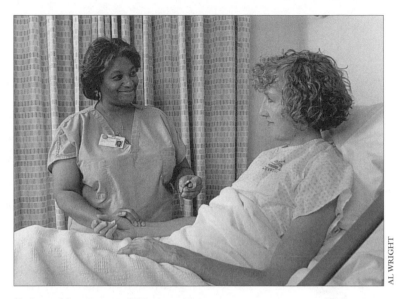

AL WRIGHT

Patient with nurse practitioner

hand holders, the explainers, the go-betweens with the family." In the hospital, the nurses will tend to your physical needs – "simple things, like, is the patient consti-pated? How is their pain being controlled? Does their left knee hurt, so they can't get comfortable to sit and talk?" Your nurses will also tend to your personal hygiene needs if necessary. And don't forget that they can answer questions. "Most patients don't know where their bone marrow is, or what a platelet cell does, or what's an immunoelectrophoresis test, or whatever. I think nurses play a very valuable role in translating a lot of that infor-mation," says Theresa Koetters.

What if you don't get along with one of your nurses? "Acknowledge the problem," says Koetters. "Inpatients on an oncology unit or a medical-surgical unit can ask to speak to a charge nurse or a head nurse. Say, 'I'm having some difficulties here – is there anything we can get fixed?' or 'Do I have any choice about this?' There are some situa-tions where patients or families will simply say, 'I don't want Robert to take care of my mother anymore,' period, amen, there's no choice about it. Many times adjustments can be made. I think most difficulties like that can be solved with compromise, communication, and just an acknowledgement that there's some conflict."

Nurse's aides assist the trained nurses by giving baths, making beds, and performing other tasks that don't require extensive training. Because there is a shortage of qualified nurses, the registered nurses in your hospital may have to confine themselves to the technical tasks for which they have been trained, while aides and volunteers do the simpler jobs.

A *dietitian* can be an important member of your health care team. Proper nutrition is critical before, during, and after many cancer therapies. You may need special help if you have dietary problems (if you need extra protein, for example) or eating problems (such as dry mouth or loss of appetite). Ask to see a hospital dietitian.

Most hospitals, especially those with oncology units, have *counselors* to help you to deal with the powerful emotions that go with having cancer. These counselors may be social workers, clinical nurse specialists, or trained volunteers. Your nurse can provide counseling, too; helping patients to recognize and express their feelings is an important nursing skill. Chaplains from the major denominations are usually on call, along with nonsectarian religious counselors. If you feel you need counseling of whatever kind, ask your nurse or doctor how to go about getting it.

See Chapter 6 for more on coping with your emotions.

If you have had surgery or radiation therapy, if your mobility or balance is impaired, if you have lost a lot of weight, or if you are very weak, you may need the services of a *physical therapist*. This professional's job is to help you to get back in shape. He or she will also teach you how to use a wheelchair or crutches if you need them, so that you will be mobile when you leave the hospital.

The latest trend in many hospitals is to begin rehabilitation early in the course of treatment–before you become disabled–and to continue it after you are discharged. The goal of long-term physical therapy is to help you to regain function and mobility, to do as much as you can with what you have. The therapist might teach you how to walk again, for example, or how to keep house and cook if you're in a wheelchair.

Once you are out of the hospital, you can draw on a wide range of home care services to help you to regain control of your life. In addition to a physical therapist, your home health team could include a nurse; an occupational therapist (who might teach you to regain the full use of your hands); a speech therapist (especially if you've had a laryngectomy); a home health aide (who helps with personal care); an in-home support service worker (who helps with the housework); and a medical social worker (who puts you in touch with all the others).

Many hospitals have a *discharge planner* on the staff. This professional, usually a social worker or a nurse, can help you to arrange for home care before you leave the hospital. Will you need help preparing your meals? Will you need a nurse? Rental equipment? Special transportation? The discharge planner can arrange it for you. Even if you don't expect to have any problems, you or someone in your family should talk to the discharge planner before you leave for home. You may not know what you are going to need. Discharge planners usually do.

Your Treatment: An Introduction

As soon as you were diagnosed with cancer, you were probably hit with a barrage of unsolicited advice. Your boss just read about a marvelous new treatment, if only he could locate the article. Your sister-in-law saw a TV special on chemotherapy. A friend down the street says all orthodox doctors are quacks; a certain clinic in the West Indies is the only place to go. All very well-meaning, but too many suggestions from too many quarters can drive you crazy, especially when you don't know very much about the different treatments yourself. Your job now is to learn. As for the unsolicited advice, when we asked Linda Sumner how she dealt with it, she said, "Earmuffs and earplugs." You might want to invest in some earplugs while you read the next two chapters.

There are basically three kinds of cancer treatment. *Standard treatment,* the one we refer to most frequently in this book, is treatment that is currently being used by physicians and that has been proven effective by scientific studies. In Chapter 1 we mentioned the four standard treatments: surgery, radiation, chemotherapy, and hormonal therapy. *Investigational treatment* (formerly known as *experimental treatment*) is clinical trials conducted with cancer patients, using the scientific method to evaluate new therapies or procedures. *Alternative treatment* is any treatment that is neither standard nor investigational. It includes everything from laetrile to herbal remedies to faith healing.

If you're considering which treatment to choose, it's crucial to get the facts—as many facts as you can—before you make up your mind. Even if you and your doctor have already decided on a treatment, we urge you to learn as much about it as possible. This will give you a greater sense of control, and it will correct any misconceptions that you, or your family and friends, may have.

Researching treatments sounds like a big job, but it's not as hard as you may think. In the next two chapters, we'll get you started and give you the sources you'll need if you want to learn more.

In order of their first appearance, the patients who contributed to this chapter are: John Chapman, Joe Dodig, Charles Fuhrman, Jeri Hobramson, Linda Sumner, and Paula Carroll.

Recommended Reading

Arnot, Robert. *The Best Medicine: How to Choose the Top Doctors, the Top Hospitals, and the Top Treatments.* **Reading, MA: Addison-Wesley Publishing Co., 1992.**

Written in a clear, concise, easy-to-read style, this excellent book tells how to choose a doctor and a hospital and how to become your own consumer advocate. Diagnosis and treatment are also covered. Part 1 is a consumer guide to operations and procedures; Part 2 deals with specific diseases, including cancer. The author is the medical correspondent for CBS News.

Larschan, Edward J., with Richard J. Larschan. *...The Diagnosis Is Cancer....* **Palo Alto, CA: Bull Publishing, 1986.**

Chapter 4: "Almost Painless Hospitalization." This chapter tells how to choose a hospital and how to make the most of the hospital you choose. It tells how to maintain good relations with the hospital staff and how to sustain a positive self-image while you are hospitalized. It tells you what to do if your rights are violated and how to handle billing errors.

Laszlo, John. *Understanding Cancer.* **New York: Harper & Row Publishers, 1987.**

Chapter 3: "Communication Is the Secret of Success." This chapter tells how to develop a good working relationship with your doctor, how to understand the doctor's point of view, and how to make sure that the doctor understands yours. Useful advice for families as well as patients.

Morra, Marion, and Eve Potts. *Choices: Realistic Alternatives in Cancer Treatment.* **New York: Avon Books, 1987.**

Chapter 2: "Deciding on Your Doctor and Hospital." This chapter includes two detailed score sheets, one for judging your doctor and one for judging your hospital.

Standard Treatments

Standard Treatments

The diagnosis has been made. You have had a second opinion. The presence of cancer has been confirmed. Your doctors have recommended a course of treatment. What do you do now?

Unless it is essential to start treatment immediately, wait a few days. Catch your breath, collect your thoughts, and focus on the therapy your doctors have prescribed. Noted oncologist Dr. John Laszlo, himself a cancer survivor, observes that while *time is important, it is even more important not to rush in with a treatment program before thinking it through carefully.*[1]

Of course, if you are like Joe Dodig, you may not need or want time to reflect. Joe, you may remember, insisted on an immediate operation; he wasn't interested in hearing about any other treatment. Most of the patients we spoke with, however, had at least some questions about the treatment their doctors had prescribed. They would have liked to learn more about it, and about the various alternatives, before they settled on a treatment plan.

The National Cancer Institute (NCI) defines *standard treatment* as "treatment or intervention currently being used [by physicians] and considered to be of proven effectiveness based on past studies."[2] There are four standard treatments for cancer–surgery, chemotherapy, radiation therapy, and hormonal therapy.

This chapter describes the four standard (also called "conventional," "traditional," or "orthodox") treatments for cancer. It explains how each treatment works and describes the potential risks and side effects of each. It also lists questions that you may want to ask your doctor. The

"I came to realize that my therapy could give me a chance for a new life, in some ways maybe even a better life than I had before."

–Charles Fuhrman

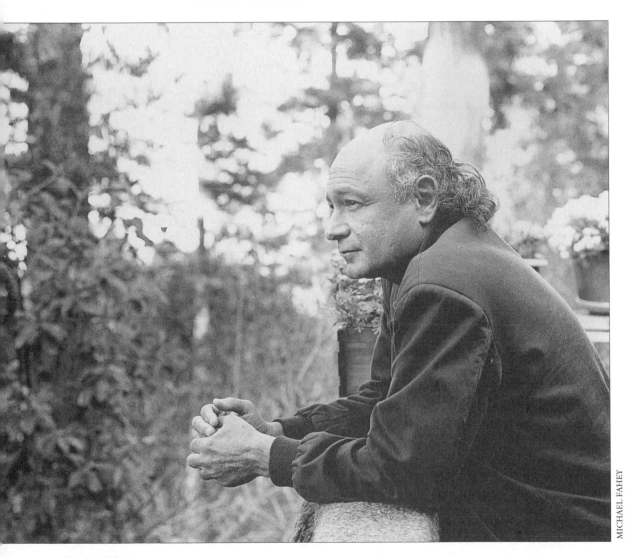

MICHAEL FAHEY

Charles Fuhrman

chapter does not rate one standard treatment against another, or recommend a specific treatment for a specific cancer. It is up to you, with the advice of your doctor, to decide which treatment would be best for you. Our goal is to take the mystery out of cancer therapy and to suggest ways of making your treatment as successful as possible.

We believe you will find our discussion factual and objective. At the same time, we must admit that we lean to the side of optimism. Cancer can be a difficult and challenging illness, and the standard treatments are not always easy to handle. But every year thousands of patients *do* handle standard treatment, *do* get through it—and in so doing, renew their hope and increase their chances of recovery.

Have Confidence in Your Treatment

Standard treatments can be applied in many ways. You may choose to leave the decision in the hands of your doctors. This can be a relief, especially if you don't feel well enough to consider the various possibilities yourself. But as we explained in Chapter 1, you will probably benefit from taking part in the decision making if you can. It will help you to feel more positive about your prospects, more in control, and better able to deal with your situation.

The first step in making decisions is to gather information. Read the section in this chapter that describes the treatment or treatments your doctor recommends. Read the list of questions in that section. Review the list of general questions that we gave you in Chapter 1. Based on what you already know—and on any previous discussions with your doctor—list all the questions that you still need to have answered before you decide on a treatment plan. Remember to prepare the questions beforehand, to try to have someone with you when you ask them, and to write down or tape record the answers. That way you won't forget what you asked or what the doctor said. Remember

For general questions about treatment, see page 27.

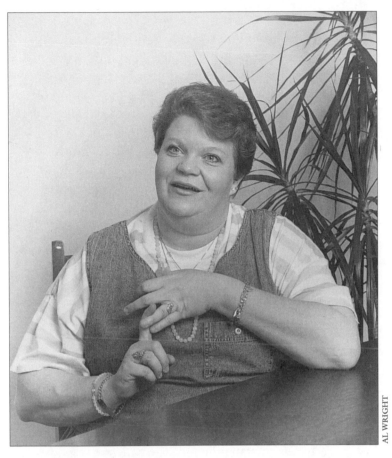

AL WRIGHT

Nancy Heitz

"There is no such thing as a stupid question. Whatever is happening is happening to you. So don't be afraid to ask."

–Nancy Heitz

too that, as Nancy Heitz, a registered nurse as well as a cancer patient, puts it, "there is no such thing as a stupid question. Whatever is happening is happening to *you*. So don't be afraid to ask."

When you have the answers to your questions, you can choose, or help to choose, a treatment plan. Once you have done so, try to think positive. It's important to have confidence in your treatment. Of course, this confidence should be based on a realistic appraisal of your situation. Given the nature of your cancer, your age, and your general health, you may have good cause to anticipate a cure. If not, perhaps you can anticipate *partial response* (a 50 percent reduction in the size of the tumor that lasts longer than one month) or *palliation* (relief from symptoms). Bear in mind too that although it may seem unrealistic to expect a cure, "miracle" cures do happen. It is fair to say that once the treatment begins, no one knows exactly what will take place. "The connotation of the term *advanced* cancer is a gloomy one," one medical researcher writes. "It implies an inevitability of death, and yet any prognostication may be confounded by the idiosyncrasies of the cancer....[A] cure may still be achieved."[3] In dire cases, as Dr. Spivack said in Chapter 1, "you should be prepared for the worst. But you should keep on hoping for the best."[4]

In any case, you can hope to sustain–or even to improve–your quality of life. Most of the patients we interviewed came to approach their treatments with this goal in mind. "As soon as I stopped feeling sorry for myself," Charles Fuhrman told us, "I came to realize that my therapy could give me a chance for a new life, in some ways maybe even a better life than I had before."

Can having confidence in the treatment actually make the treatment more effective? While we could find no studies on the therapeutic effects of confidence in cancer treatment specifically, it is widely accepted that confidence in a given treatment can influence the patient's response to that treatment. This beneficial phenomenon is known as the *placebo effect;* we have more to say about it in Chapter 6. However, we know of no research on the placebo effect as it relates to standard cancer therapy. We must therefore fall back on anecdotal evidence gathered from the physicians and patients whom we interviewed.

The placebo effect is discussed on page 182.

Many patients did believe that having confidence in their treatment had helped them to get well. They tended to agree with Nancy Heitz, who told us, "Whether it's chemo or surgery or radiation, if you say, 'Okay, this is helping,' you help yourself to heal." And Dr. Julien Goodman, who has forty years' experience in treating cancer patients, adds, "People who have a totally confident attitude that they are going to get well somehow do. I wouldn't say that 100 percent do, but such people certainly increase their chances for recovery."[5] Most of the physicians we talked to said that people with cancer are likely to do better if they choose a therapy that they have confidence in and avoid any therapy about which they have serious misgivings. "It makes all the difference when patients believe in the therapy you have prescribed," says Dr. James Forsythe. "I never try to pressure patients into something they cannot accept."[6]

Do you have fears or reservations about the therapy your doctor recommends? If so, try to think them through before you commit yourself one way or the other. A cancer counselor can help you to clarify your thinking. Your doctor, nurse, hospital social worker, or the nearest American Cancer Society (ACS) office can refer you to one. And you might want to talk the matter over with your friends and family. If you have religious reservations, talk to your minister, rabbi, or priest. But be wary of pressure from anyone who is certain that he or she knows what is best for you. "I got such insistent advice from my family," one woman told us, "that I couldn't remember what *I* thought was best."

If, after thinking it over, you still have reservations about your treatment, be sure to tell your doctor how you feel. Your fears may be based on incomplete or inaccurate information. If so, your doctor can supply the facts you need to get your thinking back into perspective. If you are still uneasy, your cancer counselor can help you to deal with any unresolved concerns. Once you accept your treatment plan, you can put all your energy into implementing it.

Surgery

The popular term is "having an operation." The formal term is "surgery." Ten thousand years ago, healers practiced skull surgery, presumably to relieve headaches (or perhaps madness), using sharp rocks as instruments. As recently as 1860, modern antiseptic surgery was unknown. Today, using the latest in advanced technology, surgeons successfully treat a wide variety of cancers. But even the most successful operation may not eliminate every trace of the tumor. For this reason, cancer surgery is often followed by chemotherapy or radiation or both.

Surgery is done for six basic reasons:

- To remove tissue or fluid or to explore an area for diagnosis (*biopsy* or *exploratory surgery*)
- To remove a malignant tumor in its entirety (*resection*)
- To reduce the size of a tumor so that further treatment may be applied (*debulking*)
- To remove a benign tumor in its entirety so that it cannot later become malignant or interfere with nearby tissue
- To reduce symptoms and make the patient more comfortable (*palliation*)
- To remove or restructure tissue and organs after the tumor has been removed (*reconstructive* or *plastic surgery*)

While some of these procedures are more complicated than others, doctors and hospitals have a way of making even elaborate surgery seem routine. To the patient, however, no operation is routine. Even if you have total faith in your surgeon, you will probably feel more confident if you know what is going to happen. Try to get answers to the following questions:

- In simple terms, what is the purpose of the surgery?
- How much surgery is being done? Why? (For example, if you are a breast cancer patient, how much of the breast, if any, will be removed? Of the surrounding tissue? Of the underarm lymph nodes?)
- If exploratory surgery is being planned, why? If the exploration reveals a tumor, will it be taken out at the same time?
- What are my chances of being cured by this surgery? Of seeing my condition improved?
- What would I risk by not having the surgery?

- Could I die from the surgery or its possible complications? How high is the risk?
- What are the possible side effects, including pain, of the surgery and the postoperative healing process?
- Are other treatments available?
- Is the surgery likely to leave me disabled or disfigured? If so, will rehabilitation or reconstructive surgery be possible?
  (Some people–like the attorney mentioned in Chapter 1–may wish to weigh the benefits of surgery against the possibility of disfigurement.)
- How long will I be in the hospital? How long will it take me to recover completely?
- Will I need further treatment after surgery?
- How much will the surgery cost?

On all of these questions, but especially on the ones about alternatives to surgery, you might also want to consult a *medical oncologist*. This is a cancer specialist who is *not* a surgeon. He or she might provide another useful perspective.

Many different specialists are qualified to perform cancer surgery. Depending on the location of the tumor, it might be removed by a general surgeon, a gynecologist, a thoracic surgeon, a neurosurgeon, a plastic surgeon, a colorectal surgeon, an ophthalmologist, an orthopedic surgeon, a urologist, or an otolaryngologist. What is important from your point of view is, first, the surgeon's expertise in a specialized field and second, his or her expertise in treating cancer.

Prepare Yourself

How soon should you have your surgery? In many cases time is of the essence. But assuming that a few days don't matter, that you don't just want to get it over with as quickly as possible, and that your surgeon's schedule permits, it's a good idea to prepare yourself mentally and

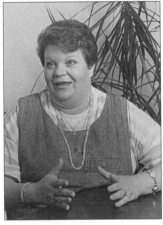

Nancy Heitz

AI. WRIGHT

"Before surgery, I prepared myself in my head.... All it takes is one positive thing to make you feel better."

–Nancy Heitz

physically. This might mean spending time with family and friends. It might mean giving yourself a few quiet days to reflect. It might mean delegating your responsibilities to others, so that you can rest and relax as much as possible. On the other hand, it might mean getting things done—checking on insurance, answering those letters, cleaning the house. However you prepare yourself, your goal is to increase your peace of mind.

For Nancy Heitz, who has had several operations, preparing for surgery meant, first of all, confronting and dealing with her fears. Above all, she feared that the surgeons might find that her condition was worse than she had thought. Nancy wanted to be ready for whatever might happen:

"Before surgery, I prepared myself in my head. I said, 'Okay, Nancy, what's the worst possible thing that can happen? Then I said, 'What's the best possible thing that can happen?' Then I just tried to make whatever was negative into something positive in my head. All it takes is one positive thing to make you feel better."

What did she mean by "one positive thing"?

"Well, take my last surgery, on my leg. I knew there was a probability they were going to find more than what the X rays were showing. But I also knew that, if they found more tumor, they'd take it out—which would give me more time on my legs. The pain, the surgery—they were the negatives. But they would lead to a positive: I would be on my legs longer; I would be healthier."

Nancy was also afraid that she would not survive surgery. She experienced this fear most keenly at a time when she was extremely ill, on the eve of an operation that was in fact a matter of life and death. She drew strength from her family and one special friend by asking them to concentrate all of their thoughts on her while she was in the operating room:

"I merely asked everyone who was going to be there—my father, my mom, my brother, and Michael—to hold me in their minds and not let me go. That eased my fear because I knew someone was holding on to me. They couldn't go into the surgery with me and hold me physically, but they could hold me mentally. That made me feel better. I didn't feel alone. Surgery is a very hard thing. It's like any treatment–it's happening to you, and you are alone in it. But you don't have to be."

Nancy prepared for her operations in another important way–by being nice to herself. Once, just prior to her fasting period the night before surgery, she treated herself to her favorite dessert, apple pie and ice cream. "I just sat there," she said, "and savored it." Her advice to others? "Do something good for yourself. Something positive. Something fun. And the treat doesn't have to be food. I mean, give yourself a facial or go for a walk in your favorite park. Whatever makes you happy."

Often, especially with an exploratory operation, doctors do not know in advance exactly how much surgery may be necessary.* This can be very frightening, but it helps to be prepared. Nancy Heitz has some advice on how to deal with this situation too:

"The doctors usually have a pretty good idea of what they expect to find. Get them to tell you what they're looking for. Ask them to be specific. That's a scary thing to do. It's really hard to say, 'Okay, I've heard about the best part; now tell me the bad part.' But that's meeting your fears–if you know the worst possible scenario, then you can prepare yourself mentally for it. If you wake up and you have lost a breast and you weren't prepared for it, you're in for a major trauma. Being prepared isn't going to eliminate all trauma, but it's certainly going to make it easier."

Here are some other ways to prepare for surgery:[7]

- Get yourself into the best possible physical condition. The fitter you are, the faster you will snap back after the operation. Lose weight, if you are overweight. Exercise, if possible, to strengthen your heart and lungs.
- If you smoke, stop smoking–at least until you are on the road to recovery. (Better yet, you might want to think about stopping permanently.) The healthier your lungs are,

*As a hospital patient, you will be asked to sign an *informed consent* form, which authorizes surgeons to act as they deem necessary in the course of an operation.

For how to quit smoking, see Chapter 8.

the less chance there is that you will develop breathing problems following surgery.

● Talk to your doctor about the possibility of storing a pint of your own blood, in case you should need a transfusion during the operation.

Some of the patients we interviewed believed that what was said in the operating room affected them, even though they were unconscious. As Dennis Brown put it, "I think that when you're under anesthesia, you're in an altered state of consciousness, and your inner mind is much more subject to suggestion." We know of no scientific evidence to support this opinion, but it is shared by some health care professionals. Some even apply the principle as the patient goes under. "As we put our patients under anesthesia, we often tell them to think pleasant thoughts," says Karin Selbach, an operating room nurse. "We may ask them to describe their idea of a dream vacation. In a calm, quiet voice, I may say things like 'You're in good hands. You're safe. When you wake up, this will all be over and you'll feel good.' I'm personally big on touch. I like to hold the patient's hand and touch his shoulder as he goes out."[8] You might want to ask your surgical team to say only positive things during your operation; this can help to give you a greater sense of control. If your surgeon replies that this is nonsense, ask him or her to humor you. Nothing that would make you more comfortable is nonsense, in our opinion.

What Are the Possible Risks?

In this chapter we define *risk* as the possibility of injury resulting from treatment. We define *side effect* as a less serious, secondary effect of treatment. In some cases the distinction is a fine one. For example, we cite secondary infection resulting from surgery as a risk, but it could also be cited as a side effect.

There are many reasons why cancer surgery is less risky now than it was even a few years ago. New techniques, such as magnetic resonance imaging (MRI) and positron

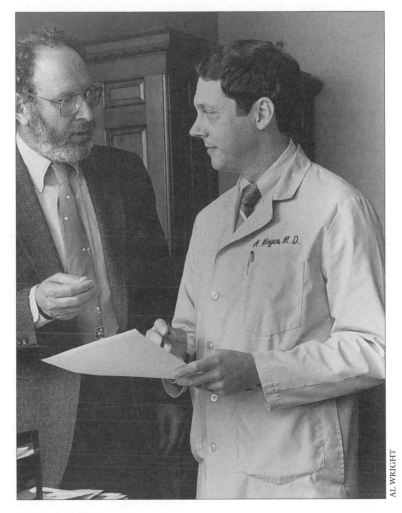

AL WRIGHT

Dr. Andrew Moyce

"Fear of treatment is often the enemy....If you allow the risks to dominate your thinking, you may leave the cancer inadequately treated."

–Dr. Andrew Moyce

emission tomography (PET), enable surgeons to locate tumors very precisely. This reduces the amount of healthy surrounding tissue that must be removed. Sometimes it also makes for a shorter operation.

Microsurgical procedures, including the use of lasers, can achieve pinpoint accuracy and have made it possible to operate on tumors that were once inaccessible. Improved equipment enables the doctor to monitor the patient's vital signs more closely. Finally, more and more surgeons now specialize in cancer cases–sometimes even in particular types of cancer. This has made for much greater expertise within the profession.

Despite all these improvements, surgery does entail certain risks. First, there are the risks that accompany any surgery: possible infection, loss of blood, the adverse effects of anesthesia. Second, in cancer cases there is a slight chance of spreading malignant cells during the surgery itself. This is a very remote possibility. Surgeons take every precaution to reduce the risk to the minimum. Nevertheless, you may wish to discuss it–as well as the other risks–with your doctor.

Dr. Andrew Moyce, one of our consulting surgeons, believes that the risk factor, especially the risk of spreading malignant cells through surgery, is greatly exaggerated. He believes that it sometimes makes patients hesitate when they should go ahead with the operation. "Fear of treatment," he says, "is often the enemy. Risks are important, but not *the* most important consideration. If you allow them to dominate your thinking, you may leave the cancer inadequately treated."[9]

So don't ignore the risk factor altogether. But remember that surgery, usually augmented by chemotherapy or radiation, remains one of medicine's most effective weapons against cancer. Every patient we interviewed who had undergone surgery felt that the benefits far outweighed the risks.

Chemotherapy

The treatment of disease with chemical agents is called *chemotherapy*. Chemotherapy for cancer involves the use of medications to destroy or immobilize malignant cells, often, although not always, when they are dividing. These medications are usually taken by mouth or by intramuscular, intravenous, or subcutaneous injection. Chemotherapy is used for one of more of the following purposes:

- As primary therapy, to destroy malignant cells in certain types of cancer

- To arrest tumor growth in the early stages of certain cancers
- To reduce the risk of recurrence or of metastasis
- To supplement surgery or radiation
- To reduce symptoms

Oncologists prescribe a wide assortment of chemotherapy drugs and combinations of drugs. Which one is appropriate for you will depend on the type of cancer you have, the stage it has reached, and your general state of health.

These factors will also determine how the drug is administered. Some patients may be hospitalized and kept under observation, especially during the first series of treatments. Others whose condition permits may be treated in outpatient clinics or in the doctor's office. Patients who are in good general health and who are receiving oral medication can often take it at home. Chemotherapy can be given anywhere from once a day to once a month. The frequency of medication may change over the course of the treatment.

To learn what chemotherapy entails, we suggest that you ask your doctor the following questions.[10] You may want to get a second opinion before you make up your mind.

- Why do I need chemotherapy?
- Are there other types of treatment for my cancer?
- How successful is the chemotherapy likely to be?
- How successful are other treatments likely to be?
- What are the risks and benefits of each option?
- What medications will I be taking? How and where will they be given?
- How long will a treatment session last?
- How long will I have to have chemotherapy?
- What are the possible long- and short-term side effects? How quickly are they likely to appear and disappear?
- Will there be restrictions on my diet, work, or other activities?
- What will the therapy cost?

What Are the Possible Risks?

Chemotherapy drugs work by destroying or neutralizing cancer cells. Usually, however, they must be prescribed in high-potency doses in order to be effective. And the higher the potency, the more damage they may also do to healthy, noncancerous cells. Especially at risk are rapidly multiplying cells, such as those found in the mouth, the lining of the intestine, the hair follicles, and the bone marrow.

Although most healthy cells recover from chemotherapy medication within a few weeks, bone marrow cells can take longer. This is important, because the bone marrow manufactures white blood cells, which help to fight infection; red blood cells, which transport oxygen and help to eliminate waste; and platelets, which help the blood to clot. While patients are on chemotherapy, frequent *blood counts* are taken to make sure that these vital components are working properly. If they are not, the medication is reduced, changed, or discontinued until they are. Indeed, part of the skill of the oncologist consists of adjusting dosages so that the maximum number of cancer cells are destroyed while healthy cells are damaged as little as possible.

Drug resistance can be another problem. For reasons that are not clearly understood, cancer cells sometimes cease to absorb a particular chemotherapy drug. It is important to discover this resistance quickly, because if the prescribed medication is continued, the body's healthy cells will be needlessly exposed to it, while the drug will no longer have any effect on the cancer. Fortunately, drug resistance is well recognized, and doctors are always on the watch for it. They deal with it by altering the medication.

In addition to bone marrow damage—which in extreme cases can immobilize the immune system and lead to death—certain chemotherapy drugs carry the risk of anemia, diabetes, liver problems, and kidney disorders. However, since 1943, when chemotherapy was first used, the risk to healthy cells has been much reduced. Powerful new drugs can be given in smaller doses. Drugs are combined in new ways that make them less toxic. Surgical implants focus drugs on malignant cells, sparing as many healthy cells as possible. Every year science is discovering new ways to make chemotherapy easier on the patient.[11]

What Are the Side Effects?

If you are considering chemotherapy, you're probably worried about the side effects. Admittedly, these can be a trial. Chemotherapy can cause hair loss, as it did in Julie Benbow's case. It can also cause nausea and other intestinal problems. However, these side effects are sometimes blown out of proportion. Not everyone gets sick from taking chemotherapy. Jay Fritz remembered being frightened by "the terrible stories going around." But he discovered that, at least in his own case, the fear was far worse than the fact. While he felt slightly nauseated for a day or two, Jay was never troubled by vomiting or diarrhea. At the end of his treatment he could honestly say, "For me, chemotherapy was quite easy."

Nor will you necessarily lose your hair. Depending on the drugs prescribed, hair loss may be total, partial, or nonexistent. And even when it is total, it is usually only temporary. Anyway, as Jay remarked, "Losing your hair doesn't hurt you." Some patients saw it as an opportunity to improve their appearance, using wigs to experiment with new hair colors and styles.

This is not to minimize the problem of hair loss. Some patients found it extremely disturbing, and one man refused chemotherapy because he could not face the prospect of even temporary baldness. Hair loss can sometimes be prevented or diminished through the use of *scalp hypothermia*. A cold cap placed on the head during and just after chemotherapy reduces the amount of medication reaching the hair follicles. Scalp hypothermia does not always work, and many patients find the procedure uncomfortable. However, it is certainly worth looking into if you are concerned about losing your hair.

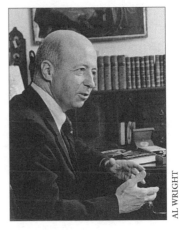

AL. WRIGHT

Jay Fritz

"For me, chemotherapy was quite easy."

–**Jay Fritz**

"The nausea is annoying and no fun for a few days. But when you look at that compared to living, or having a good chance to live, it's an easy choice to make."

–Jay Fritz

Much has been done in recent years to minimize the discomfort associated with chemotherapy. Not only has more controlled delivery made the drugs less wearing on the body, but a wide variety of preparations–including marijuana as an antinausea agent[12]–are used to help counteract the side effects of these drugs. Chemotherapy clinics have also reported some success using hypnosis, muscle relaxation, and biofeedback.[13]

Sometimes the solution is even simpler. Linda Sumner reported that her clinic kept a supply of lemon drops on hand to help overcome the side effects of chemotherapy. "When you're getting treatments, your mouth gets very hot and the saliva starts to flow," she told us. "And the lemon drops just cut it. They work great."

For Paula Carroll, apple juice was the perfect antidote to nausea. For Linda Sumner, "sucking a lot of ice." As to what to eat for your meals while you are undergoing chemotherapy, Linda suggests simply "eating what tastes good, no matter how strange it sounds. I ate mashed potatoes, sourdough toast, potato chips. Different things work for different people. I ate hot dogs for a week. You kind of go with what works."

However troublesome they may be, the side effects of chemotherapy seldom last long. A few of the people we interviewed stopped taking a drug temporarily because they could not tolerate its side effects. But none of them found it necessary to drop out of treatment permanently for this reason. The majority could echo Jay Fritz when he told us, "The nausea is annoying and no fun for a few days. But when you look at that compared to living, or having a good chance to live, it's an easy choice to make."

Dennis Brown, who suffered considerable discomfort from his many chemotherapy treatments, agreed with Jay. "I can't afford to pass up the opportunity for improvement," he told us, "just because of the difficulty of the treatment." Dennis had what seems to us a very positive way of viewing his therapy: he took a step-by-step, day-at-a-time approach. "If," he said, "I'm going to be sick for five days, I can handle that. At the end of the first day I say to myself, 'You're 20 percent done.' By the end of the second day I'm 40 percent. By the third day I'm well over half." As we suggest in Chapter 6, this step-by-step approach can be usefully applied to the entire cancer experience.

The step approach to problem solving is discussed on page 190.

We asked oncology nurse specialist Theresa Koetters what advice she would give to patients who did not share Dennis's and Jay's outlook–to people who were frankly scared to death of chemotherapy:

"I would tell them to let their doctor know they're scared to death. Let their nurse know that they have a needle phobia or that they had severe nausea or vomiting with a pregnancy or something so that we can try to anticipate and lessen the side effects as much as possible. After they've started treatment, they should tell their physician if the quality of their life is too compromised to put up with the treatment. The goal of chemotherapy is to give people time and quality of life, but if that's not being accomplished, people need to know that they can stop chemotherapy at any time. Stopping treatment is certainly not the ideal solution, especially when the physician is treating one of the very curable cancers. I believe that patients need to know when they start therapy that it may be hard, but that, hopefully, in the long run it's going to be worth it. And the job of health care professionals is to support patients through the treatment, however severe the side effects are."[14]

In the misery of the moment, the side effects of chemotherapy can certainly be hard to bear. But in the long run, we believe that the misery–if indeed it comes to that–is worth it. We interviewed one woman who had undergone two difficult courses of chemotherapy for Hodgkin's disease. Immediately after the second one she swore that she would never do it again. Twelve months later she said, "Of course I would do it again if I had to. A year ago I was simply reacting to how I was feeling at the time." She had grown to understand that her chemotherapy had given her the chance of a normal life span. Like Jay Fritz and Dennis Brown, she had come to realize that a few weeks of feeling ill was a small price to pay for that chance.[15]

Radiation Therapy

The treatment of disease with high-energy radiation is called *radiation therapy* (or *radiotherapy*). The radiation may be applied externally or internally. External radiation comes from machines; it usually consists of X rays or gamma rays. Internal radiation comes from radioactive substances such as radium, which are placed in or near the tumor.

Radiation therapy is used

- As a primary therapy, to destroy certain malignancies
- To arrest tumor growth in the early stages of certain cancers
- To reduce the risk of recurrence or of metastasis
- To supplement surgery or chemotherapy
- To reduce symptoms

Half of all cancer patients receive radiation at some point during the course of standard treatment.[16] Radiation is most often used in conjunction with chemotherapy or surgery. However, it is used as a primary treatment for some cancers, especially for fast-growing, radiosensitive tumors that can be reached without having to penetrate much healthy tissue.

While chemotherapy usually distributes medication throughout the body, radiation therapy focuses on the tumor itself. In some cases radiation is administered internally. This method delivers a high dose of radiation directly on the tumor. It is quicker than the external method, and it exposes less of the surrounding healthy tissue. Internal radiation therapy is delivered in various ways. A sealed container of radioactive material may be implanted in a body cavity (such as the uterus). This is called *intracavity radiation*. Or the container may be implanted right in the tumor (as in breast cancer). This is called *intrastitial radiation*. Or the container may be placed on the surface of the body, as close as possible to the tumor. This is sometimes called *brachytherapy;* however, the term "brachytherapy" is more often used to refer to all three methods. No matter which of these methods is used, the container is implanted in the hospital under general or local anesthesia. It is usually taken out after one to seven days, but in some cases it is left in place permanently.

Internal radiation may also be given orally (for thyroid cancer) or by injection. In the latter case, the radioactive material is injected into a body cavity or directly into the bloodstream.

In most cases, however, radiation is administered externally. Employing sophisticated electronic equipment, specially trained therapists aim powerful X rays or gamma rays at the tumor. If you are receiving external radiation therapy, you will usually have treatment sessions five days a week for a period of six or seven weeks; the exact number of sessions will depend on the nature and location of the tumor. If you are getting radiation to reduce symptoms, you will probably have it for two or three weeks.[17]

Radiation therapy is delivered by a team of specialists. The head of the team is the *radiation oncologist,* whose job it is to prescribe the appropriate treatment. The treatment is administered by the *radiation technologist,* whose job it is to run the machine. (You may also encounter the term "radiation therapist." This term can mean either the radiation oncologist or the radiation technologist.) The *radiation physicist* calculates the correct amount of radiation and makes sure that the machine delivers that amount. The *dosimetrist* calculates the number and length of the treatment sessions. The *radiation therapy nurse* will prepare you for your treatment and will tell you how to deal with any side effects. It may not be feasible to meet beforehand with every member of the team, but try to meet with your radiation oncologist before you start treatment. You will want to feel as confident in this specialist as you do in your own personal physician. Here are some questions that you may want to ask:

- Why do I need radiation?
- Are there other types of treatment for my cancer?
- How successful is the radiation likely to be?
- How successful are the other treatments likely to be?
- What are the risks and benefits of each treatment?
- Which parts of my body will be treated? Will the tissue surrounding the tumor be affected?
- How long will the course of treatment last, and how long will each treatment session last?
- What are the possible long- and short-term side effects?
- Should I take any special precautions during and after treatment? Should I take special care of my skin, for example?
- What will the treatment cost?

What Are the Possible Risks?

Radiation has to be powerful in order to be effective – many times more powerful, for example, than the radiation from medical or dental X rays. Because it is so powerful, it inevitably damages a certain number of healthy cells as it works to destroy the cancerous ones. In certain cases, the damage may not show up until long after the treatment is completed. Organs that can be damaged by radiation include the lungs, the liver, the eyes, the stomach, and the bladder. Occasionally radiation also damages the central nervous system.

The nature and degree of radiation risk is related not only to the number of healthy cells affected but also to the function performed by those cells. For instance, if disease-fighting cells are damaged, the immune system may be impaired: wounds may heal more slowly, and the body may become more vulnerable to other diseases. When radiation is directed at cells in the stomach or intestine, there is a slight risk of tissue perforation. This rarely happens, but when it does, it may take surgery to repair the damage.

The best-known risk is that of sterility. This applies, of course, only to people of childbearing age. However, unless the reproductive area is being directly radiated, it is normally shielded during therapy, and the risk of sterility is consequently low. If you have the slightest doubt about this matter, you should discuss it with your radiation oncologist. And if there is a chance that you may become sterile, you may want to ask about having your sperm or eggs frozen before you begin the course of radiation.

However, healthy cells can withstand radiation therapy better than tumor cells. This is because they recover faster. Therefore, properly spaced doses of radiation will gradually kill off the tumor cells while providing time for the healthy cells to recover. Not only is the dosage strictly controlled, but treatment is carefully tailored to the needs of each patient. The intensity and path of the radiation are precisely plotted, and everything possible is done to limit the exposure of healthy tissue. Most of the radiation patients we interviewed were aware of the intricate calculations that went into their therapy. As Linda Sumner said, " I was impressed with my radiation team, particularly with the measures they took to protect me."

What Are the Side Effects?

Most of the side effects of radiation are not serious. However, some of them can make you uncomfortable. The commonest of these are skin changes, fatigue, eating problems, and emotional distress.

Once known as "the therapy that burns," radiation causes much less skin damage today. This is due to improvements in technique—for example, the ability to focus on a tumor from several different angles. On the other hand, the skin *is* likely to react to some extent; it may darken, toughen, blister, or itch. For Leslie Haines, the worst "damage" was psychological; it took her some time to get used to the small tattoo* that was placed on her skin

*Many radiation patients are marked with removable ink. However, permanent tattoos are used when further radiation in the area may be necessary.

as a target for the X ray. Leslie felt better after she discussed her feelings with her support group. With their help she was finally able to accept the tattoo "as an honorable wound won in honorable combat against cancer."

Almost all patients experience some fatigue. This is caused by the effects of the radiation on normal cells; it is likeliest to happen when a large area—all of your lymph nodes, for instance—is being treated. Fatigue can also be caused by changes in hormone levels, by stress, and probably by other unknown factors. If you experience fatigue, the most important thing to remember is that this is *not unusual;* it doesn't mean that your cancer is getting worse. Take it easy; be good to yourself; get plenty of rest. You will get your strength back in time.

Like chemotherapy, radiation therapy tends to damage the cells in the mouth and the lining of the intestine. This can cause eating problems similar to those caused by chemotherapy.

Side effects of radiation to specific areas can include hair loss (in the area being treated); voice impairment and discomfort in the mouth, throat, teeth, and ears (from head, neck, and upper-chest radiation); loss of appetite, nausea, vomiting, and bloating (from upper-abdomen radiation); and diarrhea, stomachache, and cramps (from lower-abdomen radiation). However, nobody has all of these problems all of the time. Most of the patients we spoke with experienced only one or two of them, and that only temporarily.[18]

Perhaps as a result of the fatigue it causes, radiation can stress out the mind as well as the body. To handle both kinds of stress, try to take extra good care of yourself. Follow a healthy diet; get plenty of rest; and drink more fluids than usual. As Leslie Haines puts it, "Keep your body as healthy and your mental attitude as positive as you can."

One way to maintain a positive attitude is to use visualization. Many of our patients pictured the X rays as sunbeams, bathing their bodies with waves of healing. This enabled them to see the treatment as something that was helping them, and this in turn reduced their mental stress.

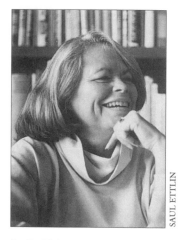

Leslie Haines

SAUL ETTLIN

For more on visualization, see page 220.

118

Speaking of positive mental attitudes, we know of one man who converted his weekly radiation treatments into flights of fancy. He dubbed the radiation machine "the Transporter…because it reminded me of the transport area and console in Star Trek." He continually bantered with the staff, awarding them symbolic Ph.D.'s in "marks-ism," not only because of their expertise in aiming X rays, but also because he liked their "Marx Brothers sense of humor."[19] This man clearly enjoyed the radiation staff; they clearly enjoyed having him as a patient.

Hormonal Therapy

Often considered a form of chemotherapy, hormonal therapy treats cancer with drugs that inhibit the production of, or duplicate, natural hormones. *Hormones* are chemicals produced in the body that regulate the activity of certain cells or organs. Although other hormones are also used to treat cancer, the most important ones, and the ones that concern us here, are the estrogens in women and the androgens (such as testosterone) in men. Estrogens are secreted primarily by the ovaries, androgens primarily by the testes. Both are responsible for the development of secondary sex characteristics—that is, of breasts in women and facial hair and voice changes in men. Estrogen also plays an important role in the menstrual cycle.

The estrogens and androgens can "encourage" the growth of certain cancers. For example, the estrogens can encourage the growth of some breast cancers and the androgens can encourage the growth of some prostate cancers. Hormonal therapy attempts to inhibit this growth-enhancing effect. When the patient is receptive to hormonal therapy, the growth of the tumor is usually slowed, and in some cases it is completely stopped. Hormonal therapy is often used in conjunction with radiation or chemotherapy or both. Hormones may also be given after surgery to destroy any cancer cells that may be left in the body.

If hormones encourage tumors to grow faster, how can

"Keep your body as healthy and your mental attitude as positive as you can."

–Leslie Haines

119

hormone therapy slow their growth? This is sometimes done by using hormones of the opposite sex. For example, female hormones are used to slow the growth of prostate cancer in men and male hormones are used to slow the growth of breast cancer in women. Increasingly, however, both sexes are being treated with *hormone antagonists*– pharmaceutical drugs that inhibit the production of male or female hormones. An example is tamoxifen, which inhibits the production of estrogen and is used to treat breast cancer. In addition to breast and prostate cancers, hormonal therapy is sometimes used to treat uterine cancer, lymphomas, leukemias, and thyroid cancer.[20]

Taking hormones, either orally or through injection, is not without risk. Depending on the hormone in question, patients may occasionally develop high blood pressure, congestive heart failure, peptic ulcers, depression, psychosis, or diabetes. However, the risk in each case is small.

The side effects of hormonal therapy are relatively minor. Men taking estrogens may experience breast enlargement, impotence, and reduced sex drive. Women taking androgens may experience an increased sex drive; their voices may grow deeper and their hair may grow in more heavily. Menopausal women may experience spotting or bleeding. Other possible side effects, including those caused by hormone antagonists, include nausea and vomiting, weight gain, fluid retention, hot flashes, vaginitis, hair loss, and itching. These side effects are rarely serious, and they normally disappear when treatment is discontinued.[21]

Investigational Treatment

Standard treatments are proven therapies. Investigational treatments (formerly known as "experimental treatments") are clinical trials. These trials are conducted with cancer patients. Patients who participate in clinical trials receive treatments that are not yet available to the general public. It is through clinical trials that standard treatments are often developed.

In this section we also discuss private research programs. These programs offer patients the opportunity to obtain experimental drugs without participating in a clinical trial.

Clinical Trials

A *clinical trial* is a study conducted with cancer patients, using the scientific method, to evaluate new therapies or procedures. Most of the breakthroughs in cancer treatment, especially in chemotherapy and hormonal therapy, have come through clinical trials.

See page 141 to learn more about the scientific method of investigation.

Clinical trials are divided into three phases. In phase one studies, a treatment is tried on human subjects for the first time. A drug may be given to a small number of patients, for example, to determine its effectiveness, its maximum tolerated dosage, and its side effects.

In a phase two study, the recommended dose and schedule for a drug, based on phase one results, are tested on various types of tumor. The drug may also be tested in combination with other drugs.

Phase three studies seek to answer several questions. Will new tests confirm the success rate found in phase two? Will the drug prove more effective than it was in phase two? Will it turn out to have unexpected side effects? Above all, how valuable is the drug compared to the standard treatments for a given tumor? To answer the last question, the new drug is given to one group of patients and the standard treatment is given to another group (called the *control* group). Both groups are randomized– that is, patients are chosen by chance to be in one group or the other. If you participate in a phase three trial, you (and possibly your doctor) may not know which group you are in, or which treatment you are receiving.

All clinical trials have *protocols*. These are guidelines that spell out the design of the project, who can participate, and what prior treatments participants should (or should not) have had. Protocols also specify the age range, sex, and condition required of the participants, as well as the type, grade, and stage of the cancer under investigation. To guarantee reliable results, patients must usually meet every requirement in order to be considered for a trial. Many clinical trials are designed to test new medications on advanced cancers. Some, however, involve patients with early-stage malignancies.[22]

Before you choose your treatment program, you may want to ask your doctor whether researchers are conducting clinical trials that apply to your type of cancer. (You can also obtain this information by calling the NCI at 1-800-4-CANCER.) If so, find out where the research is being conducted and exactly what the investigators are looking for. See whether you are qualified to take part in the trial. If you are, it's time to ask yourself whether you want to participate.

There are many things to consider before you decide to take part in a clinical trial. Distance is one. Can you afford the cost of travel if the project is located 2,000 miles away? If not, you might want to look for another suitable project nearer to home. Consider effectiveness and safety too. If you take part in a clinical trial, you will be asked to give the researchers your *informed consent*. This means that after the benefits and risks of the trial have been explained to you, you sign a form saying that you agree to participate. You will probably be given a drug that has *not been proven* safe and effective against cancer, but which researchers believe is *likely* to be both. Before you sign a consent form, ask some questions. Is the drug expected to be effective against your type of cancer? Or is it only expected to ease symptoms? Could the drug be harmful? If it could, do the protocols cover compensation and treatment for the harm? Finally, find out whether you might be placed in a control group that is receiving a standard treatment instead of the experimental drug that you hoped for. If so, are you willing to take that chance?

We suggest that you ask these questions before you decide to take part in a clinical trial:[23]

- What is the purpose of the study?
- What kind of tests and treatment are involved?

- What is likely to happen to me with this treatment? Without it?
- Are there other treatments? What are their advantages and disadvantages?
- How long will the study last?
- Will it affect my daily life? How?
- Will the treatment have side effects? What are they?
- Will I have to be hospitalized? How often? For how long?
- Will it cost me anything to participate?
- If I am harmed by the study, will I receive any treatment?
- Does the study include long-term follow-up care?

Should you take part in a clinical trial? Opinions differ. Many trials involve patients who have been diagnosed terminal. Some people feel that if you are terminal, these trials–especially phase one trials, which are highly experimental and are unlikely to benefit the patient directly–will simply waste your remaining time, time that might better be spent settling your affairs and being with your family. On the other hand, some people feel that since no other treatment has worked, you have nothing to lose–and there is always a chance that the new drug will help. Finally, some patients participate as a kind of legacy, taking satisfaction in the hope that the results of the experiment will benefit other cancer patients. As John Chapman told us, "Even if this drug never helps me, I'll feel gratified if it can help somebody else with cancer."

There is general agreement that patients can benefit from participating in phase three trials. These trials provide an opportunity to receive new and possibly effective treatments. And if, in the course of the trial, one treatment proves clearly superior to the others, *all* of the patients will receive the new treatment.

Should you take part in a clinical trial? In the end, there is no easy answer. The choice is up to you. The chance of helping yourself may not be great, but you may still find it

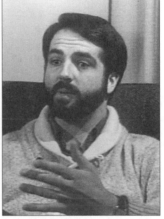

RICK SUTHERLAND

John Chapman

"Even if this drug never helps me, I'll feel gratified if it can help somebody else with cancer."

–John Chapman

worth taking. The chance of helping others may be much greater. In any case, you can always change your mind. Consent to participate in a clinical trial can be withdrawn at any time.[24]

Private Research Programs

Is there any way to get experimental drugs without being involved in a clinical trial? Yes, sometimes–but there are disadvantages. Private biotechnological companies do research to develop experimental drugs. Under current law, these companies can sell their drugs to patients who are willing to act as research subjects before the drugs have been approved for sale to the general public. Like the treatments studied in clinical trials, these drugs are promising but unproven. Note that they are *not* alternative treatments. Like clinical trials, the private research is conducted using the scientific method.

Private research programs differ from clinical trials in two important respects. First, the researchers at private companies do not work directly with the patient. The company provides laboratory services only. If you participate in one of these programs, your own doctor will administer the drug being researched.

However, the drug must be adapted to the individual patient. This is done by culturing the patient's tumor cells in the lab and then testing to see whether these cells will respond to the drug in question. Because the research takes so much time, only patients with certain types and stages of cancer are eligible to participate. Patients must usually have exhausted the options for standard treatment yet still be strong enough to tolerate the side effects of the drug. These side effects can be severe, and occasionally even life threatening.

Second, the patient pays for the treatment, and the treatment can be very expensive. Lab costs alone can easily run to $20,000, and a total cost of $100,000 (including doctors' fees and hospital fees) is not unusual. This cost is seldom covered by insurance.

In our opinion, private research programs should be viewed as a last resort. If other treatments have failed, however, and if you can afford to pay the price, you may want to ask your doctor to make the necessary inquiries.[25]

New Directions in Cancer Treatment

During the past few years, cancer research has broken new ground in many areas. In this section we describe a few of the latest techniques and present a very brief sample of studies that look promising as of this writing.

Once a highly investigational treatment, bone marrow transplantation is rapidly becoming a standard therapy for treating certain leukemias and resistant forms of lymphoma (including Hodgkin's disease). In recent years, however, researchers have discovered new applications for bone marrow transplantation. Today it is being used successfully to treat breast cancer, for example. It has also shown encouraging potential as a treatment for AIDS. As ongoing research expands the applications for bone marrow transplantation, it offers cancer patients new cause for hope.

Laser surgery is currently being used to treat swallowing problems in patients whose throats are blocked by esophageal cancer. The laser cuts through the tissue that blocks the throat, making it unnecessary to insert a tube. While this form of surgery does not cure the cancer, it greatly improves the patient's quality of life.

Photodynamic therapy (PDT) is still in the experimental stage. PDT directs laser beams at tumor cells that have absorbed light-activated drugs. These drugs encourage the laser to destroy the tissue faster. Since the drugs are concentrated in the tumor cells, the laser will destroy these cells without damaging healthy tissue. In experiments with PDT, certain throat, skin, and bladder cancers have been greatly reduced, or have vanished altogether.[26]

The search for new chemotherapeutic drugs goes on. Scientists are conducting clinical trials on several new

To learn more about bone marrow transplantation, contact the Leukemia Society of America at 1-800-955-4572.

plant products to see whether they can be used in the fight against cancer. One of these products–taxol–comes from the bark of the western yew. Another–homoharringtonine–comes from an evergreen bark that is used in traditional Chinese medicine.[27]

Researchers are also attempting to predict exactly how various tumors respond to radiation. The results of these studies will enable doctors to choose the radiation treatment that is most effective for a given patient.[28] Meanwhile, advances in technique are making it easier both to locate the tumor and to pinpoint the treatment.[29]

In hormone therapy, researchers are studying two promising new drugs–Toremifene and Ru486. Preliminary studies suggest that the latter may be effective against breast cancer.[30] And a study to determine whether tamoxifen–now used to treat breast cancer as we explained above–could actually be used to prevent it from developing in the first place was initiated by the NCI in the spring of 1992. This study, which will take five to eight years and involve 16,000 women, will also seek to determine whether tamoxifen lowers the women's risk of developing heart disease and osteoporosis.[31]

But it is in the new field of immunotherapy that the greatest strides are being made (a result, in part, of AIDS research). Immunotherapy (also called "biological therapy") attempts to stimulate the immune system to kill or control cancer cells. It uses a variety of agents, including monoclonal antibodies, interferons and interleukins, colony stimulating factors, and vaccines.[32]

Monoclonal antibodies are made in the laboratory from cells that the immune system uses to fight disease. As you remember from Chapter 2, the immune system cells in many cancer patients are impaired. They cannot recognize cancer cells–but the monoclonal antibodies can. When the monoclonals are injected into the patient, they locate the cancer cells. These can then be treated with chemotherapy. Combined with a chemotherapeutic drug or with radioactive iodine, the monoclonals also attack cancer cells directly, with very little risk to healthy cells.

On immune impairment in cancer patients, see page 58.

Until recently it was very difficult for researchers to make human monoclonals. Most monoclonals used in the laboratory were produced from mouse cells. Recent discoveries, however, have made it possible to produce monoclonals from human cells, and researchers have used these–with startling success–to treat malignant melanoma. (In one study, all of the skin tumors disappeared within days.)[33] Another recent study suggests that mouse-derived monoclonals might be used to block abnormal cell division in certain breast cancers.[34]

Other powerful stimulating agents made from the body's own cells are used to enhance the activity of the immune system. They encourage it either to identify and eliminate tumors at an early stage, or to destroy cancer cells that remain after other forms of treatment have been completed. *Interferons* and *interleukin-2* are two such agents. Each has undergone considerable experimentation in recent years, and while both have been found to have serious side effects, researchers are optimistic about their potential. Interferons have already been used with considerable success in treating one kind of leukemia, and with more moderate success in treating lymphomas and multiple myeloma.[35] Interleukin-2 has been used in a radical new procedure in which laboratory-produced genetic material is transplanted into the patient to combat kidney cancer or advanced melanoma. This treatment has been found to help about 20 percent of patients; in half of these cases, the tumors almost completely disappeared.[36]

Another recent breakthrough may help the immune system to recover from chemotherapy and radiation therapy. *Colony stimulating factors* (CSFs) stimulate the production of disease-fighting cells in the bone marrow. This enables the patient to tolerate more powerful forms of standard treatment. Researchers are currently trying to determine the best schedule and dose for administering CSFs.

Laboratory studies suggest that CSFs also stimulate certain kinds of cancerous blood cells to die, and that they can stimulate certain white blood cells to attack cancer

"Every day, there are new advances being made, and that helps to keep me going. I mean, miracles happen all the time."

–Nancy Heitz

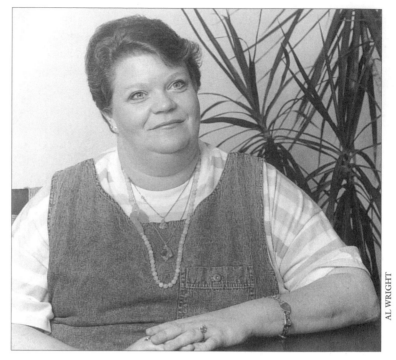

Nancy Heitz

cells in a targeted area. Researchers hope to find a way to use these properties to treat leukemia.[37]

Vaccination is the injection of microorganisms associated with a disease to bolster the body's immunity to that disease. The microorganisms are first weakened or killed. While as yet there is no vaccine that will prevent you from getting cancer, researchers have prolonged the lives of cancer patients by injecting them with killed cells taken from their own tumors. Now researchers are taking this process one step further. They are vaccinating patients with cells that have been taken from their own tumors and genetically altered to secrete extra TNF–an antitumor toxin that is naturally present in the body.[38] The researchers' goal is to learn how to immunize terminal patients against their own cancer.

Cancer cells withstand heat less well than normal cells. *Hyperthermia* involves heating the tumor–or sometimes the patient's whole body–to the point where the cancer cells are destroyed. This is done with equipment that makes use of electromagnetism or ultrasound. Hyperthermia is usually used together with radiation therapy. It is also sometimes used with chemotherapy.

Current research focuses on identifying the tumors that respond best to this treatment and on finding the most effective dose. Researchers have recently pinpointed the optimal temperatures for hyperthermia (40°C, or 104°F); now they are trying to develop the technology needed to deliver that temperature to tumors in various parts of the body.[39] (Incidentally, one study of hyperthermia treatment delivered by ultrasound suggests that the ultrasound itself may be effective against cancer.)[40]

Though at times progress may seem slow, particularly to you who are battling cancer now, it is being made on many fronts. And although, not all of the experts would agree, Dr. John Laszlo believes that we have ample reason to be hopeful. *"In all,"* he writes, *"the future is brightening up really for the first time in history: instead of the problem of cancer getting worse and worse, we seem to have turned the corner!"* [41]

For more on reasons to be hopeful see Chapter 2.

Most of the patients we interviewed shared this hopefulness. After six operations, Nancy Heitz is still genuinely optimistic. "Every day," she told us, "there are new advances being made, and that helps to keep me going. I mean, miracles happen all the time." If she could give one piece of advice to cancer patients, Nancy says, it would be "Hold on. Never give up hoping. Even as you read this, they may be discovering a new treatment for your cancer."

In order of their first appearance, the patients who contributed to this chapter are: Joe Dodig, Nancy Heitz, Charles Fuhrman, Dennis Brown, Jay Fritz, Linda Sumner, Paula Carroll, Leslie Haines, and John Chapman.

Recommended Reading

Bruning, Nancy. *Coping with Chemotherapy.* **New York: Ballantine Books, 1986.**

The author covers all types of chemotherapy. She explains when each type may be used, discusses the side effects of each, and tells how to deal with them. She also discusses emotional factors associated with chemotherapy.

Dodd, Marylin J. *Managing the Side Effects of Chemotherapy and Radiation Therapy.* **East Norwalk, CT: Appleton & Lange, 1987.**

Written for nurses, but in language simple enough for lay readers to understand, this book describes the side effects of chemotherapy and radiation therapy in detail and offers extensive suggestions for managing them. Designed to help nurses to teach self-care techniques to patients and their families, it is useful, comprehensive, and easy to understand.

Dollinger, Malin, Ernest H. Rosenbaum, and Greg Cable, eds. *Everyone's Guide to Cancer Therapy.* **Kansas City, MO: Andrews & McMeel, 1991.**

Part 3: "Supportive Care." Chapters 16 through 21 discuss the various side effects of surgery, chemotherapy, and radiation in detail and offer extensive suggestions for dealing with them.

Part 4: "Treating the Common Cancers." Forty-six chapters, each covering one kind of cancer in detail. The treatment section of each chapter includes an overview summarizing the standard treatments for the cancer in question, a detailed description of treatments by stage, a discussion of treatment follow-up, and a list of the most important questions the patient can ask. Clear descriptions, thorough coverage, and helpful illustrations make this an exceptionally useful resource.

Holleb, Arthur I., ed. *The American Cancer Society Cancer Book*. Garden City, NY: Doubleday & Co., 1986.

Chapter 10: "Coping with Problems Related to Cancer and Cancer Treatment." This chapter covers problems not discussed at length in other books, including bleeding, skin reactions, sexual dysfunction, and problems of the urinary tract. It also covers fatigue, gastrointestinal problems, and eating problems.

Laszlo, John. *Understanding Cancer*. New York: Harper & Row Publishers, 1987.

Chapter 15: "Cancer Research: The Cutting Edge." This chapter is not completely current (Laszlo's book was published in 1987), but it contains very clear descriptions of the use of monoclonal antibodies and other new techniques.

Noyes, Diane Doan, and Peggy Mellody. *Beauty and Cancer*. Marina Del Rey, CA: AC Press, 1988.

Written by a cancer survivor and an RN, this book tells you how to "look great while experiencing the side effects of chemotherapy, radiation, and surgery." Subjects covered include makeup, wigs and headwraps, skin care, and clothing. There is helpful advice on choosing post-mastectomy breast forms and bras. The book includes a list of resources and many illustrations.

Ramstack, Janet L., and Ernest H. Rosenbaum. *Nutrition for the Chemotherapy Patient*. Palo Alto, CA: Bull Publishing Co., 1990.

The authors of this book are a nutritionist and an oncologist. Part 1 explains how to use food to deal with specific problems; it includes a large selection of recipes and tables. Part 2 discusses nutrition and chemotherapy from the medical perspective; it includes a brief section on radiation therapy as well. There are four appendices on side effects and drugs.

Reich, Paul R. *The Facts about Chemotherapy.* **New York: Consumer Reports Books, 1991.**

This book is designed to help people who have cancer to become well-informed, active participants in their own care. It describes the various chemotherapy drugs and tells how they are administered; explains what they can and cannot do; discusses treatment for each of two dozen common cancers; and discusses side effects in detail. This is an outstanding book – thorough, clearly written, and readable.

Alternative
Treatments

Alternative Treatments

Your neighbor believes that prayer will destroy his tumor. Your brother gets acupuncture treatments for Hodgkin's disease. Your friend receives live-cell therapy for her cancer. And your aunt treats her daughter's leukemia with Vitamin C.

All of these people are using alternative treatments for cancer. This book deals primarily with standard treatments, which were discussed at length in Chapter 4. However, we have three reasons for devoting a chapter to alternative treatments. First, you have probably heard about the alternatives and have wondered whether they are effective. Second, you may be tempted to try them, especially if you don't believe in the standard treatments, if the standard treatment you have been receiving isn't going well, or if you have been told that standard treatment can do nothing for you. Finally, much of the available information on alternative therapy is biased one way or the other. This makes it especially difficult to reach an informed decision.

This chapter outlines the major alternative approaches now available and suggests ways to learn more about them. It briefly describes the conflict between standard and alternative practitioners—a conflict often characterized by sensationalism and lack of scientific objectivity. Drawing upon the views of patients who have undergone alternative treatment, we try to help you to form your own conclusions.

What Is Alternative Treatment?

Standard treatment is treatment that is currently being

Alternative treatments are based on the theory that cancer is best combated not by surgery, chemotherapy, or radiation, but by the body's natural ability to heal itself.

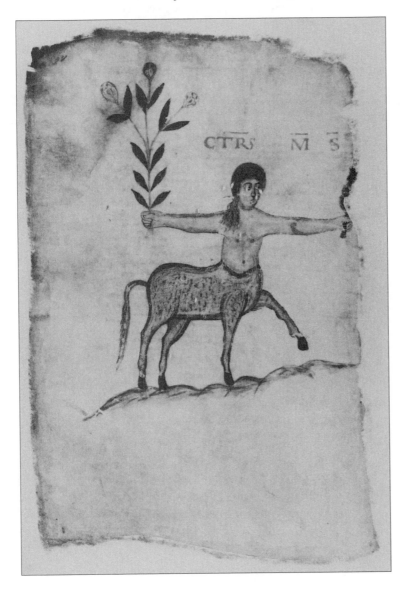

Centaur, the Master of Medicine. Mid 9th century. Manuscript. Gesamthochschul-Bibliothek Kassel. Medieval legends held that Chiron the Centaur, Aesculapius's teacher, passed herbal secrets to Apuleius, a famous Roman herbalist.

used by physicians and that has been proven effective based on past studies. There are four standard treatments for cancer: surgery, chemotherapy, radiation therapy, and hormonal therapy. *Investigational treatment* is defined as clinical trials; this definition can be broadened to include private research programs. Both are conducted using the scientific method to evaluate new therapies or procedures. *Alternative treatment* is any treatment that is neither standard nor investigational. Let's break this definition down a little further.

What is a clinical trial?
See page 121.

Alternative versus Holistic

You have probably heard the term "holistic medicine." Some people use "holistic" as a synonym for "alternative," but in fact the two terms do not mean quite the same thing.

Holistic medicine views the mind and the body as a single unit, and it treats them together as a unit. That is, it deals with the patient's physical, mental, emotional, and spiritual health. It believes that all of these things are interconnected, and that they must be treated together in a balanced way. This is the main premise of holistic medicine.

Holistic medicine, then, is one form of alternative treatment. And many other forms of alternative treatment adhere to the holistic concept to some degree. But different alternative treatments tend to emphasize different aspects of the holistic. That is, they may be primarily physical, primarily mental and emotional, or primarily spiritual. An example of the first would be treatment that consists primarily of—but is not limited to—diet and vitamin supplements; of the second, one that consists primarily of positive thinking; and of the third, one that consists primarily of prayer. Furthermore, some alternative treatments are purely physical or purely spiritual. Examples would be treatments that consist *exclusively* of injections or of faith healing. These last are not holistic therapies at all. Alternative treatment, then, includes, but is not limited to, holistic treatment.

Note too that some physicians practice standard medicine but take what might be called a "holistic approach." Their patients receive massage, psychological and spiritual counseling, nutritional guidance, and so forth *along with* surgery, chemotherapy, or radiation. These people are not getting treated with holistic medicine, which we define as an alternative to standard treatment. What they are getting is *complementary therapy*. We shall have more to say about this later on.

A Variety of Approaches

There are many alternative treatments for cancer, so many that we can highlight only a few. Most are based on the theory that cancer is best combated not by surgery, chemotherapy, or radiation, but by the body's natural ability to heal itself. Hence the stated objective of most alternative treatments is to restore this natural ability. This is done by improving the patient's overall health, strengthening the immune system, and eliminating toxins that might inhibit the body's performance. Depending on the therapy in question, "toxins" can mean anything from pesticides to waste materials in the body to mucus and fats; these last are believed by some alternative therapists to clog the tissues, leading to disease.

Alternative treatments fall broadly into seven categories. In practice, however, alternative therapists seldom confine themselves to a single method; a treatment program may use therapies drawn from more than one of the following groups.[1]

Nutritional

Most alternative therapies that emphasize nutrition call for adherence to a very strict diet. Often called "metabolic therapies," they are based on the belief that waste materials and toxins impair the body's metabolism, and that an impaired metabolism causes cancer. The diets used in these therapies are typically based on vegetarianism, with a strong preference for raw, organically grown fruits and vegetables. These are believed to be the foods most naturally suited to the human body; it is claimed that they help the body to eliminate toxins. Some nutritional programs tailor each patient's diet to his or her specific tumor and metabolic condition.

Many nutritional programs call for massive doses of vitamins *(megavitamin therapy)*. Some call for mineral supplements, such as zinc and iron. Supposedly these too help the body to eliminate toxins. Some nutritional programs call for herbal, coffee, or citrus enemas. These are said to detoxify the body by activating the liver.

Herbal

Herbal remedies are usually prescribed to strengthen the immune system. Some herbal remedies, however, are believed by their proponents to attack tumors directly. Iscador, which is made from mistletoe, and essiac, an herb tea, are among the best-known herbal remedies used in alternative treatment. Herbs used in traditional Chinese medicine, such as ginger and ginseng, are also popular. A few herbal practitioners choose to keep their formulas a secret. It may sometimes be possible to discover the names of the herbs they recommend, but not how much of each herb they use.

"Medicinal"

As we use it, "medicinal" is something of a catchall term. It refers to a number of substances that alternative practitioners use in the hope of bolstering the immune system or shrinking the tumor. Usually prescribed in the form of injections, widely used "medicinal" substances include enzymes, amino acids, polypeptides, hydrazine sulfate, live cells, DMSO, BCG, gamma globulin, and whole-blood components.

Laetrile, a derivative of apricot pits, is a well-known and popular "medicinal" substance. It is used in Mexican clinics that practice metabolic therapy, supposedly to destroy cancer cells. After extensive testing, scientists have found no evidence that laetrile is effective—or even safe. As long ago as 1977, FDA commissioner Donald Kennedy described it as "a major health fraud."[2] Today, laetrile for treating cancer is illegal, practically speaking, throughout the United States.[3]

Naturalistic

In the following discussion, the term "naturalistic" refers to naturopathic and homeopathic treatment. *Naturopathic* medicine uses only natural substances–herbs, water, sunlight, fresh air–to treat illness and rid the body of "impurities" or toxins. *Homeopathic* medicine is based on the concept that like cures like. It uses very small doses of selected substances to treat illnesses the symptoms of which could be caused by a large amount of the same substance. A homeopath, for example, might fight fever by administering a minute dose of a drug that raises the body temperature. Homeopathic remedies are believed to stimulate the body's ability to heal itself by eliminating toxins and bringing the body back into balance ("homeostasis"). Although some practitioners may use homeopathy to relieve the side effects of standard treatment, we know of no homeopathic cancer therapy. In fact, at least one homeopath warns that patients should beware of any homeopath who claims to cure cancer.

Body movement and manipulation

Most of the treatments in the next category depend on the manipulation of body energy–a term that has been variously defined as "life force," "vitality," "Innate Intelligence," or "chi." Practitioners of these treatments believe that this energy can become blocked or otherwise disturbed, and that it can be rebalanced by one or another physical means. Various forms of exercise–stretching, breathing, relaxation, aerobic dance, and certain types of yoga–are usually seen as body restorers and antidepressants rather than as primary treatments for cancer. The same is true of acupuncture and acupressure therapy, which claim to restore the free flow of energy among the various organs. The energy is believed to flow along pathways called "meridians"; pain and illness are said to

At least one homeopath warns that patients should beware of any homeopath who claims to cure cancer.

139

*Some acupuncturists consider this a dangerous form of cancer therapy. In their opinion, acupuncture actually stimulates the growth of the tumor.

More on psychological methods in Chapter 6.

result when the energy is blocked. Acupuncture restores the flow of energy by inserting thin needles into specific points on the meridians;* acupressure achieves the same effect by pressing with the fingers. Chiropractic manipulation and massage attempt to rebalance body energy by manipulating the spine or other parts of the body. These too are usually regarded as complementary therapies.

Psychological

Some alternative therapists prescribe meditation, visualization, positive thinking, and various forms of counseling. They may also use chanting, art therapy, and hypnosis. The goal is usually to improve the patient's quality of life, to facilitate problem solving, to control pain, and in general to support primary treatment. However, certain therapists believe that some of these methods can actually shrink tumors or slow their growth.

Spiritual

Like the psychological methods, prayer and religious ritual are used to help patients to improve their quality of life while they undergo standard or alternative therapies. However, they are occasionally used without other therapy. The best-known example, perhaps, is Christian Science. Adherents of this religion believe that sickness is an illusion. They believe that to cure it, the patient must develop a spiritual understanding of the Truth. Christian Science practitioners are believed to direct healing to the patient by means of prayer. Another well-known example is faith healing, which may include incantation, the laying on of hands, and the casting out of evil spirits.

In short, there are hundreds, if not thousands, of alternative approaches. And a great many alternative therapists combine several approaches in one treatment program. However, no alternative approach has been proven effective by scientific studies. And although some standard physicians use alternatives as complementary therapy to support whatever primary therapy they have prescribed, no standard physician uses an alternative approach as a primary treatment for cancer. In the next two sections, we explain why.

Why Is Alternative Treatment Controversial?

It is no secret that alternative treatment is controversial, and the controversy is often heated. But the hotter the controversy, the harder it is to determine the facts. Let's see if we can look at the issue objectively.

What Science Says

Mainstream science supports standard treatment for cancer and is generally suspicious of alternative treatment. It has two reasons for taking this position. The first is that alternative treatments are unproven; they have not stood the test of scientific investigation. The second is that alternative treatment entails the risk of delay. The National Cancer Institute (NCI) and the American Cancer Society (ACS) both support the position of mainstream science.

In order to evaluate this position, it is first necessary to understand what is meant by scientific investigation. A study is considered scientific when it meets the following criteria:

- The objectives of the study must be clearly stated.
- The methods used to achieve those objectives must be clearly stated, both in the protocol and in the report of the results.
- The study must include a control group. This makes it possible to determine whether the treatment being studied is better than the standard treatment—or than no treatment at all.
- There must be clear evidence that the subjects of the study actually have the condition in question, in this case, cancer.
- Subjects must be randomly assigned to treatment groups and control groups. This is done to eliminate bias. That is, for example, the subjects who have the best chance of getting well should

What's a protocol?
What's a control group?
See page 121.

not all be assigned to the treatment group. This might make the treatment seem to be more effective than it is.

- The subjects' response to the treatment must be objectively assessed. The methods used must be sound and well defined.
- The results of the study must be analyzed thoroughly enough to determine exactly what the effects of the treatment were.

Clinical trials are discussed on page 121.

Scientific studies are conducted by means of clinical trials. The results are published in reputable scientific journals. They are reviewed and evaluated by researchers who are experts in the field. These researchers must be *objective;* they should not be paid, for example, by the company that sells the treatment under investigation. The study must also be reviewed by a human subjects committee in a qualified medical institution. Finally, the results of the study must be replicable. That is, other researchers using the same method must be able to achieve the same results.

These criteria may seem picky and complex. But every one of them is there for a reason: to make sure that the new treatment really works.

Alternative treatments are developed using methods that in one way or another fail to meet all—or any—of these criteria. For example, the new treatment being studied is sometimes used after, or along with, standard treatment. This means that even if the patients get better, there is no way to tell which treatment caused the improvement. Sometimes there is no biopsy evidence to prove that the person had cancer in the first place. Sometimes there is no experimental evidence at all. Results are not reported in scientific journals; they are not reviewed by experts in the field. Finally, alternative researchers seldom keep good records. This means that there is no way of replicating their results—or even of knowing exactly what their results were.

Proponents of alternative treatment often make their claims on the basis of *anecdotal evidence.* That is, they claim that a treatment works on the basis of stories about people who appear to have been cured, or of testimonials from people who believe that they were cured, by the treatment in question. But no matter how sincere it is, anecdotal evidence doesn't *prove* that the treatment works.

The proponents of alternative treatment respond to these charges as follows. First, they say that their own research is adequate for their purposes. This may be true, but it is immaterial, as we have just explained, if the goal is to *prove* that the treatment is effective. Research that does not meet the criteria outlined above does not meet the standards required for scientific proof. That research into alternative treatments does not in fact meet these standards is acknowledged by some physicians with a foot in each camp. One such physician is Dr. James Forsythe, a Nevada oncologist who works comfortably with patients who are also under alternative care. "Frequently people who are in alternative medicine don't have the statistics to back up what they do," says Dr. Forsythe. "And there does tend to be a lack of scientific method. If they are giving laetrile, they may give three vials this week and four vials the next week and then reduce it to one. It's a kind of haphazard approach."[4]

Second, the proponents of alternative treatment say that they welcome investigation by their critics. Here the picture is far from clear. Many clinics do seem to welcome investigation. But some do not–especially the ones that refuse to divulge the exact nature of their therapy. And even the clinics that welcome investigation don't always have records that can be analyzed. Sometimes too their treatment programs change so rapidly that they cannot be studied over time.

Third, the proponents of alternative treatment say that mainstream science has refused to conduct research on alternative medicine. This is to some extent true. There has in fact been a lack of systematic research on the part of mainstream science, and this is not entirely due to uncooperativeness or poor management on the part of the alternative clinics. Part of the problem–perhaps a large part–is money. To do full, simultaneous assessments on a group of patients–to establish each patient's condition,

"Treating cancer is like fighting a fire. By the time you've tried out the alternative, it may be too late."

– Dr. Andrew Moyce

to track this condition during the course of treatment, and to follow it up afterward – is very expensive. Government agencies, which fund most research, have generally been unwilling to fund studies of alternative treatment when there are competing demands to fund studies that are backed by standard medicine.[5]

Even when scientific investigations have been conducted, however, alternative practitioners have not always been ready to accept the results. In the 1970s, for example, a series of studies by the NCI showed that laetrile was of little medicinal value in treating cancer. Dr. Ernest Krebs, the discoverer of laetrile, claimed that the NCI research was flawed because impure strains of laetrile had been used, and because only terminal patients were treated. However, no objective evidence ever appeared to support Dr. Krebs's assertion.[6]

Mainstream physicians oppose alternative treatment for another reason as well. As Dr. Andrew Moyce puts it, "the most important danger of alternative treatment is delay. It is not for nothing that we spend all of our time working to convince people that the key to successful treatment is early diagnosis and management." Patients, these physicians argue, often risk their lives by choosing an alternative approach over a standard one. This is especially true in cases where the standard treatment has been highly successful. "Treating cancer is like fighting a fire," says Dr. Moyce. "By the time you've tried out the alternative, it may be too late."[7]

The issue of delay is absolutely crucial. Perhaps no other single factor contributes as much to the cancer patient's chances of recovery. Bladder cancer patients who are treated promptly – before the cancer starts to spread – have a 90 percent chance of surviving five years. Bladder cancer patients with distant metastases have a 9 percent chance. The figures for malignant melanoma are 90 percent and 14 percent respectively; for colon cancer, 91 percent and less than 7 percent.[8] If you try an alternative treatment first, wait to see whether it will work, find that it doesn't, and only then resort to standard treatment, the time you spend waiting may cost you your life. Such, at least, is the position of mainstream science.

Finally, we should add that most mainstream physicians don't think all alternative treatments are equally bad. They consider some to be harmless, or even indirectly beneficial, when used as a complement to standard treatment. Examples include visualization, meditation, and the use of support groups. These promote a more positive attitude, which in turn helps the patient to deal with standard therapy. The same is true of treatments that emphasize balanced nutrition and exercise. If there is no proof that these treatments cure cancer, at least–most physicians would say–they do no harm. They are inexpensive; they improve the patient's general well-being; and they have their place as complementary therapies. It is quite another story for the person who goes to a clinic in Mexico to be injected with some unproven substance. This patient is unlikely to remain on standard treatment; the injections are usually expensive; and it is arguable whether they improve the patient's quality of life. From the standpoint of mainstream science, this form of alternative treatment is highly suspect.

What the Law Says

It is illegal under federal and state laws to treat, or claim to cure, cancer with drugs that have not been approved by the Federal Drug Administration.* The FDA approves only those drugs which have met the standards for scientific proof. Since alternative treatments are unproven, they are not approved by the FDA. Therefore under U.S. law it is illegal to use them to cure cancer.

This explains why many of the leading alternative clinics are located outside the United States. The heaviest concentration is in Tijuana, on the California-Mexico border, where a number of the people we interviewed have been treated.

Many alternative therapists do practice within the United States. Some are licensed physicians who incorporate

*FDA regulations define a *drug* as any article "intended for use in the diagnosis, cure, mitigation, treatment, or prevention of disease."

145

selected alternative methods into their treatment programs. This is legal as long as the alternatives are used only to *complement* standard therapy. Still others, who apparently offer primary alternative care, maintain legality by stating that their treatment merely helps to "combat" cancer, not to "cure" it. Clinics that do not *claim* to cure cancer, however, may *imply* a cure by pointing to people who have (presumably) been cured after undergoing their therapy. The line between claiming and implying can be a fine one.

Will the Two Sides Ever Agree?

The fight rages on between the supporters of standard and alternative treatment. But changes over the past few years have brought the two sides a little closer together. For example, mainstream science has begun to investigate the possible benefits of certain alternative therapies. In 1986 the NCI gave the New York Botanical Garden $500,000 to conduct a worldwide search for medicinal plant substances that might be helpful in fighting cancer. Researchers traveled to the rain forests of Latin America, Africa, and Southeast Asia to interview native healers about their use of indigenous wild plants. As of this writing, the New York Botanical Garden is still engaged in this research, now funded by a variety of sources.[9]

There is also a growing interest in established alternative cancer therapies. In 1990, the Congressional Office of Technology Assessment (OTA) published a detailed review of alternative treatments, the first study of its kind undertaken since the national war on cancer was declared in 1971.*

On a more general level, the NCI and the ACS have recently changed their attitude toward diet. Both organizations, which at one time paid only scant attention to the nutritional aspects of cancer therapy, now recommend reducing fat and refined sugars and increasing dietary fiber to help prevent cancer from occurring or recurring. To one degree or another, diet has also become a staple of many standard treatments. As Dr. Forsythe says, "When they talk

*You can obtain a copy of this study, or a summary of it, by writing to the Superintendent of Documents, Government Printing Office, Washington, DC 20402-9325, or by calling 1-202-783-3238. The full study, *Unconventional Cancer Treatments,* is 312 pages long and costs $14.00. The summary is 32 pages long and costs $1.75. To fax an inquiry or an order, call 1-202-275-0019.

about diet and life-style changes, I don't really consider these alternative therapies. I consider them as part of standard therapy."

There are also signs that changes may be taking place within the law. In New York, in April 1987, Dr. Emanuel Revici was convicted of malpractice for using alternative methods after the judge had instructed the jury that the law allowed only standard therapies. In what was to become a landmark ruling, a higher court overturned this decision. It concluded that there was "no reason why a patient should not be allowed to make an informed decision and go outside currently approved medical methods in search of an unconventional treatment.... [To do so] is within the patient's right to determine what to do with his or her own body."[10]

Despite these changes, alternative therapy remains in professional limbo. Doctors have lost their licenses for prescribing certain alternative therapies that purport to treat cancer. You should know, then, that if you rely exclusively on an alternative approach, you will in many cases be going not only against the medical mainstream but against the legal mainstream as well.

How to Evaluate Alternative Treatments

It is not easy to evaluate the effectiveness of a given alternative treatment. As we have just explained, the NCI and the ACS endorse only treatments that have been proven effective in scientific studies. The difficulty with alternative treatments is that they cannot be proven effective, either because no such studies exist or because the available data have not been derived using the strict scientific methods required for conventional clinical trials.

We are left, then, with a series of anecdotal success stories—stories of patients who survived for a certain period after their treatment. Alternative therapists often present these stories as case studies that (they say) demonstrate the effectiveness of the treatment in question. Unfortunately,

For more on cancer and nutrition, see Chapter 8.

they seldom, if ever, present case studies of patients who went through the same treatment and died. Without such studies, the *overall* effectiveness of the treatment cannot be evaluated.

Without hard evidence of the sort produced by conventional clinical studies, it is difficult to know how much credence to place in a given success story. Did the patient have standard therapy along with (or before) the alternative therapy? If so, could the standard therapy have played a part in the improvement? Would the patient's condition have improved without treatment? Did the patient even have cancer in the first place?

There is no easy way to answer these questions. Nor is there an easy way to decide whether a given alternative is worth considering. There are, however, guidelines that can be helpful. We suggest that you first ask the following questions of the people who administer the treatment:

- What types of cancer does the clinic claim to have treated successfully? (Be sure that your type is included.)
- What are the goals of the specific treatment that interests me? What results can I realistically expect?
- How long has the clinic been in operation? How many patients has it treated? (The longer the clinic has been in operation, the more likely it is that it has benefited some people. Similarly, the more patients it has treated, the more reliable it is likely to be. Try to find out whether the numbers have been rising or falling. If the trend is down, it may mean that the clinic's reputation is down too.)
- What kind of follow-up procedures are available?
- What is the training of the staff? How many staff members have graduated from accredited universities or medical schools?
- Are there case histories available for examination and are they in language that you can understand? If they are available, who collected them? (An independent researcher selecting randomly

from the files is preferable to a staff member putting together the clinic's own collection.)

While few alternative practitioners have been involved in clinical investigations, it might be worth raising the following questions just in case any research information is available:

- Has the clinic conducted and published the results of research projects, such as animal studies, computer models, or clinical trials? (If so, ask for a copy of the study results and ask a medical person not connected with the clinic to review them.)

- Have independent studies been conducted on this clinic or on the kind of therapy that it provides? (If so, follow the suggestions given above.)

If possible, visit the clinic that interests you. The Cancer Control Society (CCS) runs regularly scheduled tours of many Tijuana clinics. You may be able to get a sense of the operation from the way the staff respond to your inquiries. Will they, for example, let you speak to a nurse? To a doctor? To the patients? Of course, a welcoming attitude is no guarantee of medical competence.

Second, talk directly to people who have undergone the treatment that you are considering. If you don't know any, CCS provides lists of patients who have been treated by various clinics. Bear in mind that these people have volunteered their names and are therefore likely to be satisfied with their treatment. Moreover, no list of dissatisfied patients or failed cases is given.* You may also be able to get names through a cancer support group.

We interviewed over a dozen people on one CCS list and found the majority to be thoughtful and articulate about their experiences. Here are the questions we asked them:

- What was the exact type and stage of your cancer?
- How and why did you choose this clinic or decide on this form of treatment?
- Did you try standard treatments first? If so, which

*Telephone 1-213-663-7801. CCS is a private organization that promotes alternative therapies. Note that the Alpha Institute does not advocate the methods or the position of this group. A word of caution. Although we were given what was said to be an updated list, more than a few telephone numbers provided by CCS were out of service with no new number given. Whether this was the result of poor tracking on the part of CCS or whether the patients listed had died we were unable to determine. In addition, a few of those whom we did reach declined to be interviewed.

ones? For how long? What were the results?

- Was your alternative treatment used in conjunction with standard treatment?
- Did your alternative treatment have any side effects?
- Were diagnostic tests performed when you entered the program? What were they? Was an extensive case history taken?
- What was the attitude of the staff?
- Were you given access to other patients who were treated at the clinic, those who were not helped as well as those who were?
- How expensive was the treatment? How were the costs handled? Were you asked to pay the entire fee up front, or was it possible to pay it in installments?
- Were treatments covered by health insurance? If so, what type of health insurance?
- Was your family encouraged to participate in your treatment plan? If so, how?
- Was there any follow-up? Were you asked to return for checkups or further diagnostic tests? Were you invited to call for advice or support?
- Did your condition improve as a result of the treatment? If so, was it possible to measure the improvement? For example, did your tumor get smaller?
- Would you choose this therapy again?
- May I call you in the future if I have further questions?

Third, stay informed. Consult such popular periodicals as *Consumer Reports Health Letter*, *In Health*, and *American Health*. Keep up with the latest developments in research and treatment as reported in the press. The *New York Times* runs a special "Health" column on Wednesdays. Many local libraries can access recent medical literature via on-line databases.

Above all, we suggest that you maintain a healthy skepticism about unproven claims for curing cancer.

Standard medicine may sometimes be slow to welcome innovations, but its caution in accepting unsupported theories has often been justified.

Michael Lerner, a nationally recognized expert on alternative therapies, who believes that some of these therapies deserve a fuller hearing from mainstream science than they have received, has drawn the following conclusions from his research:

"There is no decisively successful cure for cancer among the alternative therapies.

"There is little credible scientific evidence with which to evaluate the more modest contributions of these therapies."[11]

These conclusions are especially significant because some alternative programs claim truly extraordinary results. For example, according to several patients we interviewed, at least one Tijuana clinic claims an 85 percent cure rate. And one alternative therapist gave us this literature from a practitioner in Japan who claims to have discovered a cancer vaccine:[12]

> *Tens of thousands of cancer sufferers have already been cured....These include a considerable number whose doctors have given them only a few months to live. Even when patients treated by other doctors using surgical methods, and those pronounced hopeless, are included, the cure rate...is 70 percent. For patients who have not been surgically treated by other doctors, the rate climbs to 90 percent.*

In our opinion, such claims—from Mexico, Japan, or anywhere else—should be looked upon with the highest degree of suspicion.

"There is no decisively successful cure for cancer among the alternative therapies."

–Michael Lerner

What Do the Patients Say?

We've given you a brief overview of common alternative therapies. You've heard what science says and what the law says. We've listed some questions for you to ask. Now let's hear what the patients have to say.

"Before I ever had cancer, I had never believed in surgery. I never believed in chemotherapy and I never believed in radiation. I was always a great believer in alternative health anyway."

–Judy Lakotas

Common Themes

In gathering information for this chapter, we did in-depth interviews with people who had chosen alternative treatment. Their cancers included those of the breast, colon, stomach, esophagus, lung, lymph nodes, skin (melanoma), thyroid, and uterus. The treatments involved most of the approaches listed in this chapter. While we did not attempt a scientific study, we believe that our findings illustrate how patients in general choose and experience alternative treatment programs. In the course of these interviews, six common themes emerged.

Dissatisfaction with standard treatment

The attraction of alternative treatment is not confined to patients for whom standard treatment can do nothing more. Research indicates that most of the people who choose alternative therapy do so not as a last resort, as one might think, but because they believe that the choice is in their overall best interests.[13]

In keeping with these findings, many of the people we interviewed said that they turned to alternative therapy because they did not believe in standard therapy, not because they had been told that their case was hopeless. As Judy Lakotas said, "Before I ever had cancer, I had never believed in surgery. I never believed in chemotherapy and I never believed in radiation. I was always a great believer in alternative health anyway." Another patient, typical of many, told us, "I just relate chemotherapy to sickness. It's my belief structure. When I hear 'chemotherapy,' all I can think of is hair loss and vomiting."

Many patients object on philosophical or emotional grounds to what they view as the "invasiveness" of standard treatment. Among the patients we interviewed, distrust of chemotherapy and radiation was especially high.

Many people are drawn to alternative therapies simply because they think that these therapies will be easier to endure. Merely altering one's diet or taking vitamin supplements can seem preferable to patients who fear that standard therapy will disrupt their lives. One man who preferred to remain anonymous told us, "I thought taking a few pills was a whole lot better than losing my hair. In my business, I need to maintain a certain image."

We also heard complaints about standard physicians.[14] Some of our interviewees said that their doctors paid too little attention to their feelings, especially when giving diagnoses; that they were not given enough information to make intelligent choices; and that they were not told enough about the risks and side effects of standard treatment. To the extent that these complaints are valid (we also heard them from patients who had remained on standard treatment), standard medicine may be partly responsible when cancer patients look elsewhere for primary care.

Some people who chose alternative treatment said they were attracted by reports of "miracle" cures attributed to the therapy in question. Most of the patients we interviewed had talked to at least one other person who appeared to have been cured by the treatment that our patient had chosen, and all had heard about people who had been "saved from certain death" by one alternative treatment or another.

Minimal research

Most of the people we interviewed did very little research before they chose an alternative treatment. As the following quotations reveal, some did almost none, and only a few did the kind of thorough analysis we recommend:

"We were so busy we didn't really do a lot of research about discovering who the quacks are. We took the recommendation of our dentist. He's a fine professional man, and I felt confident that he would send me to someone I could trust." (Sue Olitt, melanoma patient)

"I talked to a lady from this list of alternative patients. I did not look into any other clinic because she told me that she had been to three other places and they were not as good. I took her word for it." (Anne Reinke, breast cancer patient)

"The worst part of my [alternative] treatment was infinitely easier on me than the mildest chemotherapy my doctor had given me."

"I didn't read anything. I chose the program because I knew two people who had recovered on it. And to me that was better than any book—knowing somebody that did it and got well was more to me than anything I could read." (Gayle Bartolomei, lung cancer patient)

"I looked at this videotape, and they claimed 80 percent success with everybody who walks in the front door. They cited 300,000 case histories. And I thought, 80 percent sounds much better than the 20 percent odds I was hearing from conventional therapy." (Arnold Schraer, melanoma patient)

"I went to the health food store and got books. I went to medical libraries. Someone gave me the name of the Cancer Control Society. I called them right away, and they sent me a packet of information with lists of books, clinics which did alternative treatment, and people who had successfully undergone it. I think I spent two weeks sitting in a chair in my room just reading and calling people." (Odile Belladonna, breast cancer patient)

Foreign clinics

Many of the people we interviewed sought care in Tijuana. Their reactions were generally favorable. Some found Tijuana itself dirty and "dumpy"; some felt alienated by the language barrier; and one or two suggested that the treatment could have been more professional. But most patients were very satisfied with the nature of their therapy and the care, consideration, and professionalism exhibited by the medical staff:

"The place looked professional. It was very simple. They had a clinic and a hospital where people who were very sick were inpatients. Within the first twenty minutes of talking to the doctor, I just knew I was in the right place. It was not what he said, but the feeling that I had there. It was so hopeful and so uplifting." (Odile Belladonna)

"It was a very friendly place. The doctors were all visible and they talked to you whenever you wanted to. I thought it was wonderful that you could be up and about, wear your own robe, have your radio. If you get dressed, they take you in the van to the beach or to the shopping center–you know, all those things that are good for people's morale." (an anonymous breast cancer patient)

"The staff was very nice, very considerate. They pampered you. If you called to order anything, if you needed an aspirin or something, they'd bring it up right away. They let you walk through the kitchen and see how the food and juices were prepared. The doctors were very informative and answered all your questions." (Peter Hass, lung cancer patient)

Painless? Not always

Nearly all of our patients had had some standard treatment. Most of them found alternative care far easier to take. "The worst part of my [alternative] treatment was infinitely easier on me than the mildest chemotherapy my doctor had given me," said one of them. However, many patients went into it believing that alternative therapy is *always* easier, that it *never* has unpleasant side effects. As the following observations attest, this is not true:

"Drinking all those glasses of raw liver juice is terrible, completely terrible." (Gayle Bartolomei)

"You can't have any salt at all. No oils. It's very, very restrictive. And very expensive. In fact, if I had known what it was like I might not have gone with it. I'm glad I did, but it really is limiting. You have to look all over to find the right foods and then cook them in a certain way. You have to use purified water. They won't even allow you to take a bath in normal tap water." (Jeff Losea, esophageal cancer patient)

"I was a little shaky from all the stuff I was taking. You take vitamin C to the point where you get unbearable diarrhea. I could never get up to the doses prescribed. And some of those other things–polypeptides and all that–shake your body up a bit."(Fred Stugard, lung cancer patient)

Cost

Financial considerations were especially important for all of the people we interviewed. In only a few cases did

> *"Drinking all those glasses of raw liver juice is terrible, completely terrible."*
>
> **–Gayle Bartolomei**

health insurance cover even part of the cost of alternative therapy. When it came to prices and the pressure to make payments, patient reaction was mixed:

"It was $2,600 for the two weeks. We paid that up front, and that was all I ever had to pay. I mean, they didn't nickel and dime you like other hospitals." (Anne Reinke)

"The clinic was very money oriented. Especially at the beginning, everything was money, money, money." (An anonymous lung cancer patient who decided to try alternative treatment after being told she had only two to six weeks to live)

"They tell you it's $3,500 for a lifetime—all doctors' visits, prescriptions, tonics, everything. I think that's a good price, considering what you pay going to [standard] cancer doctors and clinics. I signed up for a lifetime, but I only had $1,000 to give them. They didn't complain about it. And later I went with no money at all and got everything I needed." (Arnold Schraer)

Positive response

We have no way to judge the effectiveness of the alternative therapies these patients chose. First, many of those who agreed to be interviewed had been diagnosed within the previous two years. This is not enough time to assess the long-term results of treatment. Second, in many cases standard treatment either preceded or accompanied alternative treatment, so that when the patient recovered, there was no way of knowing which therapy was responsible. However, the patients' response was overwhelmingly positive. Almost all of the people we interviewed said that they were doing well, and they attributed their good health to their alternative treatment. Some patients, however, found fault with the way the treatment was administered. We heard numerous complaints about unreturned phone calls, unanswered correspondence, and neglected paperwork. A few patients felt that their care was inconsistent and disorganized.

But overall, the patients we interviewed said they were glad they had chosen alternative treatment. Or as Bob, whom you will meet presently, put it:

"I eat heartily; I feel better than I have for years; thank God I went the alternative route."

A Risky Case

One patient in particular—we will call her Lisa—took what we see as the wrong approach to alternative treatment. We interviewed Lisa in September 1990. We present her story to emphasize the importance of thoroughly investigating any treatment that you are considering.

Lisa was experiencing a burning sensation and swelling in one breast. A standard physician told her that she required immediate surgery. Since she was totally opposed to surgery, Lisa sought advice from the proprietor of a health food store. This woman recommended a hair analyst,* a man who "just happened to be there that day." (Lisa later learned that the hair analyst, as she put it, "operated out of" the health food store.)

"He spent two and a half hours just talking to me. And I felt so good when I left him. He just reassured me that everything was going to be okay. He's a very kind man, and he made me feel like, 'Hey, life's worth living again. I'm going to be all right.'"

The hair analyst, whom we will call John, tested Lisa's hair and began to treat her with vitamin and mineral supplements. But he also gave her the name of an oncologist who, according to Lisa, strongly endorsed John's treatment program. In fact, as we later learned, the oncologist actually said that he did not object to her taking alternative treatment as long as she took standard treatment along with it. The oncologist ran the usual tests on Lisa, confirming the first physician's diagnosis of breast cancer.

Though she continued to see the oncologist, Lisa regarded him as her backup health care professional and refused to have the chemotherapy he recommended. She did agree to take a hormone medication, but she gave it up after she talked to John:

"John is quite knowledgeable. He knows about the

*By chemically analyzing a person's hair, hair analysts claim to diagnose deficiencies in certain important vitamins and minerals. This is not an accepted method of diagnosis.

drugs the doctors don't know about. When I get a drug I talk to him about it, and he says, 'Don't take that. It causes cancer.' And he's right. The medication does keep the lumps from growing, but it spreads the cancer. When I told my oncologist I wouldn't take it anymore, he said, 'Well, I'll give you something else. I'm not happy with your progress. Those tumors aren't going down fast enough.' So he gave me another drug, but I won't take that one either."

Despite her faith in John, Lisa did wonder about another alternative she had heard about from a friend—an anticancer serum offered by a practitioner in Greece. But when she called Greece, she discovered that the practitioner was on vacation, and no one was allowed to administer his serum during the three months he was gone. Lisa thought she might go to Greece sometime in the future.

We asked Lisa whether John used other treatments and what he might do if the vitamins and minerals didn't work. She said she thought he had access to laetrile. And if all else failed, she knew he would send her for the therapy in Greece, in which, she said, he had great confidence. We reminded Lisa that John had not known of the Greek clinic until he heard about it from her. We said that we wondered why he was so enthusiastic about it now. She replied that he had probably read up on it since she first mentioned it.

Is it too extreme to label Lisa's hair analyst a quack? Lisa believed that John had had medical training, although she did not know what kind, and John himself never volunteered any background information. On the other hand, John never claimed to be treating Lisa's cancer. According to Lisa, he stated specifically, "I'm not treating your cancer. I'm treating and feeding the cells what they need to be fed, and straightening out your whole system." However, this kind of qualifier could very well have been offered to protect John's legal position. From everything else Lisa reported—especially the fact that John advised her to stop taking the medication her oncologist had prescribed—it is obvious that both Lisa and John believed that he *was* treating her cancer.

Whether John was a quack is less important than Lisa's questionable approach to her own treatment. On the basis of one recommendation and a long conversation, she put herself entirely in the hands of someone who, in her words, "operated out of" a health food store and whose qualifications were dubious, to say the least. Given the seriousness of her condition, Lisa's decision to entrust this man with her medical care and probably her life strikes us as dangerous in the extreme.

Six More Years

Another patient—let's call him Bob—took what we feel is a more constructive approach to alternative treatment. Bob was diagnosed with prostate cancer in February 1979. Exploratory surgery revealed that the cancer had spread to the lymph nodes. It was too late for radiation; Bob's physicians told him that chemotherapy could give him another six months at best. Without it, they said, Bob had two months to live.

Bob knew only one thing: he didn't want chemotherapy. He had heard too many horror stories; rightly or wrongly, he believed that chemotherapy would make him sick. Bob worked hard and he played hard; he liked to coach Little League and fish; he owned and ran an auto repair shop. He didn't want to be—as he saw it—an invalid.

A friend gave Bob a book about alternative treatment. It described cures that the author attributed to the alternatives; it said that this therapy had no debilitating side effects. So Bob decided to go the alternative route. He reasoned that at this point he had nothing to lose. He hoped for a cure; failing that, he hoped to buy himself more time. Meanwhile, Bob's oncologist put him on hormonal therapy. Bob remained on hormonal therapy, complemented by alternative treatment, for the rest of his life.

Bob received his alternative therapy from a licensed MD at a small clinic in Nevada. He was given polypeptides, vitamin supplements, and several of the "medicinal" treatments described in this chapter. He was also told to give up smoking and alcohol and to follow a strict vegetarian diet. Examinations by his oncologist during the next two years showed that Bob's prostate cancer was under control.

In the spring of 1981 Bob began to feel ill. He was constantly tired; he had severe swelling in his legs; and for the first time he felt depressed. His Nevada doctor sent him to a medical clinic in Tijuana, where his alternative treatments were stepped up. Three weeks later Bob's symptoms were gone and he was his old, energetic self again.

Bob lived an active life for the next three years. Tests in 1982 showed that his cancer had spread to the bone. Bone cancer is usually painful, but Bob experienced no pain. The swelling returned periodically, but visits to the Tijuana clinic brought it back under control.

In late 1984 Bob's condition degenerated. The swelling was chronic now, and Bob was often tired. The alternative treatment no longer relieved these symptoms, but still there was no pain. It was obvious that the end was near, yet Bob remained active. He worked hard in his auto shop; he was coaching Little League two weeks before he died.

The end came in March 1985. Bob was admitted to the hospital with extreme fatigue and swelling in his legs. He died painlessly two days later. He was making plans for a new business a few hours before he died.*

*We wish to emphasize that this is not the typical course for alternative treatment. Even Bob's alternative therapists couldn't explain it. It is safe to say that another patient with an identical diagnosis could undertake identical treatment and get totally different results.

Bob's story differs from Lisa's in several respects. First, Bob's cancer was diagnosed incurable from the beginning. Therefore he had no realistic grounds for hope and nothing to lose by trying alternative treatment. Second, Bob stayed in standard treatment. Although he refused chemotherapy, he had hormonal therapy throughout the entire course of his illness. Third, all of Bob's alternative treatment was administered by licensed medical doctors—not by a hair analyst in a health food store.

And in fact Bob did enjoy six more years—six busy, productive, pain-free years. There is no way of knowing whether he owed these years to his alternative treatment, to his standard treatment, to a combination of both, or to the medical phenomenon of unexplained remission. Bob himself credited the alternative treatment. "It has worked wonders with me," he told us simply.

The Best of Both Worlds

Is alternative treatment for you? Only you can decide. But if you are considering a radical departure from standard treatment, ask yourself why. Is your choice consistent with your beliefs? Gayle Bartolomei, who was treated at a Tijuana clinic, made her choice after asking herself "belief" questions like these: Would chemotherapy or radiation be my way? Or do I believe in a more natural approach? Am I comfortable with standard medicine? Or do I want to venture out and try something different, something the American Medical Association hasn't put its stamp of approval on?

We have only one thing to add to Gayle's approach. Try to balance what you believe against what you know. Whether your belief system moves you in the direction of alternative or of standard treatment, get all the facts before you make up your mind. Ask the questions listed earlier in this chapter; read the books listed on page 163. Talk to other people who have taken the road that you are considering.

Beliefs are important, as we explained in Chapter 4. A therapy that you believe in may well have the best chance of success. But belief is only one aspect of your treatment program. When your beliefs *and the facts* support each other, your decision is likely to be the best one for you.

And now it is time to state our own beliefs. Based on hundreds of interviews with cancer patients, we believe that the ideal approach is standard treatment complemented by alternative therapy. We believe that it is generally best to go with standard treatment because standard treatment is proven. We believe that it is often best to complement standard treatment with carefully chosen alternative therapy. We make this last statement for two reasons. First, although no alternative treatment is known to cure cancer, many are known to improve the

For more on coping skills, see Chapter 6.

patient's quality of life. They do this by increasing the patient's sense of control, coping skills, and physical well-being. Second, as we have just explained, alternatives may sometimes provide the therapeutic benefits of belief.

Choose your alternative treatments carefully. Follow the guidelines given in this chapter and throughout this book. (Don't forget that while many alternatives may make you feel better, some are so rigid that they may make you feel worse.) When you have chosen your alternatives, use them to complement standard treatment, chosen with the advice of your physicians. This, in our view, is the way to give yourself the best of both worlds.

If you should decide to follow our advice, you may, if our research is any indication, find doctors who will be willing to cooperate. A few physicians, as we have explained, take a holistic approach, incorporating alternative methods into standard treatment. At present these physicians are still a minority. None of the patients we interviewed told us that his or her oncologist provided alternative treatment, and one or two said that their physicians were openly hostile to the whole idea. However, most patients received a more sympathetic hearing. Many said that their physicians—though they could not endorse alternative treatment per se—stood ready to support them if they used the alternatives strictly as complementary therapy. These doctors recognized that such an approach could make a real difference in their patients' lives. Or as a wise oncologist told Jeff Losea:

"Whatever gives you the most hope, do it."

This, in our opinion, is a strategy that every patient can take to heart. It is also a strategy that is finding more and more supporters within the medical profession.

In order of their first appearance, the patients who contributed to this chapter are: Judy Lakotas, Sue Olitt, Anne Reinke, Gayle Bartolomei, Arnold Schraer, Odile Belladonna, Peter Hass, Jeff Losea, and Fred Stugard.

Recommended Reading

Cassileth, Barrie R. "Questionable and Unproven Cancer Therapies." Chap. 13 in *Everyone's Guide to Cancer Therapy,* **edited by Malin Dollinger, Ernest H. Rosenbaum, and Greg Cable. Kansas City, MO: Andrews & McNeel, 1991.**

This chapter gives a brief history of unproven cancer treatments; it explains how the medical counterculture of today, like that of the nineteenth century, developed in reaction to medical technology and to the so-called tyranny of doctors. It describes the commonest alternative treatments and explains how to tell when a therapy is questionable. Pro standard treatment.

Fink, John M. *Third Opinion: An International Directory to Alternative Therapy Centers for the Treatment and Prevention of Cancer.* **3d ed. Garden City Park, NY: Avery Publishing Group, 1992.**

A resource book of data on treatment centers, educational centers, support groups, and information services in North America and overseas. The information provided comes from the groups themselves, and the author does not comment on particular therapies. This book is well organized and easy to use. A valuable guide for anyone who seeks resources on alternative therapy.

Gerson, Max. *A Cancer Therapy: Results of Fifty Cases.* **Bonita, CA: Gerson Institute, 1990.**

This classic of alternative medicine describes in detail the theory and practical application of Dr. Gerson's nutritional cancer therapy. It is based entirely on anecdotal evidence. The book includes fifty case histories, many tables, and extensive notes. The complex content and the heavy writing style (the author's first language is German) make for difficult reading. Pro alternative treatment.

Kushi, Michio, et al., eds. *The Macrobiotic Approach to Cancer.* **Wayne, NJ: Avery Publishing Group, 1982.**

A collection of articles by supporters of macrobiotic cancer therapy. Michio Kushi believes that cancer is caused by the patient's own attitudes, diet, and life-style; he explains how to treat it using a macrobiotic diet. There are several short chapters by physicians who favor this approach and a set of informal case histories, some of them provided by the patients themselves. Pro alternative treatment.

Laszlo, John. *Understanding Cancer.* **New York: Harper & Row Publishers, 1987.**

Chapter 13: "Experimental Therapy or Quackery: What's the Difference?" Laszlo explains in detail how new drugs are developed by means of clinical trials. He compares this methodology with the way in which "quack" remedies are developed and promoted, using the drug krebiozen as an example. He provides guidelines for identifying quack treatments and discusses some of the reasons why intelligent people find these treatments appealing. Pro standard treatment.

Morra, Marion, and Eve Potts. *Choices: Realistic Alternatives in Cancer Treatment.* **New York: Avon Books, 1987.**

Chapter 10: "Experimental and Unproven Treatments." This chapter explains the difference between experimental and unproven treatments and cites examples of each. It examines in detail the claims made for laetrile, the studies that the NCI conducted to evaluate those claims, and the legal status of laetrile in the United States and Mexico at the time this book was written. Pro standard treatment.

Olsen, Kristin Gottschalk. *The Encyclopedia of Alternative Health Care.* **New York: Simon & Schuster, Pocket Books, 1989.**

The author states that this book is not intended to be used as a source of medical advice. She describes a wide range of alternative therapies that can be used to supplement standard treatment for various diseases. These range from aromatherapy to chiropractic and from iridology to massage. She gives a brief history of each therapy, explains what it is supposed to do, and describes what it feels like. She lists applications and cautions and concludes each discussion with suggestions for further reading. Olsen is a journalist with a degree in holistic health education. Her approach is generally thoughtful and open minded, and her book is well organized and easy to read.

U.S. Congress, Office of Technology Assessment. *Unconventional Cancer Treatments.* **OTA-H-405. Washington, DC: U.S. Government Printing Office, September 1990.**

This report describes the commonest alternative cancer therapies, reviews the claims that are made for these therapies, and suggests ways of validating those claims. It covers costs and legal issues, and it tells what kind of people are likeliest to use alternative treatment. Therapies are categorized as psychological and behavioral, nutritional, herbal, and pharmacologic and biologic. There is a special chapter on immuno-augmentative therapy. This study was produced by a panel of experts in both standard and alternative cancer treatment. An excellent, unbiased resource.

Weil, Andrew. *Health and Healing: Understanding Conventional and Alternative Medicine.* **Boston: Houghton Mifflin Co., 1983.**

Dr. Weil examines both standard and alternative medicine in the context of the mind-body connection. He discusses a wide range of alternative therapies, giving the history and citing the pros and cons of each. He draws upon both clinical and personal experience and cites case histories from all over the world. A research associate in ethnopharmacology at Harvard University, Dr. Weil supports much of standard medicine but believes that alternative therapies are preferable for treating certain conditions. He does not generally support the use of standard therapies to treat cancer, but he does not go into this subject in detail. Very readable. Pro alternative treatment.

Coping: Meeting the Challenges

Coping: Meeting the Challenges

I believe there are two types of cancer patient: the cancer victor and the cancer victim. A cancer victim lets the disease take him over; he doesn't reach out into life anymore. A cancer victor, even if his case ends in death, lives his life abundantly and fully. Cancer victors are happy; they go for walks; they smell the flowers; they go for bike rides; they do the things they want to do. They don't let the disease take over their lives. They let it have certain control points, but they don't let it control them.

– John Chapman

The secret of being a cancer victor is to learn to cope. But the definition of coping is very broad. At one extreme, it can mean struggling to overcome something unpleasant. Coping can mean white-knuckling it through life.

Coping can also mean something positive and creative. It can mean finding fresh solutions to your problems. Finding ways to make your life more pleasant and more rewarding. Getting the most out of any situation. Making a positive adjustment to the changes that life brings. In this book we use "coping" to mean all of these things.

For the cancer patient, the term "coping" takes on special meanings. Andrew Kneier, a clinical psychologist who specializes in oncology counseling, defines it as mastering a series of challenges: "enduring some difficulties, reducing others, being resilient, finding positive opportunities, striving to adjust."[1] In this chapter we draw on suggestions from Andrew Kneier, other professionals, and cancer patients themselves to show you how you can meet those challenges.

"Cancer victors don't let the disease take over their lives. They let it have certain control points, but they don't let it control them."

– John Chapman

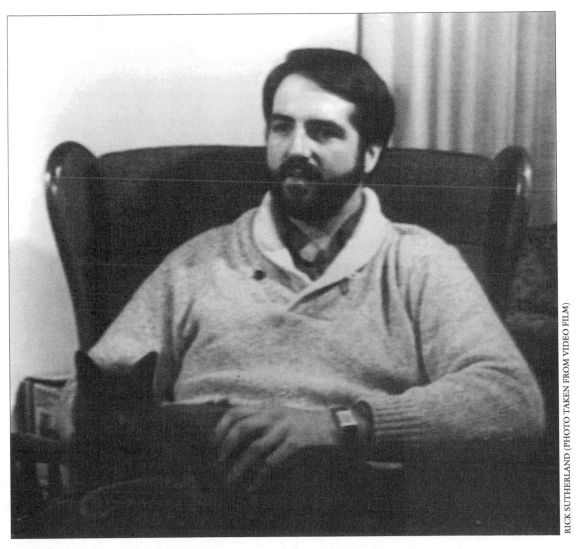

RICK SUTHERLAND (PHOTO TAKEN FROM VIDEO FILM)

John Chapman

Like John Chapman, we believe that cancer patients can be victors, and we believe that the secret is to learn to cope. At the same time, we want to emphasize that *there is no one right way to cope*–with anything, and especially not with cancer. Well-meant rules about the "right way" to cope can be just one more burden on the cancer patient. In this chapter we offer suggestions that we think you will find helpful. We believe that there is only one *rule*–the rule that you should do what is best for you.

This chapter offers suggestions, then, on how to create a coping program that is tailored to your specific needs. It suggests how to apply a variety of skills, some of which you probably already have, to open up life-changing possibilities. In this chapter cancer patients tell you in their own words how they coped with stress and powerful emotions and describe some of the ways they found to make their lives more enjoyable.

On legal and financial issues, see Appendix 2. On issues surrounding death, see Appendix 1.

In this chapter we deal with emotional issues. Of course, cancer patients must cope with other issues as well. These may include money problems and job discrimination. They may even include a terminal prognosis. You will find information on all of these issues in special appendices.

This chapter consists of four sections. In the first one we help you to examine your emotions and suggest ways of dealing with them. In the second one we discuss stress and the damage that it can do. In the third one we present general guidelines for learning to cope. And in the last one we suggest specific techniques that you may want to include in your own coping program.

Powerful Emotions Are Part of the Cancer Experience

When you're told you have cancer, you are flooded with powerful emotions. You may feel numb; you may have trouble knowing *what* you feel. It's important to realize that, however strange they may seem, you have experienced emotions like these before. Fear, anger, depression, grief–these are familiar feelings. But they may seem unfamiliar now, because they are so strong.

If you have cancer, we hope you will remember two things. One: it's normal to feel whatever it is you are feeling. There's no need to be afraid of your emotions or to hide them. And two: you can deal with those emotions. In this chapter we're going to show you how.

If you are a caregiver or a friend, this chapter should help you to understand how the cancer patient feels. We think it will help you to understand some of your own feelings too. As we said above, the emotions that we discuss are ones that everybody has experienced–though usually in a milder form.

You May Feel…

Fear

Fear–even terror–often hits first after a cancer diagnosis. Something shocking has occurred, and you don't know what's going to happen next. Will the pain be unbearable? How will you ever cope? Are you going to die? It's easy to imagine the worst, and many people feel extremely vulnerable until they are able to get answers to some of their questions. "I was totally devastated," says Paula Carroll. And Jean Mitchell told us, "My first reaction was to burst into tears."

Fear often escalates into full-blown panic. You may experience a multitude of symptoms. These include shortness of breath, dizziness, chest pains, palpitations, trembling, sweating, choking, diarrhea, upset stomach, numbness, hot flashes, chills, aching muscles, restlessness, and fatigue. You may be terrified if you believe that these symptoms are caused by the cancer. In fact, they are probably just your body's way of reacting to fear.

Anger

For some people, the first reaction is anger. As Arnold Schraer put it, "You get angry with your disease. And you get angry at people around you." These may include

Coping for families and friends is discussed in detail in Chapter 7.

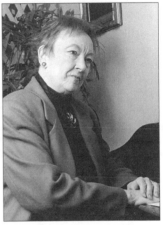

AL WRIGHT

Jean Mitchell

"My first reaction was to burst into tears."

–Jean Mitchell

the doctor who diagnosed the cancer, or who didn't diagnose it sooner. You may also get angry at your family and friends because they don't understand what you're going through, or because they are powerless to make it better. You may get angry at yourself for not seeing the doctor sooner. Or you may get angry because you have lost control over your body, or because the treatment is disrupting your life.

Sometimes just one part of your treatment triggers the anger. Nancy Heitz recalls how she felt when she learned that she couldn't wear her high heels anymore. She had to wear orthopedic shoes instead, and "I'm very lucky that there's any glass left in my bedroom window," she says, "because I had shoes with steel shanks in them, and that was the ultimate in negativity to me. I couldn't wear my fun shoes, you know. I was in these *massive* shoes. And I threw them at the window."

Grief and self-pity

Anger is often accompanied by grief. "Underneath the anger is a sadness about being sick," says Arnold Schraer. "You're grieving for being ill; you don't want your life to end right now. There are things you want to do, and you do love the planet, and you love some people, and all of a sudden, you're sick. And you're really sad." "The thing that bothered me the most was that I might not be around to watch my kids grow up," Rick Marill says.

Anger and grief turned inward breed self-pity. "I began to feel very sorry for myself," Jean Mitchell told us. "I thought, 'God! Why me? Why me? It was bad enough that it should happen to my mother. Why me?'" Elfriede Adams was angry because her friends could make plans for next year's vacation–"and I felt sorry for myself because I could not predict tomorrow."

Guilt

For other people, the first reaction is guilt. Some of the patients we interviewed blamed themselves for their illness and made themselves miserable trying to figure out what they did to cause it. These people tormented themselves by asking, "Was it my diet? Was it the smoking? Should I have quit my job when the stress got to me?" Some patients felt guilty when they saw the pain their illness was causing others. They also felt guilty about becoming a burden to their loved ones.

Depression

Any of these reactions may be accompanied by depression. Depression makes it harder to work through other emotions. When you are depressed, your energy level is low, and helping yourself or asking for help can seem impossible. At first, Arnold Schraer was too depressed to get out of bed and do a simple pain-relieving exercise. Sometimes all he could think about was his cancer. He felt small and alone, despite the flowers and other gifts in his room that reminded him that he had good friends, and a deep dread of future tests and operations immobilized him.

"I curled up in a fetal position at first," says Linda Sumner. "I think there is an initial response of just wanting to curl up, die, and hope everything will go away."

Loneliness

Cancer can make you feel very much alone, "very introspective, very self-centered and closed into your own world," says Dennis Brown. Gayle Bartolomei puts it even more strongly. "It's a real lonely disease," she says. "You're real scared."

There are three factors at work here. First, having cancer can make you feel "different." "Nobody else has to deal with this," you think; "nobody knows what I'm going through. Other people aren't in pain; they go about their lives; they plan for the future. They can't ever know what it's like for me." All of this creates a sense of isolation.

Second, you may be isolating yourself. Some people deal with trouble by withdrawing. This is understandable, but when the trouble is cancer, withdrawing is not an effective way to cope. You are pulling away just when you

For more on the reasons why people withdraw from cancer patients, see page 270.

need the most support, which makes the effects of isolation that much worse.

Third, other people may be withdrawing from you. This is not at all unusual. Coworkers, friends, and even your family may handle their fear, or their discomfort at not knowing what to do, by avoiding you, ignoring you, or rejecting you subtly. This is a fact of life, and it's important to recognize that when it happens it is not your fault. When you feel isolated, whatever the reason, it's time to reach out for new connections and to strengthen old ones.

Loss of self-esteem

Cancer can change your body and your life in ways that are hard on your self-esteem. Hair loss, weight loss, loss of stamina, ostomies, scars—all these can make you feel terrible if you think of your body as being "who you are." Loss of independence and the need to rely on others can be hard on you if you are self-sufficient, proud of your ability to go it alone. Many people base their self-esteem on their work, on what they do and how well they do it. If you are such a person, your job is "who you are." When cancer means cutting down on your schedule, or even giving up your job, you may feel like "nobody." And if you see yourself as a leader, someone who makes decisions and gives orders, the need to delegate authority can make you feel worthless.

Cancer brings changes, unavoidable changes. Sometimes it changes the very things that you believe make you a worthwhile person. If your self-esteem is based on things that cancer can damage, loss of self-esteem may be a problem for you.

Denial

People react very differently to a diagnosis of cancer. While most people go through a period of emotional turmoil, a few refuse to admit that they are ill at all. A temporary denial right after the initial diagnosis can be a normal, useful psychological defense. It keeps you functioning, and it keeps you calm. To accept what is painful and frightening, you may need time and a lot of emotional support.

Long-term denial is another matter. If you cannot accept that you are ill, you cannot deal with the problems that illness causes. You may ignore that chronic cough, that lump in your breast–symptoms that you should mention to your doctor. If you cannot accept that you are ill, you may place a heavy burden on your family. You cannot help them to help you, and you cannot plan for their future should you die. Finally, if you cannot accept that you are ill, you may refuse treatment altogether. This can have catastrophic results.

It is important to understand the difference between *denying* illness and *not dwelling* on it. Some people cope by gathering information; it helps them to learn all they can about their condition. Others, while they readily acknowledge that they are ill, don't want or need a lot of information. For these people, gathering information is just "dwelling on it." If you fall into this second group, you should know that "not dwelling on it" is OK, but that *ignoring* it is not.

Unresolved emotions

After giving themselves time to sort through and experience their feelings, get answers to some of their questions, and find some support, most of the patients we talked to started to feel better. However, this is not always the case. If you don't give yourself time to work through your feelings, or if you find that you can't, you will have to cope with what we call "unresolved emotions."

Unresolved anger is a common example. Anger is unresolved when it's continuous, when it's misdirected, when it interferes with your life. How can you tell when you're experiencing unresolved anger? "I think it's when you're feeling out of character for you," says clinical psychologist Ricki Dienst. "When you're chopping everybody's head off. When you're feeling that the *only* way to get things is to be angry."[2]

Unresolved anger has many possible origins. These

include fear, the sense that you have lost control, and pressure caused by anxieties unrelated to cancer. Sometimes it's just the way you've always dealt with problems.

Unresolved anger can interfere with your treatment program. It wastes energy; it leads to self-destructive behavior; it alienates your physicians, friends, and family; and it blinds you to your full range of options. Furthermore, it keeps you under constant stress, which may weaken your already overburdened immune system.

You'd *never* get counseling? Before you make up your mind, see page 203.

If you are experiencing unresolved anger, you will probably benefit from professional counseling. A counselor can help you to find the underlying causes of your anger, to recognize how self-defeating it is, and to learn to deal with it constructively. Cancer support groups are also helpful. Sharing your anger with others in a controlled setting can help you to put this emotion into perspective.

For more on cancer support groups, see page 201.

Unresolved guilt is painful and destructive. Guilt is unresolved when you cannot deal with it and move on; you get stuck in it. Unresolved guilt often goes hand in hand with unresolved depression, which is characterized by its intensity; by symptoms such as insomnia, weight loss, and difficulty in concentrating; and by recurrent thoughts of death or suicide. Unresolved depression makes it harder to fight illness. Patients who suffer from unresolved depression are less likely to follow their doctor's advice, to make use of their support team, or even to eat. There is evidence that unresolved depression weakens the immune system.[3]

You don't have to endure emotions that isolate you and erode the quality of your life. Many of our interviewees triumphed over guilt and depression with the help of a therapist. We highly recommend this particular option. Other options include family therapy, support groups for cancer patients, physical exercise, and short-term mild medication.

For more on issues surrounding death, see Appendix 1.

Unresolved fear is fear that you can't deal with; it controls your life. The fear that is hardest to resolve may be the fear of death. Although it is not always acknowledged, this is a normal reaction to a diagnosis of cancer and one that many patients must contend with. Furthermore, even patients who do not have a terminal prognosis may need to come to terms with their eventual death. (In this respect, cancer patients are no different from anybody else.) Here again therapy can be helpful.

Finally, unresolved dependency can be a problem. If you have cancer, you will probably need to turn certain duties over to others, but serious illness can cause a normally dependent person, or even an independent person, to become abnormally dependent. This is unhealthy. Letting others do everything makes it impossible for you to play an active role in your own health care. It puts you in a victim position in relation to your cancer. Again, we believe that the most effective way to overcome unresolved dependency is with individual or group therapy.

Unresolved emotions are often made worse by the meaning that cancer holds for you. Cancer can "mean" all kinds of things, as Andrew Kneier observes. You may see cancer as a punishment for your sins; as the price that you must pay for past good fortune; as a character fault coming out in your body; or as the result of a defective life-style. Cancer can also represent the failure of your hopes and goals; it can disrupt the "plan" that gives your life meaning. If you have had a hard life, you may see cancer as the crowning blow in a long series of blows.

Ricki Dienst recommends support groups for patients who have trouble with the issue of meaning. "Sometimes you can't recognize the meanings that *you* bring to cancer," she says. "But if you sit and listen to somebody else's meanings–that you don't believe in at all–and you say, '*That's* not what cancer is,' you begin to understand that these meanings are not inherent in the disease." A therapist who specializes in oncology counseling can help you to uncover and resolve the meanings that cancer holds for you.

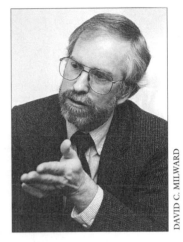

DAVID C. MILWARD

Andrew Kneier

What if you can't afford therapy? See page 204 and page 205.

Mastering Emotions

Learning to accept and express your emotions is a strong part of a good coping program. This process consists of several steps.

Identify them and accept them

Start by recognizing and acknowledging as many of your emotions as you can. This can be *very* difficult for people who tend to repress their feelings; you may want to use professional help to get the process started. Learn to figure out exactly what you feel–about other people, about your surroundings, about yourself. To start, stand back and watch your emotions neutrally. Try to stay objective and nonjudgmental. See how many emotions you can identify. You may be surprised by what you learn. What feels like anger, for example, may really be fear–fear of the thing you are "angry" at. What feels like righteous indignation may really be pain–pain caused by something that the other person did. Asking yourself direct questions ("How would I describe the way I am feeling now?") can also be revealing. Keeping a journal is another good way to learn more about your feelings by trying to describe them.

Next, recognize that all of your emotions are OK. Do you fight your feelings, especially the ones that you consider "wrong"? Do you see fear, anger, grief, depression, and so forth as your enemies? Psychologists Hal and Sidra Stone call this listening to your Inner Critic–the voice in your head that tells you that your feelings (or your looks, or your actions, or your character) are bad. "The great similarity we have noted among all the Inner Critics of the world," the Stones say, "is their ability to cripple people and to keep them unhappy and ineffective."[4]

Fortunately, you can learn to deal with this inner voice. As the Stones point out, the Critic is not you. "It is a voice in you that has developed for specific reasons. It is not a voice that has to run your life forever."[5] For a complete discussion of this subject, we recommend the Stones' book *Embracing Your Inner Critic*.

We have found that one way to quiet the Critic is simply to accept your emotions. Once you've given yourself permission to experience, say, anger, you silence the inner voice that says, "It's wrong to feel angry."

To handle her anxiety, Odile Belladonna would ask

"Instead of turning away from it, I would just look the fear straight in the face. Ride it out, and ultimately it just dissolves."

–Odile Belladonna

herself what her biggest fear was. Then, "instead of turning away from it, I would just look the fear straight in the face. Ride it out, and ultimately it just dissolves. It just dissolves when you learn to face it, to look at it, and say, 'Okay, my fear is such-and-such.'"

Accepting your emotions also means accepting your own occasional irrational behavior. For Linda Sumner, who was upset by the weight she gained under chemotherapy, this meant "realizing that you're going to go through binges, wild binges, where you eat four jars of apple butter, and that it's OK."

Then express them

The next step in mastering your emotions is to express them. It's important to do this in a healthy manner; expressing your emotions does not mean blowing up or dumping impulsively on others. Otherwise, how you express them is up to you. You can do it verbally, physically, or through creative art. Some patients said that when they talked about their anger with a friend, it was replaced with an inner calm. Arnold Schraer used art to master his emotions. "If I'm very angry at somebody–my doctor– and I do a *really* angry drawing of my doctor, after the drawing I feel like that anger that was inside of me, which was suppressing my system and bottling me up, is now expressed." Sometimes Arnold used movement too. "When I get really scared, really angry, I make myself go outside and walk, or I do tai chi, do something to move my energy through my body, no matter what it is. Just move it through the body and release it." Later in this chapter, you will learn how other patients explored various forms of self-expression to find the ones that were the most satisfying to them.

And reap the rewards

As you work on mastering your emotions, there are two things we would like you to bear in mind. First, different people react differently to a diagnosis of cancer. You may experience all or some of the emotions listed here. You

"When I get really scared, really angry, I make myself go outside and walk, or I do tai chi, do something to move my energy through my body...and release it."

–Arnold Schraer

may experience them in any order, and you may experience different versions of the same emotion at different times. This is especially true of anger. Many people react to cancer with negative anger at first (Why me? It isn't fair!). Later they learn to react with positive anger (I'll fight this thing! I'll beat it! I won't let it win!). This second kind of anger can give you focus, strength, and determination in dealing with one of life's most formidable foes.

That brings us to our second point. Mastering your emotions is rewarding. Getting rid of negative emotions makes room for positive emotions to emerge. As you learn to master negative emotions, you break their hold over you. You gain insight into yourself and into what is important in your life. As you learn to master negative emotions, you discover how much control you really have – over your own mind and over your well-being.

As you work on mastering your emotions, there may be times when you will get discouraged. If this happens, remember the rewards. It is no exaggeration to say that mastering your emotions can change your whole life.

Stress and Your Emotions

I can't find any parking – I'm going to miss my plane!
If I don't meet this mortgage payment, the bank
will foreclose!
What if that lump in my breast is cancer?

Sound familiar? If you've ever faced a situation that kept you awake at night, made your heart pound and your palms sweat, you've experienced severe stress. *Stress* is defined as a physical response to a perceived threat. You perceive a situation as dangerous; this makes you feel afraid; your fear, in turn, sets off physical changes in your body. The perceived threat need not be extreme; it can be as mild as the need to make a simple decision. And the fear can range from discomfort to overt terror.

Moderate stress can be helpful; it can motivate you to do what needs to be done. It can motivate you to clean out that overflowing closet, for example. And even more serious stress can be helpful sometimes. Let's say your cancer has been in remission, but lately you've been feeling tired. You dread visiting your doctor; in fact, you're so nervous you can't sleep. After three bad nights, you phone the doctor's office for an appointment. In this case, the stress leads to positive action.

However, too much stress is harmful. It is important to learn to handle stress-producing situations in a healthy, constructive way. It is especially important if you have cancer, because cancer patients experience a great deal of stress.

The Mind-Body Connection

Does the mind affect the body, and if so, how? This is a complex and often controversial topic. Your emotions can set off changes in your body, as we have just explained. This is the mechanism of stress. Studies in the new field of psychoneuroimmunology (PNI) suggest that stress can directly affect your health.[6]

Excessive stress suppresses the immune system in a variety of ways, one of which is to decrease natural killer (NK) cell activity.[7] Natural killer cells play an important role in the body's defense against various diseases, including cancer, and a decrease in NK cell activity has been associated with malignant growth.[8] Stressful life events that can be related to suppression of the immune system include the death of a spouse, divorce, test taking, waiting for surgery, and unemployment.[9]

Some studies suggest that there may be a direct relationship between cancer and psychological stress.[10] It is important to emphasize that stress is not believed to *cause* cancer, only that some researchers feel that it may influence the progress of the disease.[11]

Some studies suggest that by changing how you deal with your emotions, you can alter the way in which your body fights illness. For example, one study found that group therapy increased the survival time of women with breast cancer by almost 100 percent.[12] The therapy

It is important to learn to handle stress-producing situations in a healthy, constructive way.

We discuss relaxation
on page 221.

consisted of weekly meetings at which the women were encouraged to express their feelings, discuss their problems, deal with issues of grieving and loss, and find meaning in their illness by using their experience to help others. They were also encouraged to develop close ties with one another in order to counter feelings of isolation and loneliness. Relaxation has also been shown to reduce the effects of stress on the immune system.[13]

One famous case demonstrates the effect of emotions on illness. Norman Cousins was diagnosed with a severe collagen disorder that paralyzed his neck and limbs. He was told that his chances for a full recovery were 1 in 500. Instead of resigning himself to being one of the 499 chronically ill patients, Cousins dealt with his prognosis by deciding that he would be the one person who would recover. He set up his own treatment program, a key part of which was daily doses of *laughter*. He "made the joyous discovery that ten minutes of genuine belly laughter had an anaesthetic effect and would give me at least two hours of pain-free sleep."[14] Cousins made a complete recovery. Recent studies of laughter as both a pain-reliever and a stress-modifier support Cousins's results.[15]

What can be learned from Cousins's experience? We think the most valuable lesson is his emphasis on the will to survive and the use of positive emotions to cope with illness. He described his experience in *Anatomy of an Illness*, a popular book that also stirred great interest in the medical community. It led clinicians to reconsider seriously how beliefs and emotions affect physical health.

Some physicians attributed Cousins's recovery to the *placebo effect*–that is, to an improvement that occurs not because of the treatment itself but because the patient believes that the treatment will work. However, this is a circular argument. The placebo effect depends on one's faith in the treatment–in other words, on one's emotions and beliefs. And the influence of positive emotions and beliefs is exactly what Cousins credits with his recovery.

What does the mind-body connection have to do with coping? Simply this. If it is true, it is another reason for learning to cope. There is no doubt that your emotions affect the quality of your life, but there is good reason to believe that they may also affect your physical health, and specifically that they may influence your fight against cancer.

The battle against cancer is fought on two fronts: the physical and the emotional. In the following pages you will learn how to fight that battle on the emotional front.

Special Stresses on Cancer Patients

Any illness creates stress, but cancer is especially stressful. First, there are the diagnostic tests. Trying to understand the nature of these tests places a heavy burden on the cancer patient. Then there is the waiting. Part of taking tests is waiting for, and worrying about, the results. Clocks seem to stop when you are waiting for news; meanwhile, you imagine the worst. All of this creates more stress.

Once the diagnosis is made, there are other stresses. Now you may face the fear of pain, of disfigurement, of loss of control, of death. (This last fear may be completely unrealistic. The overall cure rate for cancer is over 50 percent, and cure rates for some cancers top 90 percent.[16]) All this stress can terrify you even more if you believe that stress causes cancer. This belief is not supported by the evidence, as we have just explained.

Soon after the diagnosis, you may well receive an outpouring of support. Family and friends cannot do enough for you. Unfortunately, support itself can cause stress. People who care about you may offer you unasked-for, and unwanted, advice. They may be reacting to their own fears, or they may really believe that their advice will help. The advice may be merely annoying or downright disturbing, and the other person's anxiety may be contagious. Some supporters may try to impose their own rigid belief systems on you. One cancer patient received a letter from a well-meaning relative informing him that he must

But even if stress *did* cause cancer, you can gain a sense of control over your circumstances, and this can help you to reduce stress. See below, and Chapter 8.

convert to her religion if he hoped to save his eternal soul. All this did was depress and agitate the patient, who already had his own beliefs.

Health care professionals can also contribute to your stress. Overworked doctors and nurses may not be able to spend much time with you, or to give you all the information you want. They may seem cold and insensitive when you need a great deal of comfort. Although there are few truly unpleasant health care workers, there are a lot of tired, harried, and indifferent ones.

In fact, the whole health care system can be stressful. Bills, insurance, paperwork, red tape, receptionists who forget your name and secretaries who lose your file—all of these can send your blood pressure soaring.

For more on how to overcome the fear of recurrence, see Chapter 8.

Finally, cancer is more stressful than most illnesses because it can recur after it has been treated. Most patients have to work hard to control their fear of recurrence, particularly before they reach the five-year plateau discussed in Chapter 1. Fortunately, this fear, like others, can be overcome.

One final point. The whole idea of managing stress causes stress in some people. If you're one of those people, honor *your* needs. If the idea of having to manage stress is a source of anxiety for you, then you shouldn't feel that you have to manage stress in order to cope. There is no one right way to cope. The best coping program is the coping program that works best for you.

We repeat what we said above: there is no good evidence that stress causes cancer. It is not even known for certain whether stress influences the progress of the disease. Furthermore, countless people have beaten cancer even though their lives were full of stress. We don't suggest that you must manage stress in order to keep your cancer from recurring. And we don't suggest that stress was what gave you cancer in the first place. But stress does affect your general health, and it does affect your quality of life. For both of these reasons, we think it is well worthwhile for most cancer patients to learn how to manage stress.

Learning to Cope: 15 Good Ideas

Managing stress is an important part–but by no means the only part–of a good coping program. This section offers ideas for constructing a coping program tailored to your own needs.

1. Obtaining Information

It helps to learn all you can about what you are facing. This will make it easier to see the problem clearly and to manage your fears. When you don't have the facts, you may exaggerate the negative and overlook the positive. Facts can improve your perspective; they empower you; and they show you what your options are. And almost always there *are* options.

A mountaineer who embarks on a climbing expedition knows that he may encounter a blizzard or even an avalanche. He checks out the weather before he starts and studies maps of the routes he'll be taking. He learns all he can about where he is going. Knowledge is one of his survival tools.

Information is a survival tool if you are dealing with cancer too. For example, right after your diagnosis, you can help yourself to cope by looking for information on your type of cancer. This will help you to know your adversary. It will enable you to participate in making decisions about your treatment. It will help to build up your confidence, and it will give you a sense of control.

There are a number of ways to get the facts. Start with a trip to the bookstore or the library. Many books include bibliographies that direct you to further sources of information. Make sure that the books you consult were published recently. Information on cancer can go out of date very quickly. When Elfriede Adams was diagnosed with Hodgkin's disease, she told us, "I immediately looked up Hodgkin's in a twenty-five-year-old medical book and read that it was fatal within three to fifteen years. I was, of course, devastated." Had she consulted a current source,

To learn more about your type of cancer, contact the American Cancer Society at 1-800-ACS-2345.

> *"When you're dealing with cancer, it's like you're in a room without any way to get out.... But the vast majority of the patients I know are always on the lookout for a door or a window in that room."*
>
> **–Ruth Swain**

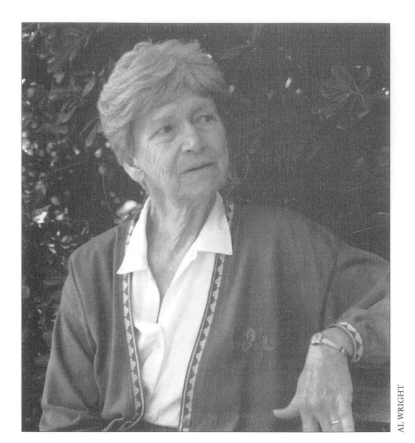

AL WRIGHT

Ruth Swain

Elfriede would have learned that in 1990 the *seventeen-year* survival rate for *advanced* Hodgkin's, with appropriate therapy, was 56 percent.[17]

Talking with well-informed people is another excellent way to discover exactly what you are dealing with. Suppose, for example, that you are the mother of a child with cancer. You might join a group for parents in your situation. Through discussions with these other parents, you will learn what resources are available to you. You can get the facts about tutors, medical plans, and family counselors—facts that will help you to make good decisions.

A word of caution. When gathering information, don't accept the pronouncements of friends and relatives as gospel. Remember: misinformation abounds. One way to deal with this is to include your friends and family in your fact-finding missions. Take your daughter with you when you go to talk to your doctor, for example. That way she–and you–will get the facts straight.

2. A Positive Attitude Helps

"When you're dealing with cancer, it's like you're in a room without any way to get out," says Ruth Swain. "You're very vulnerable and helpless. And some people withdraw and say, 'Well, there's nothing much I can do, so I just have to fold up my tent and live with it.' But the vast majority of the patients I know are always on the lookout for a door or a window in that room."

It's easier to cope if you think positive. Thinking positive means looking for answers rather than giving up hope. It's believing that you have the resources within you to confront a challenging situation. For Paula Carroll, thinking positive is "not running from things. It's not denying them." On the other hand, as Brad Zebrack points out, "a lot of people misinterpret a positive attitude for, 'I always have to be up; I always have to look good in front of my friends; I can't let them know I'm sick.' A lot of deception. Having a positive attitude doesn't mean I'm always happy, or I'm always going to feel good." Therapist Ricki Dienst agrees. "That leads to people being down on themselves when they feel bad. I don't think it's helpful to say that one needs to go through cancer with a happy face on. That you aren't going to survive cancer unless you have a happy face. There are times for crying. It's normal. It's appropriate." Thinking positive, then, is "not always to express the happy thought, but to really work through and express the sad one. To confront it and feel it and express it. And then move on."

A positive attitude can be learned. Two of the best books on this subject are Martin Seligman's *Learned Optimism* and David Burns's *Feeling Good Handbook*.[18] Seligman believes that pessimists tend to blame themselves for unpleasant events and to overestimate the effect of

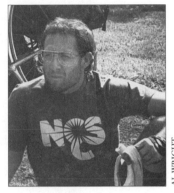

Brad Zebrack

> *"Having a positive attitude doesn't mean I'm always happy, or I'm always going to feel good."*
>
> –**Brad Zebrack**

For more on keeping a journal, see page 213.

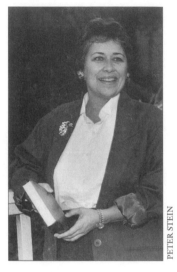

Nancy Heck

those events. He explains how to reverse these beliefs, using a five-step process. Burns, a psychiatrist in the field of cognitive therapy, also describes specific techniques for changing negative attitudes, and other forms of what he calls "twisted thinking."

To develop a positive attitude, start by noticing when you are thinking negative. Are there certain pitfall times that seem to trigger negative thinking? Does it happen when you're tired? Hungry? Under too much stress? See how often you can catch yourself thinking negative. You may even want to keep a running record and watch yourself improve.

Next, "emphasize what you have going for you," says physical therapist Nancy Heck. "Identify your strengths and use them. Set goals and achieve them. Notice every little bit of improvement." Some people, she adds. like to log their progress in a journal or a chart.[19]

All this may seem difficult at first, but you will improve with practice. Just trying to think positive is an important first step. Simply by trying for a positive attitude, you are already achieving it to some extent. An effective coping program makes it easier to develop a positive attitude.

3. The Power of Humor

People with a positive attitude can often see the light side of a dark situation. They know that life is often comic, and they welcome the opportunity to laugh. Laughter is a release for everyone; it allows people to let down their barriers and to draw closer to one another. Sometimes it miraculously transforms pain into opportunity or challenge. When Paul Ryder told his family that he had cancer, his wife's immediate comment was, "Other than that, Mrs. Lincoln, how did you enjoy the play?" Paul's condition *was* serious, but her response gave everyone a chance to pull away from the initial shock. Humor helped them to relax a little, and when it was time to discuss a course of action, they felt a greater sense of unity.

The night before her mastectomy, Jeri Hobramson and

her family ate dinner in a Chinese restaurant. The next morning, before she was wheeled into the operating room, Jeri taped the message from her fortune cookie to her breast, so that it was the first thing her surgeon saw: "You never appreciate what you've got until it's gone." Sharing this joking camaraderie with her doctor boosted Jeri's spirits and helped her to accept a difficult loss.

Most people know what makes them laugh. But few people regularly treat themselves to the funny movies, TV shows, books, or even people who cheer them up and help them to forget their struggles, at least for the moment. Sarah Glazer succeeded in taking her mind off a serious upcoming operation by watching old Woody Allen movies with her best friend. "It wasn't even my idea," she told us. "One night Debby just showed up with *Take the Money and Run*."

Humor is a fine coping mechanism, but occasionally it can be a defense behind which the person conceals hard-to-accept emotions. Bear in mind Sharlynn Crutcher's warning: "Laughter is great—but not as a coverup."

4. Good Communication Is Important

Good communication is telling other people how you feel in such a way that they understand you. Poor communication can create stress by creating misunderstandings. That is why learning to communicate helps to reduce stress.

For some people good communication is extremely difficult. But good communication is a skill that can be learned. It consists of expressing your feelings clearly and calmly and allowing the other person to do the same. *This means that good communication includes listening.* Listening is more than just waiting for the other person to take a breath. If you find yourself doing this, try refocusing on what is being said. Ask questions; don't assume that you can read the other person's mind; restate in your own words what you believe the other person said. ("What I think I heard you say is, you don't like me doing that. Is

> *"Emphasize what you have going for you. Identify your strengths and use them. Notice every little bit of improvement."*
>
> **–Nancy Heck**

that what you really meant?") Other helpful techniques include making "I" statements to express your feelings (*"I* feel inadequate when you interrupt me" versus "You shouldn't interrupt me") and looking for something to agree with in what the other person said. Sometimes you can even agree to disagree. Above all, learn to recognize when you are becoming defensive, critical, sarcastic, or martyred. ("Well, I only *asked*. Excuse me for living.") These are all ways of not saying what you really feel, and they are the enemies of good communication.

5. One Step at a Time

Most problems become more manageable if you try to solve them one step at a time. This reduces your anxiety because it helps you to feel more in control. It is a very effective way to solve a difficult problem or to achieve a complex task or goal. The idea is to see one big task as a series of many little tasks. Focus on each little task individually, complete it, and go on to the next. Some patients actually reward themselves for completing each small task; they treat themselves to a rented movie, a special dinner, a nap. The satisfaction that you derive from each small accomplishment will increase your sense of mastery and your motivation to achieve your long-term goal.

Admittedly, this approach is not always easy. Newly diagnosed cancer patients, especially, are often afraid to delay decisions. They want to take all the steps at once; they think there are lots of vital things that they must do *right now*. If this sounds like you, remember that it is always best to start with an overall strategy. It helps to start by viewing the problem as a series of tasks. No matter what you do after that, this will give you some sense of control and will help you to manage your fear. But remember: the most efficient way to get everything done is to slow down and take one step at a time.

As a newly diagnosed cancer patient, you might apply the step process as follows. At first perhaps you're in shock;

you're too terrified to focus at all. Give yourself as much time as you need to adapt to the situation. Take a deep breath and realize that you're probably going to be panicky for a while. Try to acknowledge your fear and to realize that it's natural. Try to be really good to yourself. Do things that you think might calm and nurture you: take a hot bath, listen to music, talk to a friend. When you feel that you are able, sit down and list all the things you will need to do. (You might ask a relative or a friend to help.) Then number them in the order in which they must be done. You might decide that you should begin by getting information. You would find out exactly how the diagnosis was made, and you might get a second opinion. You would also find out what kind of cancer you had, whether it had spread, what further tests you would need, and how soon you would be notified of the results. Then, depending on your priorities, you might start to build a support team or to investigate treatment options.

The people we interviewed who took this approach told us that they got through each step more successfully than they felt they would otherwise have done. Also, they worried less about the future. Taking action in this way gave them a sense of control over their illness.

The step approach is a valuable part of the problem-solving process. In the following discussion we give another example of how to use it.

6. The Problem-solving Process

You must have some confidence that your problem can be solved, and that you can solve it, before you can take effective action. Sometimes your very first step will be to silence the inner voice that whispers, "You can't do that." "You aren't smart enough." "It will never work." As we have explained, you can learn to quiet this voice. There are many ways to do it; we have found that one of the most effective is exaggerating the voice to expose its absurdity: "That's right. I'm too dumb to tie my own shoes."

Other people can also discourage you from believing

"Nobody is more qualified than you to make decisions about yourself, for what feels right to you."

—Odile Belladonna

that you can solve your problems. This is especially true if you have not yet developed much self-confidence. But remember, as Odile Belladonna says, "Nobody is more qualified than you to make decisions about yourself, for what feels right to you."

Honest communication is essential here. When other people try to discourage you, you need to be able to make them understand how you feel. Tell them plainly how you want them to help you. This might mean asking your father to stop offering you advice, for example, or asking your wife not to criticize your ideas.

Let's see how the problem-solving process works. Suppose that you have undergone surgery for an early-stage melanoma. Your doctor says that you are doing well and should have no further trouble, but you are terrified that your cancer may recur. Your doctor tells you that you need to learn to relax and have some fun.

At first you feel hopeless. "How can I learn to relax," you think, "with death staring me in the face? This is no good. I've got to get my life under control. What can I do right *now* to make myself feel better?"

Well, you could eat ice cream. You could go to that movie you've been wanting to see. You could make an appointment for a massage tomorrow morning. Make a list of small goals—anything that you think would comfort you.

As you achieve these goals, you begin to feel a little better. You begin to see the task of learning to relax as a challenge. You realize that you can use the step approach to meet that challenge.

Listing options

First you take out a sheet of paper and begin to brainstorm. You think of all the sports and activities you used to enjoy. Put them down on your *option list*. You used to like to play cards with friends; you went bowling every Friday night; you once loved to go fishing with your kids; and you and your wife enjoyed hiking when you were young. As you list your options, you start to think about other activities that you were once attracted to, even though it's hard now to imagine doing them. You remember how a young business associate once spoke enthusiastically about rock climbing and piqued your curiosity in the sport. This becomes another item on your option list. As your list grows longer, you begin to see how much there is to life *besides* cancer. You begin to think, "I really do have options. I actually could do some of these things."

Making an action list

Next make a list of specific, immediate goals. This *action list* includes calling up two friends you used to play cards with, seeing whether you can find your bowling ball, talking to your wife about taking some short hikes, getting information on rock-climbing classes, and checking out the fishing tackle stored in the basement.

You like the idea of hiking, and you decide to test it out by walking for fifteen minutes every other day. You decide that rock climbing might be too strenuous for now, so you put a question mark beside it.

Taking action

Mapping out the steps of a plan is helpful, but you still have to act if you want to get anywhere. Two obstacles to action are procrastination and the Inner Critic. (Sometimes they work hand in hand: I procrastinate and the Inner Critic blames me for it, or I hear the Inner Critic and that makes me procrastinate.) The first day you leave your office for a fifteen-minute walk, the voice in your head says, "Are you trying to kill yourself? You're a sick man, remember? Save your strength. You've got an important meeting this afternoon."

Fortunately you recognize that this is the voice of your Inner Critic, and you're learning how to deal with that voice. "Right," you respond. "I'll probably fall dead in the first block. Then I'll miss the meeting. And then our company will lose the account and go bankrupt."

You start walking, and within a few minutes you become absorbed in looking at the architecture, which (had you forgotten?) was once another interest of yours.

Two obstacles to action are procrastination and the Inner Critic.

193

When you get back to the office, you have won two small victories: you have managed your powerful Inner Critic, and you have taken the first step of your program. You reward yourself by buying a bunch of daisies for your desk.

If you keep the steps small, as in this example, it's much easier to deal with big problems. Cancer in particular—its treatment and its aftermath—cannot be handled all at once. Doing what you can at the moment and appreciating each small accomplishment will help you to get through the toughest times.

Dealing with setbacks

What if you're hit with a setback? Again, make a list. First write down all the possible solutions to the problem. Next consider the pros and cons. That is, ask yourself, "If I use this solution, what is the best thing that could happen? What is the worst thing?" Write down your answers next to each solution. Finally, list the options in order of priority, based on the pros and cons. Be flexible. If new information comes in, readjust your priorities accordingly.

Even in the worst situations, this process gives you a measure of control. If option A doesn't work out, you can fall back on option B. Since you're prepared for the worst, you're free to hope for the best.

7. Managing Your Time

To avoid getting sidetracked from your goals, it's important to make good use of time. One way to do this is to plan out your week. Keep a book calendar by the telephone. At the top of each page, write down what you'd like to accomplish that week. Start with the things you absolutely must do. Try to schedule appointments at the times that are most convenient for you. Give yourself some freedom and flexibility, especially if you aren't feeling well. You may want to schedule in some time just to do nothing.

Be willing to make small adjustments when necessary. If you are truly determined to exercise every day, you may need to get up fifteen minutes earlier. If you really want to limit your phone calls, set a timer for five minutes. If you want to get your errands done by noon, wait until evening to take that long, relaxing bath.

From week to week, notice which tasks are the hardest for you and which are the easiest. If you find yourself procrastinating a particular chore, try writing down all your thoughts about that chore. This can yield valuable insights. For example, let's say you find yourself putting off yard work. You write down your thoughts. *Every time I go out there lately,* you write, *it seems like Sid Jones comes out and wants to talk about cancer.* Suddenly you realize that this is why you are so reluctant to do yard work. Now that you know what the real problem is, the solution is obvious. Tell Sid that you prefer not to discuss your medical situation.

When you organize your time effectively, you achieve a better balance between work and play. This improves your quality of life. If you take care of the necessities first, you can fit in more pleasures afterward. Most important, you learn that you have some control over your life. You can *make* time for pleasant things to happen.

8. Reaching Out

"I need help."

Are these the three words you most hate to say? If you have cancer, learn to ask for help. Failing to do so may actually jeopardize your recovery.

Self-reliance can be carried too far. There are times when you can't get what you need–practically or emotionally–unless you are willing to turn to other people. You may need help for as little as an hour or as long as several years. You may need one person, or you may need a network of supporters. The important thing is to recognize your needs and to allow others to lighten your burden.

It is often easier to ask for practical than for emotional support. If you are bedridden after an operation, you

Imagine that you are a sixteen-year-old boy. There is no way that you could tell your aunt how you feel—so you volunteer to water her garden instead.

will need someone to shop and cook for you. If the medication you're taking prevents you from driving, you will have to let someone else drive. This kind of support is straightforward; you know exactly what you are asking for. But even asking for practical support may make you feel dependent. If it does, there are several things that you can do. Ask a variety of people for help so that you won't feel too dependent on any one person. Ask yourself what you can do for the other person in exchange. ("I'll order in Chinese food for both of us after he's done my wash.") This has the added advantage that it takes you out of yourself; it gets you thinking creatively about what you can do for others.

Doctors and other health care providers can often tell you where to find practical help. But you might want to start by enlisting your friends and family. The people closest to you often welcome the chance to help out in practical ways. Having a definite job to do, such as picking up a prescription, allows them to show their concern. This is especially true of people who have trouble expressing their emotions. It gives them a concrete way to show they care. The tasks they perform take the place of the words they cannot say.

Imagine that you are a sixteen-year-old boy. Your favorite aunt is undergoing chemotherapy. She taught you to drive; she helped you to get your license. Now she's lost all her hair and she's too weak to stand. There is no way that you could tell her how you feel—so you volunteer to water her garden instead.

It can be especially hard to ask for emotional support. Many people have difficulty expressing their emotional needs. Even under stress, they don't want to appear too needy. But there is a big difference between being too needy and simply reaching out for help. Asking for help (we want to emphasize this) is not a sign of weakness. But *not* asking for help when it is appropriate *can* be a sign of weakness and a major obstacle to a speedy recovery.[20]

Unresolved conflicts sometimes create barriers that prevent you from asking for help or from allowing someone to help you. Let's say I've always been jealous of my older brother. He was smarter than I was, and more popular, and better at sports. We're both in our fifties now, but we never talk. When the doctor tells me that the diagnosis is cancer, I need all the support I can get. But I don't tell Steve. Instead, I still resent him for being the strong one.

It's best to resolve these conflicts if you can. We will have more to say about that presently. But realistically, resolution is not always possible. When a conflict cannot be resolved, it is usually best just to accept the limits of the relationship. Try not to agonize over it, or force yourself to do something that will make you uncomfortable. Some families cannot cope; in fact, they may need support themselves. Some families are estranged; some patients have no family. In these cases, friends and others can offer comforting support. It is optional—it is not essential—to resolve family conflicts. There are many other ways of reaching out.

9. Resolving Strained Relationships

Is there anyone you feel angry with right now? It's natural to cling to grievances, even petty grievances. But is that what you really want? In working with cancer patients, many of them terminal, Dr. Paul Brenner found that "invariably the most important thing in their lives was their relationships. It wasn't the car they owned; it wasn't the house; in fact, to a large degree, it wasn't even their illness. They just wanted to resolve incomplete relationships."[21]

Resolving strained relationships is one of the best things you can do for yourself. It lowers stress, and it increases your quality of life. In this section we list a few ways to get started.

Empathize

Many things can strain a relationship. Often it's the memory of something that the other person did. Try to see the conflict through the other person's eyes. Can you

For more on the importance of relationships, see Chapter 8.

197

feel what he or she may have felt? If you talk to the other person, try explaining how you feel, rather than criticizing or assigning blame. These techniques can promote mutual understanding and pave the way for a better relationship.

Compromise

Knowing how to compromise can resolve a past grievance or a current conflict. It can also nip a quarrel in the bud. Compromise, like empathy, is easier with honest communication. Brad Zebrack and his girlfriend, Joanne, had been looking forward to a weekend getaway trip. At the last minute Brad came down with a cold. He was still weak from chemotherapy; he knew he should stay home and rest. He also knew that Joanne really needed to get away. Should he disappoint her or not? If he went, he would be miserable, but she would be miserable if they stayed home.

Finally Brad sat down with Joanne and talked. He was upset at first, and she was frustrated and angry. But each of them respected the other's needs, and they were both willing to be flexible. So they compromised: Joanne took a trip by herself; Brad stayed home; and they both enjoyed themselves thoroughly. Their willingness to compromise enabled them to find a solution that pleased them both and drew them closer together.

Forgive

To resolve strained relationships, it helps to be able to forgive. To forgive is to see the person apart from what he did. To focus on the love that existed once between the two of you, the love that is still there, down deep—or perhaps that you only wish were there. To forgive is to put the common good of the relationship above your need to hold a grudge.

It's easier to forgive if you get the anger out of your system first. One way to do this is to write a letter addressed to the other person. Tell him exactly what he did to you; tell him exactly how you feel. Be as harsh and critical as you like. When you have it all down on paper,

For more on communication, see page 189.

tear the paper up. The important thing is to express your anger, not to convey it.

Forgiveness is healthy. It frees you from emotions that add stress to your life. If forgiveness comes hard for you, you're not alone. But even trying to forgive is a step in the right direction.

Set boundaries

Another way to improve strained relationships is to set boundaries. If you know that bringing up certain topics–politics, say–sets off a quarrel, you can deliberately avoid those topics. Another way to set boundaries is to limit the amount of time you spend with the person. Whenever you visit your parents, you get along fine for the first two days. By the third day you're starting to get on one another's nerves. You solve the problem by leaving after one or two days.

A third way to set boundaries is by choosing where to meet and what to do. If lunch with your in-laws is fun when you go to their favorite Italian restaurant and always a hassle when they come to your house, recognize this fact and make the restaurant your "official" meeting place.

Focus on the positive

When you find yourself in a strained relationship, it helps to focus on the positive. Sometimes this means looking back to a time when you and the other person were on better terms. Remember the good feelings that you had toward that person then? How can you recapture those good feelings now?

Today perhaps you and your sister Katy are estranged. But remember how, when you were twelve, you'd go shopping together? You'd clown around in the dressing room, trying on clothes that you had no intention of buying. Call up your sister and suggest a shopping trip. Give your adult self permission to clown around. By the end of the day, you may feel closer to Katy than you have in years.

Or maybe you never did get along, and you haven't

If forgiveness comes hard for you, you're not alone. But even trying to forgive is a step in the right direction.

On resolving family conflicts, see Chapter 7.

seen each other since your father died. Write your sister a note and invite her to lunch. Remember: you are a different person now. So, perhaps, is she. When you meet, look for things to appreciate. Concentrate on Katy's good points. Focusing on the positive will help you to a new understanding of your sister and maybe of yourself as well.

One last point about resolving relationships. It's important not to have any expectations. That is, your goal is to tell the other person that you love him. Don't expect that he will necessarily love you back. If he doesn't, it doesn't mean you've failed. The important thing is to resolve your own feelings.

10. The Team Approach

Dealing with cancer is much easier if you have many sources of support—a team, as it were. This team might include your doctors, your nurses, your family, your friends, a cancer support group, members of your church or temple, and perhaps a counselor. It is to your advantage to have as many people pulling for you as possible. The more people you have on your team, the more you will benefit from individual variations in personal interests, job specialty, and personality. Having a team not only ensures that your medical and support needs will be met but also helps to turn your mind away from yourself and makes your illness easier to endure. It's helpful for your helpers too. No one team member has too much to do, and members can turn to one another for support.

It is best to have a specific plan, with a leader or coordinator to manage the details. (Don't expect your doctor to do this, however. Doctors have more than enough to do already.) You can lead the team yourself, or you can appoint a leader, or someone may fall into the position naturally. Some teams share the responsibility by having a different leader each week. Some teams function without a leader.

Choose team members whom you feel comfortable with—people who support you and understand you; people who are flexible, cooperative, and upbeat. People with a good sense of humor can help you to see your troubles in a different light. Include people whom you enjoy doing things with. Remember that your goal is to give yourself access to information, comfort, and support. You want people who are part of the solution, not part of the problem. Try to avoid people who drain your energy, chronic complainers, people who just don't see things your way. Stay away from people who seek to control any situation that they find themselves in (unless you need or want a controlling member).

How do you deal with "helpers" who aren't helpful? Remember: they probably mean well. Don't alienate them; just limit the time they are around. Give them jobs to do that take them out of your presence; limit their visits; set up a strategy for dealing with these people in advance. Don't frustrate their good intentions except as a last resort—but never forget that *your* welfare comes first.

The rigid ones can pose a special problem. What about team members who insist that you *never* stray from your strict diet, for example? Some caregivers try hard to make you do what they think is best. Esther Joyce told us about a friend who had this problem. "Her caregiver suddenly started bringing her quarts of carrot juice to drink. And so finally she cut her loose, and rightly so. I mean, she was making her life a living hell. All very well-meaning." If you have this problem, remind your caregiver that although you appreciate the concern, *you* are the one who is in charge of your recovery.

Many of the patients we interviewed spoke highly of cancer support groups. To Linda Sumner it helped just to be with people who were going through "the same fears, the same pain, the same whatever-it-is you're going through." "It's like a second family in the group," John Chapman told us. "We cry on each other's shoulders, or we push the other person up, give them the strength to go on for treatment. It's the kind of togetherness that only people in life-threatening situations can share."

If you have never been in a group of this kind before,

> *"It's like a second family in the group.... It's the kind of togetherness that only people in life-threatening situations can share."*
>
> – John Chapman

you may feel nervous about joining one. Most of the other people in the group probably felt the same way to begin with. Get a few of these people's names from the hospital staff and talk to them informally before you come to your first meeting. Knowing what to expect will make you feel a lot better.

When you participate in a group, look for similarities, not differences. "Most people," says nurse Karin Selbach, "walk into a support group with an attitude, saying, 'I'm different; I'm unique; these people don't have the same problems I have.' People start off by making judgments on people, noting a lady's funny hairdo, for example." What makes a support group work, she adds, is finding common things that you can share. Listen to the other people's physical and emotional experiences. See which ones you can identify with, she suggests.[22]

Finally, many patients said that doctors and other health care professionals gave them first-rate emotional support. They listened to their fears and offered reassurance; they steered them toward other people who could help them; and they tried to identify with their feelings and give them coping tools. Or, as Esther Joyce put it in describing her oncologist, "He doesn't believe in deserting a patient, and he has a great deal of respect for me. Everything we handle is on a mutual basis. He's a great support."

Where can you turn for practical, as distinguished from emotional, support if you have no family or close friends? That is, whom can you ask to help with your errands, for example? Start with your neighbors and perhaps the members of your church or temple. Then call the local chapter of the American Cancer Society (ACS). Ask them to recommend volunteer services, county services, and appropriate commercial services. Under certain circumstances, hospice can help out too.

One of the most surprising and gratifying aspects of building a support team is the way one person leads you to another. For example, your doctor puts you in touch with another patient whose diagnosis is similar to yours; a member of your support group recommends a nutritionist;

To learn about hospice, see Appendix 1.

your friend's mother gives you the name of a good nurse. Following up on leads can be rewarding if you remain open-minded about each new contact. Be patient and persistent; when you can't reach someone by phone, write a note. If one person can't see you, ask to see someone else. In short, keep trying.

You may be surprised to see who ends up on your support team. Its strongest members may be people you never would have thought to ask. On the other hand, some of your closest friends—even family members—may be so frightened by your illness that they just disappear. We have more to say about this in Chapter 7.

Unfortunately, support teams do not appear out of nowhere. They develop, sometimes slowly, after you express your needs as honestly as you can. Reach out and ask, "Will you…?" Try to find out how much time and effort each person is able to put in. Sometimes others will sense your needs and try to fill them. But in the last analysis, building your team of supporters is up to you.

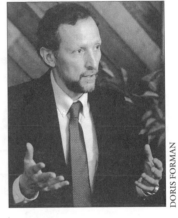

Robert Fuhr

DORIS FORMAN

11. The Benefits of Counseling

A counselor can be a vital member of your support team. Psychotherapists, marriage and family counselors, certified social workers, psychiatrists, and the clergy—all can provide effective counseling.

Some of the problems that call for therapy were discussed earlier in this chapter. Of these, depression and anxiety are especially common. So are issues of dependency and sexual problems. With regard to the last, "there are many therapists who specialize in counseling for sexual problems," says clinical psychologist Robert Fuhr. "They would feel very comfortable seeing cancer patients and helping them through the experience."[23] To obtain the names of qualified counselors in this field, contact the Sex Information and Education Council of the United States (1-212-673-3850).

Many people are reluctant to go to counselors.

"There are many therapists who specialize in counseling for sexual problems."

–Robert Fuhr

Sometimes they are afraid that therapy will take years. In some cases it does take considerable time, but most good therapists like their clients to resolve their problems as quickly as possible. Short-term therapy, which is limited to an agreed-upon number of sessions (usually between five and twenty), focuses on specific problems. Many of the people we interviewed were surprised by the help that they received in just one or two sessions.

Some people resist going into therapy because they are afraid of being overwhelmed by powerful and confusing emotions. In fact, therapy doesn't necessarily consist of expressing deep emotions at all. It depends on the client's needs and goals and on how the therapist works. In any case, you are the one who decides; you set the limits on what you want to deal with. Remember too that professional therapists are trained to create a safe environment for expressing emotions. Unfortunately, many people believe that therapy has to be painful. Fortunately, this is not the norm. And the rewards of therapy can be enormous.

Finally, some people resist going into therapy because they think that it's shameful, or that it means you're crazy, or that you should be able to solve all your problems yourself–and if you can't, it means you're weak. This reflects a very old-fashioned view, one that associates therapy with mental illness. It is more accurate, and more useful, to view going into therapy as a way of maintaining good mental health.*

How do you go about finding a counselor? In some ways, it's like finding the right doctor. Look for someone you can trust and be open with. Look for someone who has experience with cancer patients if possible, as well as with your particular problem. Look for someone with a proven track record. Above all, look for someone whose personality meshes with your own. Give yourself time to find a counselor who really understands what you are going through, someone with whom you can communicate.

Get the names of recommended counselors from your

*And if your circumstances make counseling impossible for you, just talking things over with a friend can help. Simply acknowledging the problem can make it easier to deal with.

doctor, from other patients, from the ACS, from your County Psychological Association. Interview one or more candidates before you make your choice. Ask them how they work, how long they think your therapy will take, and what they charge. This introductory session is sometimes offered free or at reduced cost. If you are uncomfortable with any part of it, you are under no obligation to proceed any further.

Find out whether the counselor is licensed or board certified. Most states have licensing laws that govern psychotherapists, social workers, marriage and family counselors, and so forth. Contact the local office of the state licensing board for the profession in question. You will find this board listed in the yellow pages under Licensing Boards or Professional Associations; or phone the State Office of Consumer Affairs and ask to be put in touch with the licensing office. The State Board of Psychology or the State Board of Behavioral Science Examiners can also provide information on licensed counselors. If your state is one that does not require licensing, contact the National Board of Certified Counselors (1-919-547-0607) and find out whether the counselor is board certified. You can also ask the counselor to show you his or her license or certificate.

The cost of therapy varies a great deal–anywhere from $40 to $125 an hour at this writing. Some insurance plans will pay only for counselors who are on their preferred list. Few insurance plans will pay for a counselor who is neither certified nor licensed. If your medical insurance does not cover counseling, look for someone whose fees are based on a sliding scale. Certified social workers may provide counseling at no charge. So, of course, do members of the clergy.

Many of the patients we interviewed told us how much they had benefited from counseling. But it was Dick Elliot who gave us the final word on reaching out. "Therapy has made me realize," he told us, "that I need more than myself to deal effectively with myself."[24]

"Therapy has made me realize that I need more than myself to deal effectively with myself."

– Dick Elliot

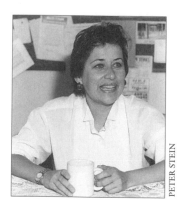

Nancy Heck

"It's better to do a little bit consistently than to expect yourself to do so much that you do nothing."

–Nancy Heck

12. Sometimes Compromise Is Best

An overambitious coping program, and a rigid determination to carry it out, can do you more harm than good. Unrealistic expectations create stress. In other words, you can hurt yourself by trying to do *too much too often* or *too perfectly.*

Long-standing habits, such as smoking or overeating, can be difficult to change, despite your high motivation and your doctor's orders. Many people we talked to succeeded best when they were gentle and patient with themselves. Lowering your expectations or finding a compromise is far better than rigidly adhering to a program that feels like a straitjacket. If, for instance, cutting out *all* sugar makes you feel deprived, you might allow yourself desserts twice a week. If you find yourself getting obsessive about exercising every day, try loosening up your schedule. "It's better to do a little bit consistently," says physical therapist Nancy Heck, "than to expect yourself to do so much that you do nothing."

Dennis Brown had been forcing himself to follow a strict program of meditation. Every day at exactly 4:00 P.M. he made himself meditate for one hour—no exceptions. Far from reducing stress, this regimen made him even more tense. Eventually Dennis realized what was going on. "It felt so good when I got out to a cocktail party or a business meeting," he told us. "I noticed that I welcomed an excuse to take a break from my program."

If you insist on rigidly sticking to your routine, your very efforts to relax may backfire. When you don't give yourself permission to be flexible, you start to view your choices as burdens, and this produces stress. In short, an occasional break is good medicine.

According to Dr. Douglas Brodie, who has treated many cancer patients, a good coping program should be practical and balanced. "It has to be something a person is willing to do and can continue to do," he told us. "It can't be an unworkable program. It won't be stuck to. They'll drop the whole thing if it's too strict."[25]

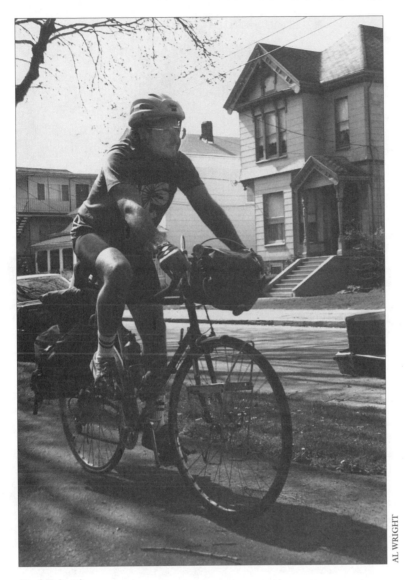

AL WRIGHT

Brad Zebrack

"I just had to believe that at some point in the future I'd be able to do something more active. The bike trip became a goal to shoot for."

–Brad Zebrack

13. Testing New Waters

One way to cope with cancer is to set new–even big–goals and dreams. This gives you a sense of purpose, something to focus on; it takes your attention off yourself and your problems. You discover new abilities and learn new skills, and this in turn increases your self-confidence.

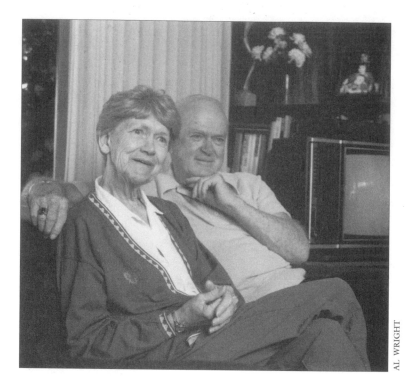

Ruth and Fred Swain

AL WRIGHT

> *"There are certain TV shows that we watch regularly. And we write those down, and we look forward to them. And then the week has a look-forward-to-it-ness."*
>
> **– Fred Swain**

Starting new dreams can make you enjoy life more.

Brad Zebrack had to take a year off to undergo treatment for Hodgkin's disease. During that time, he began to dream of taking a year-long cross-country bicycle trip. "I just had to believe that at some point in the future I'd be able to do something more active. The bike trip became a goal to shoot for." With the treatment completed, he did take his trip; he saw it as a celebration for beating cancer. Brad hoped that his trip might help other cancer patients as well. "The idea being that they could say to themselves, 'Well, if this guy can ride his bike around the country after having that cancer, maybe I'm going to be able to do x, y, or z again in my life once this treatment is all over.'" Knowing that he would be honoring himself and giving to others with his trip helped Brad to see that "I could still have this vibrant, productive life ahead of me."

Exploring an old interest more fully is another way to test new waters. Let's say you enjoy listening to your local jazz station at home. Your friend wants you to go with him to a jazz club. You're up to it physically, but you're shy; all your life you've felt self-conscious in crowds. Finally you agree to accompany your friend to a small jazz concert. You've never seen a string bass up close before. You watch as the bass player takes the lead, and a whole new world opens up for you. Before long, you're going to jazz clubs every Saturday night and making plans to attend the upcoming jazz festival.

Many people—not just people who have cancer—stop themselves from actually doing the things they might enjoy. The young woman who loves art but who won't take an art class because she thinks she isn't good enough misses a chance to gain pleasure from her efforts and from her increasing skills. The gardener who never plants a rosebush because he has heard how difficult it is to grow roses deprives himself of the very beauty he loves. Active coping means taking risks now and then. It means pushing yourself to overcome your insecurities and fears. According to the patients we spoke with, it's well worth it.

14. Setting Small Goals

We have already explained how to solve a big problem by breaking it down into little ones. A different, but related, coping technique is to set yourself small, specific goals. A *small goal* may be something that you can do right now, such as going to the library and finding one book on cancer. Every day offers you the chance to set and meet at least one such goal. For one patient, eating a nourishing meal might be a small goal. Another patient's small goal might be to listen to a relaxation tape. Some cancer patients said that calling a member of their support group was one of their daily goals.

A small goal can also be something to aim for. It motivates you to action, even if it is only in your thoughts. When you are feeling ill, small goals help you to concentrate–even briefly–on what you want to happen, what you plan to do. Setting it as a goal helps to remind you that you intend to take a friend to lunch, attend the homecoming game, update your photo album. Dennis Brown set himself two such goals: to hand his daughter her diploma at her high school graduation and to go fly fishing in the spring. If you feel too ill to work toward the goal right now, you can still plan what you want to accomplish as soon as you feel better.

A small goal can simply be something that you can look forward to. "There are certain TV shows that we watch regularly," says Fred Swain. "And we write those down, and we look forward to them. And then the week has a look-forward-to-it-ness. And that makes life more meaningful."

15. Don't Forget Pleasure

In developing a coping program, don't forget pleasure. You won't do anything that you don't enjoy for very long. Pleasure motivates you; it gives you a reason to keep going; it makes the hard times easier; and it serves as a reward.

Always try to meet your needs in the way that gives you the most pleasure. Let's say you need to exercise. You decide to spend twenty minutes a day riding a stationary bicycle, but you soon discover that this bores you silly. Find another form of exercise–one that you enjoy. How about swimming? Low-impact aerobics? How about riding a real bike on the street, out in the sun and rain, watching the people? How about taking a leisurely walk? Be flexible. Remember: if you don't enjoy it, you won't keep it up.

Work on an option discovery list of things you can do to give yourself pleasure. Treat yourself to a trip to the zoo, buy yourself a magazine, call that one certain friend who always cheers you up. Use your imagination; see how many ideas you can come up with. Do you like writing poetry? Building model planes? Do you like making friends via ham radio or computer modem? One of Paul Ryder's great pleasures was baking bread. What kinds of things do *you* enjoy? You might like to ask a family member or a friend to help you make out your list. He or she can remind you of old pleasures that you had forgotten or suggest new ones that you might not have thought of. Anything that you can do for you will help in your total coping-healing program.

When Dennis Brown learned to make time for pleasure, he found the experience therapeutic in and of itself. It nurtured him and broadened his horizons. "I think you have to set a priority each day for doing something that you enjoy doing," Dennis told us. We think Dennis is right. In developing your coping program, make pleasure a top priority.

Developing Your Own Coping Program

There is no right or wrong way to cope. Your choices will depend on your personality and on your interests. Keeping journals, participating in support groups, developing new hobbies, exercising, laughing—these are only a few of the countless options.

In choosing techniques, keep an open mind. People who remain open to discovery are often happily surprised to find how much they enjoy doing something new.

It's best if you have a variety of ways to cope. Sometimes what works one day won't work the next. Choose techniques that are tailored to your situation at the moment. When your mood and your energy are high, take a long walk or go to dinner with friends. When your mood and your energy are low, stay home and listen to music. If you have been shut in for days, ask somebody to drive you to the country. If there's no one around to talk to, telephone, or write a friend a letter.

Choosing the best techniques for *you* may be the most challenging part of developing a coping program. In this section we offer a few specific suggestions.

> *"I think you have to set a priority each day for doing something that you enjoy doing."*
>
> **–Dennis Brown**

211

Fresh Air and Sunlight

On the first sunny day after a week of rain, even a short walk feels especially good. The sun warms your face, and the air smells sweet. It's tempting to stop somewhere and give in to the pleasure of the experience. But do you? Probably not. Instead you remember the "reason" for your walk and trudge on. Later, when you do have a little free time, you've forgotten how wonderful it felt being outdoors.

Try including more fresh air and sunlight in your life. You can enjoy small doses of this pleasure no matter how busy you are. Park the car a few blocks away from the office. Eat your lunch at an outdoor cafe. Read your magazine on a park bench. These are some of the ways that the people we interviewed brought the outdoors into their lives. Those who were too weak to walk liked to sit in a wheelchair on the lawn, or simply to keep the window open in their bedroom.

Walking and Hiking

We highly recommend walking and hiking. Walking gives the body an excellent workout and subjects it to very little strain. Once your doctor gives you the go-ahead, you can walk almost anywhere. Explore your own neighborhood or discover new ones. Circle around a track; stroll through a shopping mall; hike in the woods. Go alone or take a friend along.

At first you may be able to manage only a few steps. Give yourself credit for those steps and increase your distance as your strength permits. Rest as often as you need to. Set your own pace each day according to how you feel. As it gets easier for you, you'll probably want to walk longer. Again, be sensitive to your body's limitations.

Once you've established a comfortable walking pace, you may find that your senses are sharper. You notice colors, sounds, and smells more readily when you're in the relaxed, receptive state that walking creates. With your senses fully engaged, focusing on the beauty of your surroundings and away from your problems, you are better able to enjoy your life and to open your mind to new possibilities.

Listening to Music

One of the best ways to engage the senses is to listen to music. Music can help you to remember good experiences and to forget bad ones. Some people can visualize their favorite places as they listen to music; they "visit" the seashore where they spent their childhood summers, for example. You don't need to be able to visualize in order to enjoy music, however. It can be deeply relaxing simply to let the sounds envelop you.

For more on visualization, see page 220.

Music is widely used in modern clinical practice to reduce stress, and its beneficial effects have been documented.[26] But you don't need the experts to tell you that music is good for you. It cheers you up; it calms you down; it helps you to sleep; it helps you to get in touch with your emotions. By putting your mind in a relaxed state, it decreases pain. You can listen to music alone or with your friends, in a concert hall or in your living room. Invest in a set of headphones and listen to music while you exercise. Take along those headphones and enjoy your favorite music in your hospital bed. Savor the happy memories it evokes (This was always "our" song). And then look forward to feeling better—well enough to attend that band concert in the park.

Keeping a Journal

Whether it's written in a notebook or recorded on tapes, a journal can be a valuable coping tool. In it you can record events and your responses to those events. You can use your journal as a trusted confidant, telling it what makes you happy, what irritates you, and what you want to accomplish. Keeping a journal is a good way to clarify your thoughts and feelings.

When you are going through a rough period, you can use your journal to help you to identify and dissipate powerful emotions. Simply writing, *Today I feel frightened, but I don't know why* can help you to step back from the feeling and view it objectively. This helps to break its hold on your mind. Writing down your feelings can give you new insights about yourself as you focus on and deal with your fears.

Many patients reported that keeping a journal helped them to develop problem-solving techniques. "I'm finding more solutions for myself," Anne Reinke told us. "I'm writing down thoughts, and then after I write them down I'm thinking, 'Well, was this really important? Or could I have handled it a different way?'" You can record your good thoughts too. Later, when you are going through a bad time, go back and read them to give yourself perspective.

In a journal you can rehearse a conversation by writing out what you plan to say, how the other person might respond, how you might deal with each possible response, and what you would hope to gain from the exchange. You can list all the possible solutions to a problem and write down how you feel about each one. When you are working toward a goal, you can record your daily or weekly progress in your journal. Finally, no matter what you record—feelings, activities, or thoughts—read back over your journal every now and then. Notice the ways in which you have grown, count your achievements, and give yourself full credit.

Keeping a Pet

A cat, a bird, an aquarium—all these can help you to cope in a variety of ways. Pets are good company, but they provide other benefits as well. Whether it's a poodle or a simple hamster, having something to care for can be good for you. It takes you out of yourself, and it gives you a

"My cat, Precious, became an important part of my life. She was an outlet for me because she didn't expect anything."

–John Chapman

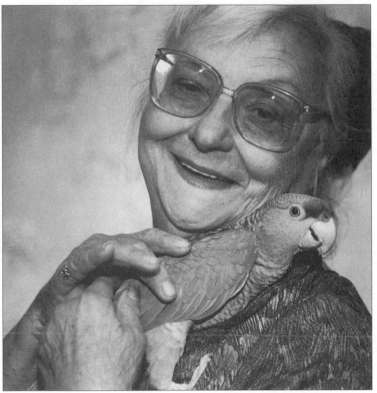

AL WRIGHT

Pets are good company.

sense of purpose. It feels good to be needed, and pets need love. Birds and fish require very little care, but they can be rewarding too. Keeping pets has physical benefits as well; you can take your dog for a brisk walk or calm yourself down just by watching your tropical fish. Pets are a source of many pleasures—the pleasure of playing with them, of talking to them, of learning about them, of reliving happy times (remember that puppy you had as a child?). The beneficial effects of pet therapy are well documented.[27] It's no accident that more and more hospitals and nursing homes have pets on the visiting, or even on the regular, staff.

Keeping a pet can broaden your perspective. "They look at things quite differently," says Fred Swain. "And once you begin to realize why your pet is doing what it's doing, it sort of alters your attitude towards life. It adds another dimension. And I think the more dimensions you have, the more it keeps you from focusing unduly on the cancer."

Perhaps most important for cancer patients, a pet is something to love. "My cat, Precious, became an important part of my life," John Chapman told us. "She was an outlet for me because she didn't expect anything. I was able to give her an outpouring of caring and love and attention where I wasn't always able to do that to a human. I'll never forget what that little outlet of loving an animal has meant to me."

Prayer

Many of the people we interviewed prayed. These people felt that they possessed a powerful tool. They told us that praying calmed and strengthened them. It helped them to feel less isolated and to approach challenging situations with a sense of trust. For many, the very act of reaching out was a way to bring their emotional needs to the surface and clarify them. One cancer patient who asked for courage to deal with her illness told us that through prayer she was able to acknowledge how scared she really was, and that this helped her to deal with her fear.

People who pray do so in many ways. Some pray aloud; others pray in their minds. Some kneel; others pray sitting in the park or even standing at the stove. And there are many forms of prayer: prayers recalled from childhood; formal prayers; spontaneous, spur-of-the-moment prayers—all have helped cancer patients through hard times. "I'm not one who gets down on her knees," says Nancy Heitz. "I could be in there doing the dishes and I'll talk to Him. But I talk to Him like I talk to you, my dad, or my brother, or anybody else that's my friend. I just talk to Him. I say, 'Hey, this is what's bugging me. Why are you doing this to me now or letting this happen?' Then I get calmed down, and when something good happens, I say, 'Thank you.'"

Some patients seemed to live in a prayerful state. These

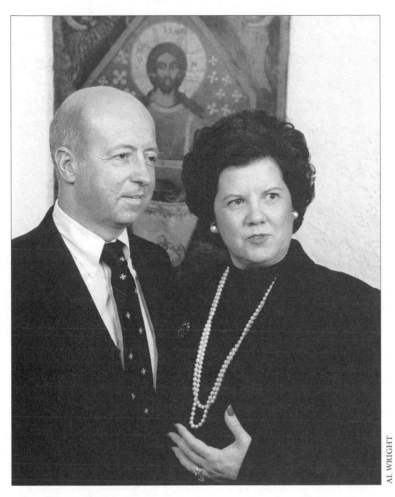

Jay and Barbara Fritz

people felt a sense of gratitude each day—for the beauty of the world, for their families and friends, even for mundane tasks and activities. Their thankfulness for the present and their hope for the future was their way of communicating with a power of life beyond themselves.

To learn more about prayer and faith, see Chapter 8.

Meditation

There are many ways to define meditation. You might define it as reflection, or as clearing the mind, or as detaching yourself from your emotions. Or you might prefer Dr. Herbert Benson's definition. Benson defines meditation simply as a "relaxation response," a "natural and innate protective mechanism against 'overstress,' which allows us to turn off harmful bodily effects."[28]

There are also many ways to meditate. One way is simply to keep your mind as free of thought as possible, focusing on your breathing or repeating a word or a sound over and over. Another way is to reflect upon an image in your mind—for example, the image of waves crashing on the beach. Another way is to focus on a phrase that holds meaning for you, perhaps part of a hymn or psalm. Another way is to focus on a question or an idea and explore what comes up. Another way is simply to watch the thoughts pass through your mind without holding on to them.

If you are a religious person, you may already be meditating without knowing it. Many people who would never think of "meditating" in the usual sense actually do meditate, using the words and phrases of their own religion.[29] Roman Catholics might use Hail Mary, full of grace; Orthodox Jews might use the daily fixed prayers, for example. People who use some form of simple, repetitive prayer elicit Benson's relaxation response. Their breathing and their heart rate slow; their blood pressure goes down; and they feel a sense of inner peace. Meditative prayer has been shown to reduce insomnia, hypertension, and the pain of angina.[30]

People who meditate using prayers gain spiritual benefits as well. One woman who took up meditative prayer to reduce her high blood pressure found that it reinforced her faith. It led her to feel closer to God, to read the Bible, and to attend church. And it made her feel more thankful for the good things in her life and less concerned about the negative things.[31]

The proponents of meditation claim that it reduces stress, improves concentration, and helps you to relax. They claim that it reduces oxygen consumption, slows heart rate and breathing, lowers blood pressure, and increases alpha wave activity in the brain.[32] Not everyone benefits from meditation, but those who do recommend it highly. People who can surrender to the experience do best, but you might want to try it if you can accept even the possibility of its being helpful.

If you decide to try meditation, choose a quiet place where you will not be disturbed. Make yourself comfortable, relax, adopt a passive attitude, and practice one method for ten to twenty minutes. Do this once or twice a day. You may need to give yourself time to explore the different methods until you find one that works well for you. Many books, tapes, and classes are available, or you may even want to take private instruction.

Affirmations

An *affirmation* is a simple statement in the present tense that puts into words a change you would like to make. You repeat this statement ten or twenty times, several times a day. The idea is that whatever you say to yourself over and over has a self-hypnotic effect. For this reason, you can use affirmations to correct negative thinking patterns. When your Inner Critic says, "You can't do it," for example, you can repeat, "I can do it," over and over. To use affirmations effectively, you must say them with strong, positive feeling. You must also word them in a positive way. For example, you might say, "I eat to make my body healthy," rather than saying, "I won't pig out on junk food anymore." Finally, you must word affirmations in a way that is tailor-made to your specific problem. For example, you might say, "I have the courage to undergo surgery." This is more effective than simply saying, "I am strong." Experiment until you find the wording that is exactly right for you.

Affirmations are also used for dealing with such emotions as worry, fear, and guilt. Set aside a specific time (or specific times) each day to say something like "I am letting go all fear of...." Proponents claim that this diminishes the power of your fear.

Sometimes it helps to write your affirmations down.

Do this several times a day for several weeks or months until the message is embedded in your subconscious mind. You might want to post the written affirmations in a conspicuous place, such as your mirror.

We interviewed several cancer patients who used affirmations either while they were undergoing treatment or while they were recuperating. These people told us that affirmations helped them to feel that they were in control. For some patients, repeating the phrase "I am healing" had an effect similar to that of meditation or prayer.

Visualization

There is nothing mysterious about visualization. It's actually something you do every day. You picture in your mind's eye the results you hope to achieve when you undertake almost any project. Say, for example, that you are remodeling your house. You visualize how it will look with the remodeling completed. In your imagination you walk through the rooms, "seeing" them, trying to get the feel of them. How will it be to have the bathroom tile in this design? Will this room look bigger if it is painted white? When it's time to do the actual work, you know exactly what you want to accomplish.

To practice *visualization* means simply to focus on a mental picture. Also called "imagery," visualization can be used to get in touch with your emotions, to lower stress, to solve problems, and to increase self-confidence. Some therapists and physicians recommend it for these purposes. There is no firm evidence to suggest that visualization actually strengthens the immune system or reduces the size of the tumor. But many patients told us that they believed it did, and that it gave them a greater sense of control over their cancer. This in turn reduced stress and helped them to feel better.[33]

You can use visualization to help you to achieve a goal. For example, you might picture yourself walking into the doctor's office to get your lab results, sitting down, and listening calmly to what the doctor says. You practice

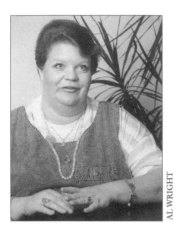

Nancy Heitz

AL WRIGHT

this image once or twice a day for a week. When you actually do go to get the report, you find it easier to talk to the doctor.

You can also use visualization to help you to relax. To do this, you create a calming picture in your mind. It might be a remembered or an imaginary scene—waves breaking on the beach, perhaps, or your grandmother's kitchen when you were a child. It might be a simple image—a religious symbol or a hawk wheeling in the sky. Some people like to add sounds and smells to their visualizations; they might "hear" the roar of the waves or "smell" the bread baking in grandmother's kitchen.

The images used in visualization are often symbolic. You might visualize your radiation treatment as the radiant light of healing energy, for example. When her treatment was especially stressful, Nancy Heitz would visualize putting her negative emotions in a box, gift wrapping the box beautifully, and sending it up to God. This helped her to feel that she had contained her anger and moved it out of her life.

Therapist Lily Kravcisin stresses the personal nature of these images. She had her Catholic mother, for example, visualize the blood of Christ flowing through her body, washing the cancer away. She had a dog trainer visualize white blood cells as white German Shepherd border patrol dogs, retrieving the cancer cells and tossing them into a nuclear reactor, where they were destroyed.[34] Carol Landt had her mother, who had always loved gardening, picture her radiation as strong, wonderful, warm sunshine: "Close your eyes, relax, feel it, picture it shining down on any of the old leaves that might be in your garden, burning them up yet helping the flowers to grow up strong and beautiful."[35] If you decide to try visualization, use images that are powerful for *you*.

Relaxation Exercises

If you exercise, you have probably noticed the beneficial effects of stretching and moving your body. Relaxation exercises, which often involve very simple techniques to

Nancy Heitz would visualize putting her negative emotions in a box, gift wrapping the box beautifully, and sending it up to God.

loosen the muscles, can help you to silence the chatter in your mind as well. Clenching and releasing various muscle groups is one quick, simple method. Try it right now: make two hard fists and hold them for a few seconds; then relax your hands and feel the difference. Try this with other parts of your body to achieve a tranquil feeling. Some people find it more effective simply to focus on each part of the body and concentrate on relaxing it, without tensing the muscles first.

Intensive relaxation is similar to the fist-clenching exercise, except that it uses the same technique on every part of the body. You might begin with tensing your toes and end with squinting your eyes, and the complete session could take an hour or more. A variation consists of first getting as relaxed as possible and then saying over and over, "Let the tension drain from..." as you visualize the tension flowing from each part of your body.

Relaxation exercises have been successfully used by cancer patients to relieve the anxiety and nausea associated with chemotherapy. They work especially well when combined with visualization.[36] They are most effective when they are done during and after (rather than before) the chemo, and when they are done with the help of an experienced therapist.[37] If you want to learn how to do these exercises, we suggest that you read the books listed at the end of this chapter or look for an instructor in your area. Excellent relaxation tapes are also available.

Massage Therapy

Massage is one of the oldest forms of therapy. It uses kneading, stroking, friction, and pressure to relieve a variety of stress-related symptoms. These include tight muscles, headaches, backaches, general tension, and fatigue. Massage makes the joints more flexible; it increases blood flow; and it reduces pain. It acts as a natural tranquilizer; one study has shown that it reduces anxiety better than many forms of physical exercise.[38]

Massage is nurturing; it satisfies the need to be touched.

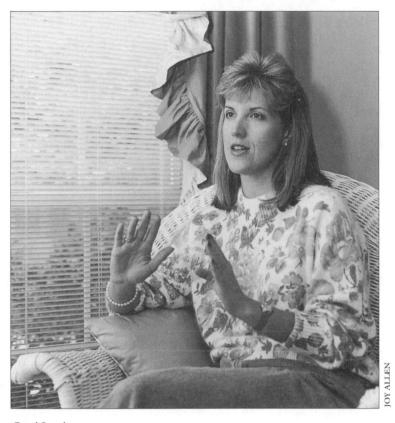

JOY ALLEN

Carol Landt

Carol Landt had her mother, who had always loved gardening, picture her radiation as strong, wonderful, warm sunshine.

More than most people, cancer patients need this kind of comfort. Being touched helps you to feel good about your body, and it helps you to feel connected with other people. Massage is good for you physically and emotionally.

Therapeutic massage is nonsexual; it has nothing to do with so-called massage parlors or escort services. A qualified massage therapist is licensed by the state and is usually certified through a professional school. To find one, ask your doctor, a local health club, or a large teaching hospital for a list of names. Or telephone the American Massage Therapy Association at 1-312-761-AMTA.

Prices for massage therapy range from $30 to $75 an hour. The cost is seldom covered by medical insurance (unless it is prescribed as physical therapy), but a professional school may charge less, or you may even have a friend who can give massage. Many massage therapists will treat you in your own home.

Breathing

Every time you breathe, you are caring for your body. As you breathe in, oxygen passes through the fine inner tissue of the lungs into the bloodstream. The bloodstream carries the oxygen to nourish every cell in your body. At the same time, body waste in the form of carbon dioxide passes out of the bloodstream into the lungs. The carbon dioxide is expelled when you breathe out. You feed and clean your body, then, with every breath you take.

Breathing helps you to care for your body in other ways, as well. For example, you can use it to manage pain. Pain is caused by muscle tension and by increased activity of the sympathetic nervous system. Deep-breathing relaxation techniques decrease nervous system activity (as measured by blood pressure, pulse rate, and respiration rate). They also relax muscle tension and lower anxiety, which contributes heavily to your perception of pain.[39] The next time you are in pain, try the following exercise. Close your eyes. Inhale deeply and exhale through your mouth, blowing out all the air. Now inhale slowly and deeply through your nose. Put your hand on your belly; feel it lift up as you breathe in. Breathe out slowly and gently through your mouth. Feel your belly flatten. Continue to breathe in and out; let your mind go blank and concentrate on your breathing. Continue this exercise for a few minutes and see what effect it has.

Deep breathing is also good for reducing stress. Fast, shallow breathing is part of the stress response; it upsets the balance of oxygen and carbon dioxide in the blood. This in turn creates muscle tension. It can also make your head ache and your heart pound. Try the deep-breathing exercise the next time you feel tense and anxious. As your body relaxes, notice how your mind relaxes as well.[40]

On meditation, see page 217. You can combine deep breathing with other coping techniques. Focus on your breathing as you meditate or combine deep breathing with visualization. Inhale and "see" yourself breathing in positive energy. Exhale and "see" the negative energy leaving your body with each breath. You can also breathe healing energy into a specific part of your body—into your sore back, for example. Deep breathing is an integral part of many relaxation exercises too.

Just as it helps to calm you down, so breathing can help you to energize yourself. Take a few quick, deep breaths the next time you're feeling droopy and lethargic and notice how your energy picks up. You can also use your breath to initiate action. Take a deep breath in; let it all the way out; and then walk straight into that meeting or that doctor's appointment.

Of all the coping techniques that we recommend, breathing is the simplest and the most versatile. It costs nothing; it requires little or no effort; it is always available; you can use it no matter what your present state of health. Do you run five miles a day? Focus on your breathing while you run. Are you building yourself up after chemotherapy? Focus on your breathing while you walk. Are you in a wheelchair? Are you flat on your back in bed? You can still focus on your breathing. No matter what condition you are in, deep breathing offers you a way to reduce stress and make yourself feel better.

A Final Thought...

Over the past seven years, hundreds of patients have described to us in detail how they coped with cancer. Over and over we have been moved by these patients' hope, their courage, and above all their extraordinary personal growth. People who at first were deeply depressed by their diagnosis have told us that learning to cope with cancer changed their lives. It taught them to explore new horizons and to appreciate their own potential. It taught them to value other people and to trust in their own strength. All of this gave their lives—during and after the cancer experience—a new and sometimes very rich dimension.

In Chapter 8 you will hear what some of these patients have to say. For now, if you are a patient we hope that what you have just read will help you to become a cancer victor. Whether or not you are a patient, we believe you can learn to cope—in the best, in the most positive, sense of the word.

In order of their first appearance, the patients who contributed to this chapter are: John Chapman, Paula Carroll, Jean Mitchell, Arnold Schraer, Nancy Heitz, Rick Marill, Elfriede Adams, Linda Sumner, Dennis Brown, Gayle Bartolomei, Odile Belladonna, Ruth Swain, Brad Zebrack, Paul Ryder, Jeri Hobramson, Sarah Glazer, Sharlynn Crutcher, Esther Joyce, Dick Elliot, and Anne Reinke. The family members who contributed to this chapter are: Lois Ryder, Fred Swain, Lily Kravcisin, and Carol Landt.

Recommended Reading

Beck, Aaron T. *Love Is Never Enough.* **New York: Harper & Row Publishers, 1988.**

The founder of cognitive therapy shows how patterns of distorted thinking create problems in couples relationships and explains how those problems can be resolved. Issues of communication are discussed at length. Easy to read, with checklists, questionnaires, and many examples drawn from Dr. Beck's clinical practice. Related topics: Mending relationships, Good communication.

Benson, Herbert. *Your Maximum Mind.* **New York: Times Books, 1987.**

Written by one of the pioneers of mind-body research, this easy-to-read, practical book goes beyond basic stress management. It teaches you to "rewire" old thought patterns, utilizing the Relaxation Response in the context of your own personal beliefs. It contains an excellent bibliography of scientific and popular works on the mind-body connection. Related topics: Mind-body/Stress, Thinking positive, Mastering emotions, Meditation, Relaxation.

Borysenko, Joan. *Minding the Body, Mending the Mind.* **Reading, MA: Addison-Wesley Publishing Co., 1987.**

A lively and very readable discussion of the mind-body connection. The techniques for improving your own physical and emotional health were developed at the Mind-Body Clinic, Behavioral Medicine Unit, New England Deaconess Hospital. The author is one of the founders of psychoneuroimmunology and a close associate of Herbert Benson. Related topics: Mind-body/Stress, Mastering emotions, Meditation, Visualization, Relaxation, Breathing.

Burns, David D. *The Feeling Good Handbook: Using the New Mood Therapy in Everyday Life.* **New York: William Morrow & Co., 1989.**

We describe this book on page 187. Related topics: Thinking positive, Mastering emotions.

Carroll, Paula. *Moment to Moment.* Merced, CA: Medical Consumers Publishing, 1993.

A cancer survivor offers practical and inspirational advice to readers who are coping with cancer. She explains how to deal with your diagnosis, how to live with the illness, how to look for and receive the support you need. Above all, she shows you how to activate your own ability to cope with potentially terminal illness. Related topics: Thinking positive, Problem solving, Mastering emotions.

Chopra, Deepak. *Quantum Healing: Exploring the Frontiers of Mind-Body Medicine.* New York: Bantam Books, 1989.

This book is on the cutting edge of mind-body medicine; it is controversial, but well written and provocative. The author synthesizes the Western and ancient Indian approaches to the mind-body connection, with special emphasis on cancer. Dr. Chopra is a practicing endocrinologist and founding president of the American Association of Ayurvedic Medicine. This book will appeal especially to readers who take a nontraditional "spiritual" approach to health issues. Related topics: Mind-Body/Stress.

Cousins, Norman. *Anatomy of an Illness.* New York: W.W. Norton & Co., 1979.

We describe this book on page 182. Related topics: Mind-body/Stress, Thinking positive, Power of humor.

_____. *Head First: The Biology of Hope.* New York: E.P. Dutton, 1989.

This sequel to *Anatomy of an Illness* describes the author's search for scientific proof that the patient's attitude affects the healing process. Based on Cousins's ten years of research at the School of Medicine at UCLA, the book is full of personal anecdotes and insights. Well written but not especially easy reading. Related topics: Mind-body/Stress, Thinking positive, Power of humor.

Davis, Martha, Elizabeth Robbins Eshelman, and Matthew McKay. *The Relaxation and Stress Reduction Workbook.* 3d ed. Oakland, CA: New Harbinger Publications, 1988.

This self-help workbook teaches you to recognize your own stress reactions and offers a wide range of relaxation and stress reduction exercises. There are chapters on time management and assertiveness training. The book is clearly written, well illustrated, and very easy to use; it is designed for the general reader, but professionals will also find it valuable. The authors are two clinical psychologists and a licensed clinical social worker with a broad shared experience in stress reduction and related fields. Related topics: Mind-body/Stress, Mastering emotions, Meditation, Visualization, Relaxation, Breathing, Time management.

Johnson, Judi, and Linda Klein. *I Can Cope: Staying Healthy with Cancer.* **Minneapolis: DCI Publishing, 1988.**

This short, highly readable book outlines the coping skills that are taught in the ACS I CAN COPE program. Written in a clear and lively style, it is packed with valuable information, illustrated with examples drawn from the lives of nine cancer patients. Chapter 6, "Enhancing Self Esteem and Sexuality," is particularly useful. There are also excellent discussions of communication and of day-to-day physical and emotional problems. Judi Johnson is an oncology nurse and cofounder of the I CAN COPE program. Related topics: Mastering emotions, Mending relationships, Good communication, Team approach.

Lakein, Alan. *How to Get Control of Your Time and Your Life.* **New York: Signet, 1974.**

Lakein teaches you to decide how best to use your time and what to do with your life. He explains how to set priorities and goals, how to make a schedule, how to decide which jobs are worth doing, and how to deal with avoidance and procrastination. This popular book is full of concrete, practical advice. The author is a time management expert whose clients include homemakers and students as well as major corporations. Related topics: Time management.

LeShan, Lawrence. *How to Meditate.* **New York: Bantam Books, 1984.**

This commonsense guide explains clearly what meditation is and describes a wide range of meditation practices drawn from Christian, Jewish, and various Eastern traditions. It tells you how to set up your own meditation program and mentions pitfalls to avoid. An excellent guide for beginners; more advanced students will also find it useful. The author is a practicing psychotherapist and an experienced meditator. Related topics: Meditation.

Matthews-Simonton, Stephanie, O. Carl Simonton, and James L. Creighton. *Getting Well Again.* **New York: Bantam Books, 1978.**

Discusses the mind-body connection in relation to the development and treatment of cancer. Provides excellent, detailed instructions on visualization and relaxation techniques. However, the authors' claim that these techniques can increase survival time in cancer patients remains unproven. For a clear discussion of the reasons why scientists consider this book controversial, see Laszlo, *Understanding Cancer*, 207-13. Related topics: Mind-Body/Stress, Visualization, Relaxation.

Moos, Rudolph H., ed. *Coping with Physical Illness.* **New York: Plenum Medical Book Co., 1977.**

This collection of articles by physicians, nurses, social workers, and psychologists describes the techniques that people use to cope successfully with physical illness. It provides an excellent overview of patient adaptive tasks and coping skills. There is a special section on cancer. Although it is intended for health care professionals, many patients and their families will find this book useful. Related topics: Thinking positive, Problem solving, Mastering emotions, Goal setting, Good communication.

Ornstein, Robert, and David Sobel. *Healthy Pleasures.* **Reading, MA: Addison-Wesley Publishing Co., 1989.**

How positive thinking and physical pleasure can improve your health as well as your quality of life. A brain researcher and the regional director of preventive medicine for Kaiser Permanente discuss the new science of mood medicine. Easy reading; excellent notes and references. Related topics: Mind-Body/Stress, Thinking positive, Power of humor, How to get the most out of life.

Pelletier, Kenneth R. *Mind as Healer, Mind as Slayer: A Holistic Approach to Preventing Stress Disorders.* **New York: Delacorte Press, 1977.**

A classic book on the physical effects of stress and on stress control techniques. Discussion is complete, detailed, and accurate as of 1977. The author is a clinical psychologist who has published extensively on behavioral medicine and psychoneuroimmunology. This book is not easy reading, but it repays the effort. Related topics: Mind-body/Stress, Meditation, Visualization, Relaxation, Breathing.

Rossman, Martin L. *Healing Yourself: A Step-by-Step Program for Better Health through Imagery.* **New York: Walker & Co., 1987.**

A simple, practical handbook that explains how to use visualization techniques to stimulate the body's natural healing processes. It also discusses the role of visualization in preventing illness, in controlling pain, and in overcoming addiction. The author stresses that these techniques should be used as a supplement to, not as a substitute for, medical treatment. Dr. Rossman is a Clinical Associate at the University of California Medical Center in San Francisco. Related topics: Mind-body/Stress, Visualization, Relaxation.

Samuels, Michael. *Healing with the Mind's Eye: A Guide for Using Imagery and Visions for Personal Growth and Healing.* **New York: Summit Books, 1990.**

The author of the *Well Body Book* explains what visualization is and how it affects your body and your mind; he gives detailed instruction in various visualization practices. Personal myths, inner guides, and the concepts of healing energy and inner light are all clearly discussed. This book is based on twenty years of scientific research into the medical benefits of visualization; it contains the exercises that Dr. Samuels has developed for use with his own patients. Related topics: Mind-body/Stress, Meditation, Visualization, Relaxation.

Seligman, Martin. *Learned Optimism.* **New York: Alfred A. Knopf, 1991.**

We describe this book on page 187. Related topics: Thinking positive, Problem solving, Mastering emotions.

Stone, Hal, and Sidra Stone. *Embracing Your Inner Critic.* **San Francisco: HarperCollins Publishers, 1993.**

We describe this book on page 178. Related topics: Mastering emotions.

For Family and Friends

For Family and Friends

When Paul Ryder developed cancer, his wife, Lois, his daughter, Vickie, and his son, Brent, were stunned—and not just because they were afraid of losing Paul. Part of the shock came from not knowing what to do. "We were totally unprepared," says Brent. "We wanted desperately to help, but we didn't know where to begin."

Brent soon learned that cancer is a *family illness*. That is, it involves the whole family; dealing with cancer means meeting the physical and emotional needs not just of the patient but of other family members as well. The Ryders learned how to do this—over time and not without making mistakes. With some thought and a little creativity, and with the help of others who have been there, we believe that your family, like the Ryders, can learn how to deal with cancer. —That your family may even emerge from the cancer experience stronger, more close-knit, and more loving than it was before.

Admittedly, some families never were strong. The cancer experience can tear these families apart. Guilt and denial on the part of family members can make the patient feel abandoned and angry. In the following pages we deal with this situation as well. We hope that the ideas we present in this chapter will help even the most troubled family to cope a little better.

This chapter is addressed to *you* the family member or *you* the patient's friend. It explains how to establish a workable, supportive, problem-solving relationship with the patient and with one another. How well you handle this difficult situation, how well you support your loved one, can alter the impact that cancer has on all

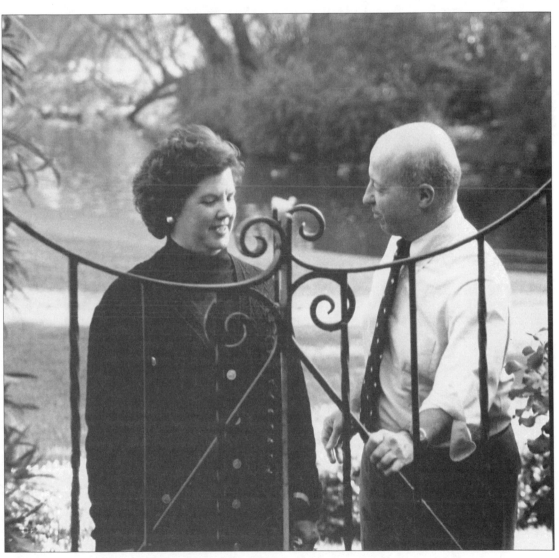

"In the beginning, the cancer experience is almost tougher on your wife and your family than it is on yourself."

–Jay Fritz

Barbara and Jay Fritz

AL. WRIGHT

of your lives. In this chapter you will learn that you *can* make a difference.

The chapter consists of five sections. In the first two we describe how families are affected by cancer and how they can deal with their own problems. In the next two we describe how they can help the patient. In the last section we explain what friends can do.

How the Family Feels

How a family deals with cancer depends on many things–on the stage of the patient's illness, on how family members deal with stress, on how well they communicate with one another, on their religious beliefs, on how well they adapt to change.[1] But when they first heard the diagnosis, all of the families we interviewed were shocked. Indeed, Lois Ryder said that the word "shock" was "far too commonplace." "Kicked in the stomach" was more like it, she told us.

Because they are so stunned, families often feel totally helpless at first. They want to "do something" immediately, but they don't know what to do. Jay Fritz told us that while he came to terms with his illness rather quickly, his family took longer. In the beginning, he said, the cancer experience "is almost tougher on them than it is on yourself. You deal with it. You have to deal with it. They have no effective way of dealing with it. They are living with the doubt just as much as you are. And they may be hurt just as much as you, because you're facing your own death, but other people face the fact of living a life without somebody that they love."

Part of the family's shock may be due to grief, as Jay suggests, grief for a loss that has not happened–and may never happen. This grief, which stems from the belief that cancer is an inescapable death sentence, can make the family feel depressed and powerless in the face of what they take to be "the inevitable." "He's going to die," they think, "so what's the use?" And if the family's grief depresses them, imagine how it makes the patient feel!

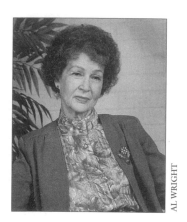

Lois Ryder

AL WRIGHT

Lois Ryder said that the word "shock" was "far too commonplace." "Kicked in the stomach" was more like it, she told us.

As Nancy Heitz observed, "It can be awful. They look at you as if you're already dead."

Cancer does *not* necessarily mean death, as we have stressed throughout this book. In fact, over half of all cancer patients get well again. However, most of the families we spoke with weren't able to grasp this fact until they had recovered from their initial shock and had learned just what they were facing.

Once the first shock has passed, family members, like patients, may experience other powerful emotions. Don't be surprised if you're swept away by feelings you aren't prepared for and don't understand, feelings that seem to come and go for no good reason. These feelings may include anger, guilt, anxiety, denial, and emotional numbness.

Just as patients often feel angry, so do many families. Just as patients sometimes curse their fate and ask, "Why me?" so some family members ask, "Why my husband?" "Why my daughter?"–and, perhaps unconsciously, resent the person who has "caused" their lives to be turned upside down. If you are the main caregiver, don't be surprised if you feel this way.

Anger can sometimes be an expression of fear. Annette Pont-Gwire, a cancer survivor and a clinical psychologist, told us that her husband wrote her a letter so angry that she has never forgotten it. "Not until years later was he able to identify what he really felt. He felt very abandoned and terrified that I was going to leave him. Die and leave him."[2]

Anger is often accompanied by guilt. You feel guilty *because* you feel angry. Sometimes you aren't really angry at the patient at all. Carol Landt, a licensed therapist who nursed her mother through cancer, points out that caregivers sometimes "displace their anger and their frustration and their great concern over a very stressful situation onto the patient."[3] And then they feel guilty.

You may also feel guilty if you blame yourself for your relative's illness. Why didn't I see this coming? Why didn't I suggest a checkup when the symptoms first appeared? Were we eating too much fat? Should I have made her stop

Carol Landt points out that caregivers sometimes "displace their anger and their frustration and their great concern over a very stressful situation onto the patient."

"In a way, you dismiss it. You kind of pretend. 'No, Mama's not ill. I mean, it's something she has, but it's going to be okay.' You don't want to believe it."

– Denise Manning

smoking? Stop drinking? I fought with him sometimes; did I give him cancer by putting him under stress?

Or you may feel guilty simply because you're afraid of what lies ahead. You're afraid of the work that is going to be expected of you. You wonder whether you're up to it. Then you begin to tell yourself how "selfish" you are.

One way or another, you are almost sure to feel anxious and afraid. You fear for your loved one. Like Annette's husband, you may fear for yourself as well. Perhaps you fear that your own life will never be the same again. Or you fear coming face-to-face with your own mortality. Your loved one has cancer; suddenly you sense how fragile life is. All of these fears may be reinforced by a general fear of the unknown. Cancer has invaded the household. Who knows what might happen next?

Anxiety leads many families to engage in denial. In extreme cases they deny the very existence of the disease and behave as if nothing has happened. Usually, however, they just refuse to accept some part of the new reality, or they accept it at some times but not at others. "I think the whole time you're scared," says Denise Manning. "You associate cancer with death, and immediately you think about people who died of the same disease. So I just thought, 'Not Mama. My mother's strong. Everybody else, but not her.' In a way, you dismiss it. You kind of pretend. 'No, Mama's not ill. I mean, it's something she has, but it's going to be okay.' You don't want to believe it."

Families that engage in partial denial may want, like Denise Manning, to believe that the diagnosis is not as serious as it sounds, or that they won't have to make very many changes, or that the reappearance of symptoms isn't significant. Sharlynn Crutcher's husband refused to talk about her symptoms at all. "I think he's in his own form of denial," Sharlynn told us. "Every time I say, 'Well, I've got this,' or 'I'm going to have another seizure,' he tells me, 'You'll be okay. You'll be fine.' And finally I got angry, and I said, 'Every time I say that, you tell me I'm going to be fine; but somewhere down the road I am not going to be fine, you know, and you just shut that door when I'm

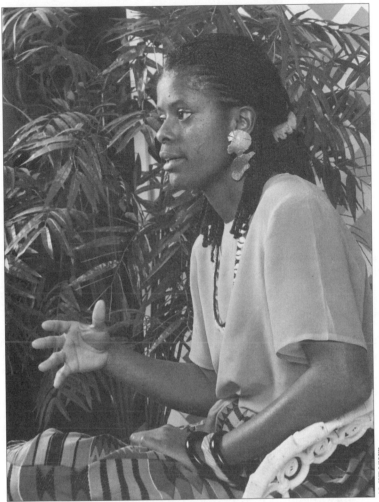

Denise Manning

trying to tell you something is hurting me.'" Persistent denial, even partial denial, can make it difficult for patients, as well as families, to cope.

Denial can have tragic results when the patient is terminal. Clinical psychologist and oncology counselor Andrew Kneier describes one such case. This patient wanted to talk with his family about his impending death, but his family refused to accept that he was dying. "Consequently the patient was unable to share what he was going through with those who meant the most to him, which

239

greatly added to the tragedy of his death. And his family was left unprepared and missed the precious opportunity to be with him in his dying and to say goodbye."[4]

But perhaps in some sense all denial is related to the fear of death. We all know that we will die someday, but most people try not to think about it. They hope and plan, often well into old age, as if death could be indefinitely postponed. So it isn't surprising that the families of cancer patients are sometimes tempted to engage in denial. June Heitz confessed that her daughter's cancer made her keenly aware of her own mortality. But she added that she deliberately refused to think about it. Echoing what may be a universal sentiment, she said, "I would like to think I'm going to be here forever."

For some people, the initial shock is followed by a kind of numbness that, at least for a time, dulls all their feelings. This is a common reaction to adversity, as Andrew Kneier points out. "You feel emotionally detached, as if it weren't really happening to you." (This is not the same thing as denial, because you acknowledge what is happening.) Carol Landt describes it as "feeling that I'm in a cocoon. I'm able to do what needs to be done, but my feelings, and some of my thoughts, are on hold."

How the Family Can Learn to Cope

All of the emotions that we have just described are normal reactions to a diagnosis of cancer. The first step in coping with them is to accept them. "I was over-whelmed by my emotions," the wife of one patient told us, "until I stopped trying to hide from them. Under-standing my feelings helped me to find the strength to go on." Denise Manning said that simply letting her feelings out helped her to feel better and more in control. "I just cried until I felt like I had no more tears in my body. I'd be sitting down watching TV and just cry, and I wasn't even aware that I was thinking about Mama. I just cried. And all the time I was crying, all this was coming out. And each time I cried, I came closer, I guess, to that calm. To that resolve."

It's easier to accept your emotions when other people accept them too. It also helps to know that you are not alone. Telling your family how you feel can bring you closer to others who feel the same way. If, on the other hand, you keep your feelings to yourself, "walls of emotional isolation develop. And this would be a bad time for emotional isolation," says clinical psychologist Robert Fuhr.[5] In short, it's important to share your feelings with others, starting, if possible, with the other members of your own family.

Use the Family as a Support Group

Some members of your family may want to join an outside support group, and we discuss this option on page 247. But before you seek outside help, consider the family itself as a possible group, one whose members already know the patient and one another. The primary caregivers will probably need the most support. For them it can be a great relief to share their thoughts and emotions with the rest of the family. But everyone can share in the group experience. Members who simply listen, who provide support and feedback, can make an important contribution too.

To solve practical problems

How does a family form itself into a support group? The simplest way is to start by focusing on practical problems. Most families have an established way of doing things. But with cancer, family life is frequently disrupted. Mealtimes may be altered, routine tasks rescheduled, sleeping arrangements changed. Even if yours is a very small family whose members are in constant contact, it might be helpful to sit down and talk about these day-to-day issues first. Make a list of practical questions. Will the patient need a special diet? What does the medical insurance cover? The family may not be able to deal with everything in one meeting, but it should help to get the main concerns out on the table.

Think of the family as part of the health care team. Discuss who can take on various responsibilities and how each person can help the others out. Who will do the shopping? Would it be better to take turns cooking or to have one person do it? Should someone go with the patient to the doctor's office? In assigning tasks, consider each person's individual resources (time, money, other obligations) and especially each person's preferences and skills. As far as possible, it's a good idea to give people the jobs that they do best and that they most enjoy. Negotiate to see who does what, how to share, and how to take turns.

You may want to discuss how you can use time more efficiently. Start by listing the household's, and each person's, priorities. What were they before the cancer was diagnosed? What are they now? How will you strike a compromise between the patient's needs and those of the family? It may help to have each family member keep a diary of his or her daily routine. Try to do this for a week or so. Then have the whole family sit down together to coordinate everyone's new schedule and assign tasks. Finally, write all of the tasks down on a calendar. That way each person knows when he or she is scheduled to do what.

If you want to use time more efficiently, it helps to be innovative. Where can you save a few extra minutes? Is it necessary to do that time-consuming low-priority task? Don't forget to allow for your own needs as well as the patient's. If you get up half an hour earlier, for example, you can give the patient a fifteen-minute massage and give yourself fifteen minutes to eat a good breakfast.

Think about possible life-style changes that might benefit the whole family. Can vacuuming be done less often? Would it be possible to change vacation plans? Can money now being spent on extras be used to pay for outside help? This last is especially important. It takes some of the strain off the family and gives each person some time to live his or her own life.

If there are new expenses, discuss how the family can save money. Can you use less heat? Less air conditioning? Can you postpone planned purchases? Do you really need to make them at all? Here again you may need to reassess your priorities. You might want to set short- and long-term goals corresponding with the course of the treatment. You can revise them as the treatment progresses. You might even turn the need to economize into a game—the person who thinks up the best way to save money gets a whole day off or the right to choose a favorite dinner.

It's useful to have a plan of action. This plan might list the family's general goals—solving practical problems, using time effectively, dealing with medical professionals, managing expenses, dealing with emotions, and so forth. The plan might also list each person's individual tasks. It might include a schedule for family meetings and suggest agendas. Try to set up the plan in a way that allows for the unexpected by including a variety of options.

It's good to establish a trial period for your plan. When the period is over, adjust the plan as necessary. You will probably need to reevaluate it periodically as the family's circumstances change.

Who attends family meetings? That depends on the family. Most of the patients we interviewed wanted to participate. Include everyone who lives with the patient and anyone else who can help make decisions and, when possible, lend a hand. You may even want to include family members who live some distance away, if they would like to participate.

Who leads the meetings? Again, it depends on the family. In most families one person tends to be the leader. In Denise Manning's family, that leader was her mother. When Mrs. Manning developed cancer, her husband and one of her daughters took her place. In Lily Kravcisin's family, there were also two leaders: Lily herself, who is a clinical psychologist, and her uncle, a Czech immigrant, "who made a lot of money in construction," Lily told us. "And he's kind of a powerful guy. And he'd call me and say, 'Lily, you call those doctors; you talk like they. Call them. Find out what's going on.'"[6] In some families, members take turns acting as leader. This works especially well when several people want the job. If you haven't

In some families, members take turns acting as leader. This works especially well when several people want the job.

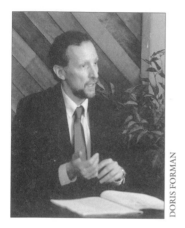

DORIS FORMAN

Robert Fuhr

"Try to encourage others to talk by expressing your own emotions first."

–Robert Fuhr

decided who your leader should be, you might make this your first order of business.

Try to hold family meetings regularly. At least hold them often enough to discuss any changes in the patient's or the family's situation. Have each person keep a list of suggestions to bring to each meeting.

Some family members may feel threatened by the prospect of a formal meeting. They may worry that people won't get along. This is especially true in families where there have been conflicts in the past. These people may feel safer with a dinnertime discussion or a chat over coffee. Or if family decisions have always been made at a particular time and place–over Sunday breakfast, say, or after work on Friday–they may find it less threatening to stick to the status quo. It is often easier, in times of stress, to do things the way the family has always done them.

Whether or not you hold formal meetings, work to keep the lines of communication open. Never assume that you know what other people want or need. Let them tell you. Unless all family members are included in the discussion, misunderstandings can occur. The Ryders learned to minimize this risk by keeping a nonstop, three-way discussion going–through person-to-person contact when they were together, by frequent telephone calls when they were not.

To express emotions

Family meetings are an excellent place to express emotions and concerns. If this doesn't happen naturally as you discuss practical problems, try to encourage family members to describe what they've been feeling. This may be awkward at first, especially for those who are either unused to dealing openly with feelings or unaware that they have any feelings to express. You might begin by bringing up your own anxieties or concerns. Then ask if anyone else has been feeling like that too. One family member told us how surprised and relieved she was to discover that her brother and two sisters were just as frightened and confused as she was.

Be prepared to deal with strong emotions. Anger and guilt have a way of surfacing when they are least expected. Remember too that not everyone experiences the same emotions at the same time. For example, some family members may be working through their fears while others are still in a state of denial. When this happens, it's important not to push. People will usually face the facts when they feel comfortable dealing with them, and with the powerful emotions that the facts evoke. Watch for signs that the person is getting ready to discuss his or her feelings; try to be open and accepting, not judgmental, when he does. It's a good idea to keep those first discussions short and let the other person decide when to change the subject.

In short, then, encourage everyone to express his or her emotions. But don't be discouraged if not everyone wants to participate at first. It's hard to talk about your deepest feelings. It may be weeks or months before some family members are ready to say how they really feel.

In fact, some people may never be ready. In a few families it is impossible to talk about emotions at all. The members of these families often feel threatened by their emotions. The reason usually goes back to their childhood. Perhaps they associate emotions with violence. Perhaps they believe that it's wrong to "burden" others with their feelings. Perhaps they don't think they have the right to feel bad. Perhaps they sincerely believe that emotions "don't matter." Whatever the cause, we believe that professional therapy can help.

For suggestions on how to find a therapist, see page 204.

What can *you* do to help? Not much, perhaps. If the members of your family have refused to discuss their feelings in the past, it may be too much to expect them to begin now. Don't insist. However, if you want to do something, therapist Robert Fuhr offers the following suggestions.

Try to encourage others to talk by expressing your own emotions first. It helps to set ground rules that encourage mutual respect. ("We may be discussing painful emotions here, so let's all be especially considerate of each other.")

"There's a camaraderie that you get from them and they from you.... You're in the battle together."

– Fred Swain

For more on keeping a journal, see page 213.

Comment on obvious nonverbal cues in a nonjudgmental way ("You look upset"), but let the other person decide whether to respond. If the problem involves only one or two people, you might ask someone who feels comfortable with those people to talk to them individually, in private.

The families that have the most trouble learning to cope are often the ones whose members never did get along, or who harbor unresolved grudges against one another. Should these families even try to hold meetings? A few of the people we interviewed said no, that trying to hold meetings would simply make matters worse. But most people felt that the attempt was worth making, if only to see whether old problems might be resolved and new lines of communication opened. If your family doesn't get along, we suggest that you test the waters to see whether anyone else is willing to give the meeting idea a try.

Keep a Journal

Some family members benefit from keeping a journal, either written or on audiocassette. You can use it to record routine data, such as doctor's appointments. You can use it to record your thoughts, your feelings, how the patient is getting along, how other family members are adjusting. You can use it to record problems and to describe how they were solved or might be solved. You can even use a journal to vent emotions that you cannot express in any other way.

The hardest part of keeping a journal is getting started. Begin with one or two entries and build from there. If you have trouble sticking with it, try to make at least one short entry every day. As long as they are honest observations and not ways of procrastinating, entries such as *I have nothing new to report* or *I just can't face writing today* are perfectly acceptable and will help to maintain the habit of keeping a journal. But you will benefit most if you enter more than the bare minimum. If you make keeping a journal a regular part of your life, you may learn a great deal about yourself, the patient, and your family.

246

Get Outside Help

Whether or not your family forms its own support group, you may want to join an outside group. Most cancer support groups welcome family members; we know some people who attended group meetings even though the patient involved chose not to. We also know family members who lived hundreds of miles from the patient who attended support groups in their own area.

In a cancer support group, you are likely to meet other families who are going through experiences similar to your own. You can learn to talk openly about your mutual concerns. The leaders of these groups understand your special problems and are trained to help you to deal with them. Often they can suggest solutions that you never would have thought of. They know what resources your community has to offer and can help you to get the most out of those resources.

Many of the family members we interviewed spoke highly of cancer support groups. Fred Swain, whose wife has lung cancer, put it like this:

"There's a camaraderie that you get from them and they from you. You don't feel that you're all alone. You're in the battle together. You've got people lined up beside you."

To find the cancer support group nearest you, inquire at the patient's hospital or call the local office of the American Cancer Society (ACS).

You may want to talk informally with other cancer families too. Try to find families who have experienced the form of cancer that you are dealing with. Check with the nearest cancer support group or ACS office for the names and addresses of such families. We know of one family who did this and ended up creating a cancer support group *just* for family members.

Of course, there are limits to what you can accomplish through a support group. If family members can't deal with their emotions—if they seem to be suppressing them, or if the problems persist or become debilitating—it may be time to consult a psychotherapist who specializes

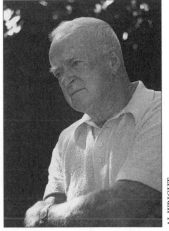

Fred Swain

AL WRIGHT

Are you nervous about joining a support group? See page 201.

*"She separated
my emotions
from the cold,
hard facts....
And basically
just told me
things I could
have figured
out on my own
if I'd had the
clear mind
to sit down
and do it."*

in working with cancer patients and their families. You may need to interview several candidates before you find just the right one. Get a list of names from your local ACS office or from the oncology social worker at the patient's hospital, and make your choice following the guidelines on page 204.

What if the family refuses to work with a therapist? In that case you might want to consider getting individual counseling. A family member who preferred to remain anonymous and whom we will call Art told us what individual counseling did for him. Art's mother was emotionally unstable. When Art's father developed cancer, his mother became hysterical and remained so for the next several years. This put enormous stress on the whole family. Family counseling was suggested, but Art's mother refused to cooperate. As his father's illness progressed, her behavior grew more and more erratic. She accused Art, who was helping to care for his father, of not loving him enough, and blamed him for trying to remain calm. Art grew angrier and angrier. "I was so overwrought," he says, "that I couldn't think straight or function properly. My blood pressure was something short of death." Finally he made his own appointment with a therapist:

"She separated my emotions from the cold, hard facts. Saying, 'Look, there's nothing you can do, and there's no reason you should feel bad for being the way you are.' And basically just told me things I could have figured out on my own if I'd had the clear mind to sit down and do it." In short, the therapist got Art to see his family situation in a realistic light.

Counseling for an individual family member can sometimes ease tensions within the family too. Once one member of the family is able to start working toward constructive solutions, the whole dynamic of the family may change.

One of the things you are likely to discover—through counseling, through a support group, or even on your own—is that emotions such as anger, guilt, and fear tend to diminish over time. If you can maintain perspective,

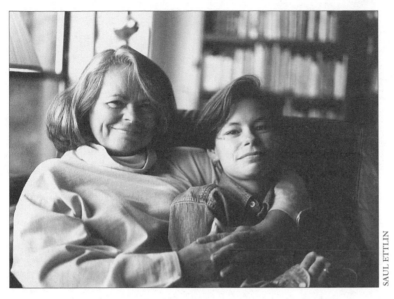

Leslie Haines and her daughter Malinn

Children can usually adapt to cancer in the family as long as you tell them what is going on.

you may be able to slow down the emotional roller coaster. This in turn may help you to feel more in control of yourself and of your situation. The more you feel in control, the better able you will be to deal with difficult emotions in the future.

Helping the Children to Cope

Children can usually adapt to cancer in the family as long as you tell them what is going on.[7] However, if you keep them in the dark, they tend to worry. They also tend to jump to the wrong conclusions. They may think that Grandma's illness is too awful to talk about, or even that they themselves did something to cause it. If you don't talk about it, you may give them the idea that it is wrong to talk about certain subjects. This leads them to bury their fears, as we shall explain presently.

It is important, then, to be honest with the children. Above all, reassure them, says Andrew Kneier, "that nothing they ever did, thought, or felt had anything to do with Grandma's illness."

249

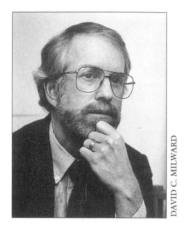

DAVID C. MILWARD

Andrew Kneier

Being honest includes accepting their feelings. If you tell them, "Don't say that" or "You shouldn't feel that way," they may bury their fears. This makes the fears stronger and harder to deal with. If Peter is afraid that he somehow made Grandma sick, it is important to accept his feelings and at the same time to explain that he is not responsible. (Note, however, that accepting his feelings does not mean telling him how he feels. Encourage *him* to tell *you*–and listen to what he says.) Bear in mind that children's buried fears may surface in the form of negative behavior. If Peter is told, "Don't feel," he may express his feelings by picking on his sister. An older child might drop out of school or start using drugs. Negative behavior, then, can often be a clue that the child is frightened or angry and needs help.

Try to explain the situation to each child individually. Be as truthful as you can, given the child's age. It is useful to have these talks as soon as possible after the diagnosis so that the children will know what to expect and will not pick up misinformation from their playmates. Make sure to explain that cancer is *not* contagious.

Try not to make it sound too frightening. You might say that cancer is like other illnesses, only more serious. If the child already knows a little about cancer, point out that many patients get well again. If the child is very young, you may prefer not to mention cancer at all. It may be enough to say that Mommy is ill but that she still loves you, or that Grandpa is sick and tires easily, so we can spend only a little time with him.

Children who are old enough to understand should be told about treatment–what all these medicines are for, why Susie's hair fell out, why Dad's radiation makes him tired and cross. Dennis Brown relied on his wife to let their children know "if I'm having a bad day or if I have a lot of pain or sickness or happen to be depressed or whatever, so that they can understand if I might be short-tempered or impatient." Though they all had busy schedules, the Browns made it a point to have dinner together every night. That way, as Dennis put it, "we always had a chance to sit down and let *everybody* know what's going on."

It's a good idea to take small children to the hospital before the patient is admitted. (Check with your doctor about the risk of infection first.) This keeps them from imagining the hospital as a house of horrors where terrible things are done. A quick chat with a friendly staff person can do much to reassure a frightened child.

If the children are very young, explanations may not help much. They may need more tangible support, perhaps extra attention from Grandmother or Uncle Ted, or extra care on their parents' part to make sure that their daily routine–story time, mealtime–is disrupted as little as possible. (Older children can usually benefit from added attention as well.) This kind of support can help to keep children from becoming too frightened by seeing mother ill in bed or big brother suddenly looking different. It can also be comforting for them to see that these things don't frighten you.

Children usually play a role in the family reorganization that we discussed earlier in this chapter. Exactly what role they play depends on the family. Most of the families we talked to had the children, especially the older ones, help in the decision making. They said that this made the children feel important and involved. On the other hand, you may feel that the illness itself is enough for the children to fret about. In this case it may be best simply to assign them specific tasks. This can be a therapeutic way to focus their attention and to keep them from worrying too much.

When cancer strikes the family, children, like adults, may be deeply upset. With your help they can usually adapt, but at best this will take some time. Meanwhile they may show their anxiety by withdrawing, acting up, or becoming depressed. If you follow the suggestions given above, these reactions are generally short-lived. If they persist–if the child remains withdrawn, downcast, or angry for several weeks–you should probably seek professional help. Many therapists specialize in helping families with young children to deal with the disruptions caused by a serious illness. Ask your doctor, nurse, or social worker to refer you to one.

Children who are old enough to understand should be told about treatment.

Caretaker: Take Care of Yourself

If children need special consideration, so does the *primary caregiver*, the person who spends the most time looking after the patient. If that person is you, you may neglect your own needs, sacrifice them, or rationalize them away. But your needs don't go away. And taking time to care for yourself is not selfish. It's vital. If you give until you start to burn out, you will do yourself, your family, and especially the patient a disservice. You can be far more effective if you take time off to maintain your strength and peace of mind.

Time off doesn't have to mean a cruise in the Bahamas. Maybe all you need is a change of pace. Make a list of things that sound refreshing: sleep late one morning, go to a movie, take a quiet walk, have time to reflect, visit that special friend who always cheers you up. Make it a point to do one of these things each day. Set taking care of yourself as a priority.

When it comes to taking care of yourself, your friends can be a valuable resource. But like the patient, you may find that some of your friends avoid you. For cancer patients and their families, this is an unfortunate fact of life. We have more to say about it later in this chapter. For now, we simply want to say that it can happen, and that it's not your fault. It probably isn't really your friends' fault, either. They may avoid you because they don't know how to deal with their fear, or because they can't express their feelings. Try not to hold it against them. Reach out, instead, to make new connections and new friends.

This brings us to the larger issue of support. To find time for yourself, you may need to enlarge—or if you are the sole caregiver, to *create*—your support system. You may also need to delegate responsibility. If, for whatever reason, you cannot call on friends or relatives, look for public or private assistance. Ask other cancer families, local cancer support groups, and the nearest ACS office where to go for help.

Above all, remember that it's essential to look after yourself. This can make you feel guilty, especially if you're

Have your friends stopped calling? Turn to page 270.

already feeling down, and most especially if the patient is getting worse and needs more and more care. Try to keep things in perspective. You are *one* member of the health care team. No one person can do it all—not all of the time, not even most of the time.

Even if you have plenty of support, there may be times when you're close to the edge of burnout. Lois Ryder told us that she sometimes felt "lonely, bewildered, unappreciated, and very much unloved," especially when everyone was showering sympathy on the patient. She said that when this happened, "I usually turned to a special friend or my minister—someone who knew just the right thing to say. When there's no one to unload to, you have to try to keep from feeling sorry for yourself. I discovered that self-pity just makes you feel worse. It makes you feel less loving."

With this in mind, let's look at one heavily burdened family member who preferred to remain anonymous. We will call her Jeanette. Jeanette's daughter has Hodgkin's disease, and Jeanette looks after her alone. When we asked her who helped her to take care of her daughter, she said, "I do." In fact, the rest of the family have told Jeanette that she is taking on too much. "But," she insists, "it is my decision, and I choose to do what I'm doing, and I don't do it as a martyr." A nurse practitioner recommended that Jeanette get involved in a cancer support group, but she says she doesn't need one. "Anyway," she says, "I'm not comfortable expressing private problems with people."

Jeanette's only relief comes from praying at night and occasionally allowing herself to cry. "Once in a while," she says, "I feel real sorry for *me*, and I may have a crying session. Crying doesn't solve the problem. It makes very puffy eyes, and that's about all."

Although Jeanette does not see herself as a martyr, she certainly seems to be taking on too much. She says she doesn't need help, but she also says that she has difficulty sleeping, and that she is getting her migraine headaches more often. She says she feels old (in fact, she is in her late fifties), and she is depressed much of the time. Jeanette is enraged that her two adult sons aren't doing more to

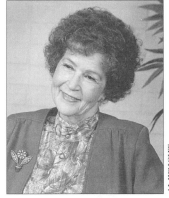

Lois Ryder

"I usually turned to a special friend or my minister— someone who knew just the right thing to say."

–Lois Ryder

AL WRIGHT

help. She has never asked them for help, but she insists that they should have provided it on their own. "It makes me furious," she says. "I should think they would be more compassionate to me as well as their sister."

"I just hang in there," says Jeanette, "so far, anyway." But Jeanette is already showing symptoms of burnout—and things could get worse. If they do, she may start to forget things, she may feel emotionally "dead," she may grow more and more resentful and depressed and less and less able to function. Eventually she may simply fall apart.

It's essential to ask for help before you get to this stage. You need to take care of yourself if you're going to take care of the patient. Here are some questions to ask yourself:

- Am I getting too little sleep? Too much?
- Do I dread getting up in the morning?
- Am I feeling more and more anxious or irritable?
- Am I feeling resentful? Overburdened?
- Am I performing poorly at work?
- Do I have time for my friends? Do I enjoy their company?
- Have I lost my appetite? Am I overeating?
- Do I cry a lot? Do I feel sad much of the time?
- Am I drinking too much? Smoking? Taking drugs?
- Am I desperate to get out of the house every day?
- Does my health seem to be deteriorating?

If you answer yes to any of these questions, you certainly could use help. This is true even if you are used to doing everything for yourself, and even if you feel uncomfortable asking for support. We strongly urge you to ask for it anyway.

How to Talk with the Patient

If you want to provide the patient with attention, understanding, and support, it helps to know how to communicate. This is how you find out what the patient is thinking; what he or she needs, or wants, or would like to talk about. This is how the patient and the family can work together to make life better for everyone.

It's important to be as natural as possible. Your loved one is still your loved one even though he has cancer, so as far as possible, try to talk just the way you always have. This can be reassuring for the patient; there's comfort in doing things the old, familiar way. At the same time, things have admittedly changed, so look for approaches that seem appropriate to the new situation. Members of cancer families and professionals offer the following advice.

Set aside enough time to talk comfortably. This shows the patient that you care about his or her concerns, and that you are willing to take the time to discuss them. It also prevents you from becoming so rushed that you only have time to get, or give, information. This can make you seem cold even when you really do care.

Listen carefully. Is the patient trying to lead the conversation? Where? Is the patient trying to change the subject? Why? The ability to listen well, to *hear* the other person, is a critical part of communicating. It helps to listen *actively* by repeating to yourself what you heard. Are you sure you understand what the patient is saying? If not, ask him or her to say it again. Remember: whether you agree is less important than whether you are truly willing to listen – and whether the patient knows that you are willing.

Try not to be overcautious or self-conscious. "Sometimes," says Lois Ryder, "I was so careful that I ended up saying nothing when I had something important to say." Family members often make this mistake. They tend to assume that the patient doesn't want to, or isn't able to, talk about certain things. In fact, the patient may well be eager to talk about them. If you have something important to say, ask the patient whether he is willing to discuss it. If you yourself feel uncomfortable discussing it, try to explain why. Then let the patient decide whether or not to pursue the subject.

This brings us to another important issue. "Too often," observes Andrew Kneier, "family members and friends play a cheerleading role with the patient. For example, if the patient expresses concern over an upcoming test, they might say, 'Oh, don't worry; it'll be fine.' Or if the patient

> *"Too often, family members and friends play a cheerleading role with the patient."*
>
> –**Andrew Kneier**

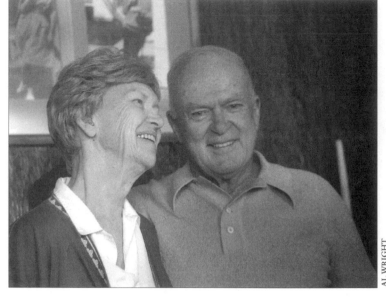

Ruth and Fred Swain

"He encouraged me to have a good cry and maybe just talk about what was bothering me. And afterwards I'd feel great."

–Ruth Swain

is afraid that the treatments are not working, they might say, 'Come on, now; it's too soon to tell.' While such comments are intended to be supporting and encouraging, in fact they usually make the patient feel that the other person is uncomfortable hearing about his or her fears." If you do this, the patient may well stop confiding in you. Worse still, he may feel that he is to blame for feeling the way he does, or that he is all alone with his fear.

"Providing emotional support," says Kneier, "does *not* mean only offering encouragement, optimism, and hope. It also means conveying to the patient that his or her reactions are understandable, and that you share them. For example, if the patient expresses a legitimate worry, you might say, 'I'm worried about that too. But no matter what happens, I'll be here with you, and we'll face it together.'" In most cases, Kneier adds, this is much more supportive, and more genuinely encouraging, than the cheerleader approach.

"He encouraged me to have a good cry and maybe just talk about what was bothering me. And afterwards I'd feel great," says Ruth Swain. And Carol Landt told us how she offered her mother the kind of support that Andrew Kneier describes:

"She reached out her hand for me, and I took it. And she squeezed my hand and said, 'What if I don't get well? What if I can't beat this thing?' And I just paused, and I know we both became rather tearful. And I just squeezed her hand back and said, 'I don't know. I just don't know, Mom. But we have to try.'"

Try to strike a balance between your need for self-assertion and the patient's needs. In order to work together effectively, both of you need to express your thoughts and feelings, neither of you needs to feel pressured or squelched. Encourage the patient to express his or her feelings; respond sincerely to those feelings, and express your own. This may take a bit of trial and error at first, but be patient and keep trying; the results can be well worth it.

Be as warm and loving as you can. If you and the patient have always had trouble talking intimately, you might try to overcome that problem now. One way to do this is simply to tell the other person that you want to do it. ("We've never really talked about these things. I'd like to. How about you?") This may not work, however, if your relationship is strained. If you have a real problem with communication, you might want to consider short-term therapy with a counselor who specializes in this field. Even one or two sessions can be helpful. If you're simply tongue-tied, here's a useful tip: practice in your mind what you want to say before you say it. This can help you to get the words out when the time comes.

Do you want to resolve that strained relationship? See page 197.

 Physical contact is important too. Sit close enough to touch, as long as this doesn't make either of you uncomfortable. Hug, if that is what you usually do. Even if it isn't, even if you haven't touched much in the past, you might want to try it now. People who have cancer need to be touched. As Julie Benbow put it, "You need to be held, because you have something wrong with your body. You begin to dislike this thing that you've taken years grooming and making the best of. And to walk up to somebody who you know and have them hug you because

Emotional reactions to a diagnosis of cancer are discussed at length in Chapter 6.

For more on humor, see page 188.

you're you is great." As a way to communicate, a hug may be worth a thousand words.

Try to be supportive. Without being artificial about it, keep disagreements to a minimum. Above all, don't lay a guilt trip on the patient. Don't say, "If only you'd stopped smoking. If only you'd seen the doctor sooner. If only you hadn't worked so hard." This is not constructive, to say the least, and the patient doesn't need to hear it. He may already be struggling with fear, depression, and guilt. Whether or not he says so aloud, he may already be thinking, "What did I do to make this happen?" This is a terrifying question. The patient may not talk about it–but not talking about terrifying things is one of the ways in which people protect themselves.

Humor helps. A good laugh, like a hug, can bring comfort to the patient *and* to you. A laugh makes it easier to lower the barriers, to say the things you can't say otherwise. Above all, laughter can help the patient to enjoy life, to feel that life is still going on around him. "My brother was laughing," Denise Manning told us, "–one of those from-the-heart kind of laughs. And my mother just sat there, and she said, 'I love to hear Sean laugh like that.' And I wanted to cry, because these are the things she wanted. Everybody just being who they are. Just living."

Shared reminiscences can comfort the patient too. They help to strengthen his or her connection with others. "Sharing happy memories tends to dilute the bad memories and make them seem less important," says Andrew Kneier. He adds that reminiscing can be especially valuable for dying patients. As they look back, it can comfort them to see how their life has enhanced, and been enhanced by, other people's lives.

Reminiscing sometimes brings tears, and this can be a good thing. Crying can help to ease pent-up emotions. On the other hand, says Lois Ryder, "if the patient has always disliked a tearful display, don't open the floodgates now." Once again, follow the patient's lead.

Watch for signs that the patient is growing tired. Is he or she restless? Withdrawn? Constantly changing the subject?

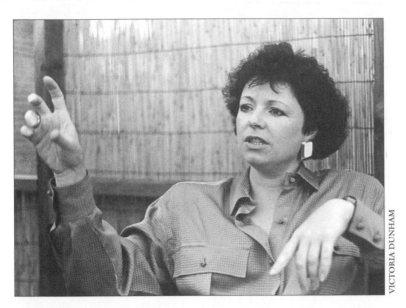

Julie Benbow

Julie Benbow remembers sitting in her chair, waiting for people to telephone. "But when the phone rang, I didn't really know if I wanted to talk to them."

If so, it may be time to stop talking. Cancer patients tend to tire readily, and some medications cause drowsiness. (Visitors especially need to remember this. They are usually less familiar with the patient's condition.) On the other hand, many patients said that they found it comforting just to have someone sitting quietly nearby while they rested. If you aren't sure whether it's time to stop talking, ask. ("Would you like to rest now?" "Shall I go, or shall I sit with you while you take your nap?")

When the Patient Doesn't Want to Talk

Sometimes the patient just doesn't want to talk. Some patients told us that there were moments when they found it impossible to talk to *anyone*, even close relatives. Sharlynn Crutcher was "very quiet around close family members, because I could see their hurt and pain." This is one reason why patients sometimes don't want to talk. (It is also one reason why they may sound unnaturally optimistic when they do talk.) Another reason why patients sometimes don't talk is that they are afraid of an insensitive response. "When I spoke about what was going on with me, they told me it wasn't as bad as I thought," says Annette Pont-Gwire. "Sometimes they even told me about others who had it worse." Annette tells us that she stopped talking about her feelings because these responses hurt her so much.

Temperament can make a difference too. Patients who are naturally introverted may simply prefer to be alone with their thoughts, while extroverts may prefer to talk them out. Some patients said that they had mixed feelings about talking. Julie Benbow, whose family lived in England, remembers sitting in her chair, waiting for people to telephone. "But," she says, "when the phone rang, I didn't really know if I wanted to talk to them."

Finally, dying patients may stop talking as they start to detach from their friends and family. This detachment is natural; we discuss it further in Appendix 1.

If the patient doesn't want to talk, try to honor that wish. This can be harder than it sounds; it's easy to feel hurt when your overtures are rejected. Try not to take it personally. Bear in mind that the patient may simply be tired. Respect his wishes and make it clear that you are ready to talk whenever he feels like talking.

Part of good communication is learning to tolerate silences without filling them with small talk. Small talk can actually be a barrier to deeper communication. If you are a talkative person, keeping quiet may take some getting used to. Start by allowing brief silences to occur. If you feel nervous doing this, you might bring along something to do or something to read. You might also like to hold the patient's hand without speaking. As you learn to feel comfortable with silence, you may discover that your presence in the room is all that the patient really needs.

Silence can be as comforting as speech. It is often easier to express your thoughts after you have mulled them over quietly for a while. (This is not the same thing as sulking and then exploding.) A kind of emotional healing can take place during silent meditation or prayer, as you and the patient calmly reflect on the issues at hand. After his cancer diagnosis, Jay Fritz and his family prayed silently together every night. "It was a positive experience for the family," says Jay, "because it gave the kids and all of us something we could feel and a way of developing hope."

For more on meditation and prayer, see Chapter 6.

However, too much silence is not a good thing. When is silence "too much"? When there's a sense of tension in the room, says Robert Fuhr. This can mean that important thoughts and feelings are not being expressed. It can mean that the patient—for whatever reason—is withdrawing. One way to deal with this problem is simply to say how you feel about it. "I enjoy being with you, but it seems to me that we hardly ever talk anymore. Does it seem that way to you?" Saying something like this expresses your feelings in a nonjudgmental way. It also allows you to acknowledge that you share the responsibility for keeping the conversation going.

When You Don't Know What to Say

You want to find ways of communicating that will bring you and the patient closer together. Most patients told us that they appreciated honesty. In any case, as Paula Carroll points out, "you have to be honest because patients can see through pretense." However, being honest does not mean telling the absolute truth no matter what. Even the most realistic patient doesn't want to be told, "You're certainly looking worse than you did yesterday."

With tact and common sense, you can learn to express your own feelings without hurting those of the patient. From what they have told us, patients can accept strong, even negative, feelings if they are communicated honestly, directly, and with compassion. Sometimes all it takes is a little consideration. Let's say you feel that the patient is asking too much of you. Instead of ignoring his request or demanding, "Can't you do some of these things yourself?" you might say, "I know you'd like me to call the doctor. But don't you think you know what to tell her better than I do?" In this way you acknowledge the patient's needs and express your own without being confrontational about it.

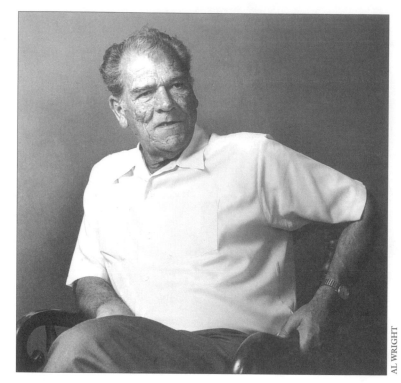

AL WRIGHT

Joe Dodig

"I know this is here, man; it's with me every minute; it's coming out of my ears, man; I feel like it's putting me in the bye-bye box. I don't want to discuss this damn thing. Let's talk about something different."

–Joe Dodig

Talk about things that the patient wants to talk about. This doesn't mean focusing *only* on what the patient wants to discuss; occasionally you may have to bring up an unwelcome subject. But when you don't know what to say, it can be helpful to follow the patient's lead. Does he want to talk about his illness, for example? Some patients do; others, like Joe Dodig, don't:

"Talk about something else. I know this is here, man; it's with me every minute; it's coming out of my ears, man; I feel like it's putting me in the bye-bye box. I don't want to discuss this damn thing. Let's talk about something different."

Not every patient is as outspoken as Joe Dodig. But by paying attention you can usually tell which subjects the patient really wants to discuss.

Sometimes when you "don't know what to say" it's because it means dealing with subjects *you* would rather not talk about. These may simply be subjects that make you feel self-conscious. For example, you might not want to talk about the patient's hair loss. Yet all of the chemotherapy patients we talked to knew that they would probably lose their hair, and most of them felt comfortable discussing the subject.

Of course, the most difficult topic of all is death. If the patient doesn't bring up death, should you? There is no one correct answer to this question. You will have to weigh your own needs against those of the patient. Much depends on the patient's frame of mind. Follow your own instincts. If the patient has said nothing, but *you* feel the need to address the issue, you might want to say something like this: "Cancer makes me think about my own death, and I'm having trouble dealing with that. Is this something we can talk about together?" This can be a good way to break the ice without forcing the patient to talk.

Although it's not always advisable, talking about death can be rewarding for all concerned. For one thing, if the patient is probably going to die, avoiding the topic can make his or her fear that much worse. Many patients and caregivers have told us that they feared death much less when they were able to talk about it openly. Then too, if you don't raise the issue, you may miss out on a last chance for intimacy. Twenty-eight years after her father died of lung cancer, Johana Garrison recalled, "When my father was dying in the hospital, I was too nervous and scared to really talk with him. I wish so much I had talked with him quietly about living and dying, about how he felt and what he thought."

In Appendix 1 we offer advice to the dying patient's family.

How to Care for the Patient

Caring for someone who has cancer can be rewarding, but it's seldom easy. Here again there are no set rules; do what works best for you and the patient. Much of the advice in this section was provided by the patients we interviewed and their families. It is based on their own experience of what works.

"We need a special balance between, on the one hand, people calling and checking on us, and on the other hand, room to live our day-to-day lives, as our own persons."

–John Chapman

Most patients benefit from being with other people. They tend to do best when they are not isolated, physically or emotionally. You can help the patient just by being there. However, it's important not to be *too* helpful. At first you may be tempted to do too much, to take care of the patient's every need, when all he needs from you is an occasional smile or an encouraging word. Family members can help a lot, but they shouldn't interfere with the patient's need for independence. As John Chapman says:

"Their concern can sometimes be overbearing. It's all good intentions, but it's almost suffocating–their goodwill and wanting to help. I believe other patients also have that problem. We need our families, but we also need space. We need a special balance between, on the one hand, people calling and checking on us, and on the other hand, room to live our day-to-day lives as our own persons."

It's usually best to take a direct approach. Ask the patient, for example, "Is this something you'd rather do yourself?" "Is this a good time to visit, or would you rather be alone for a while?" "Do you want me to come with you or not?" It's best not to assume that yesterday's answer is still good today. Ask again. The situation, or the patient's feelings, may have changed.

Even patients who are confined to their beds need not be totally dependent. They may still be able to discuss treatment options, help to make financial decisions, help the kids with their homework. As a family member, you are a critical part of the health care team. *But unless the patient cannot, or prefers not to, make the decisions, he or she remains the leader of that team.*

Your objective is to promote health, not illness; active involvement, not passivity; the fight to recover, not the urge to give up. Think of ways to reinforce the patient's self-sufficiency–by asking her to look up information in a health book, for example, even when you might find it faster yourself. Think of ways to build the patient's self-esteem. Find something to compliment. If he's wearing a good-looking sweater, say so. Let him do something for *you*–fix a meal for you or read to you—instead of the other way around.

Do things together, things unrelated to cancer. This is a way of affirming that cancer is not in control, that there's still more to life than going to the hospital once a week. As far as possible, keep doing the things you always did: playing cards, going to the beach, driving in the country, watching TV. But don't forget to try new things too, especially if the patient isn't up to some of the old ones. If a vigorous hike in the woods is out, go for a leisurely walk in the neighborhood. If the patient can't go to the stadium, watch the game together on TV.

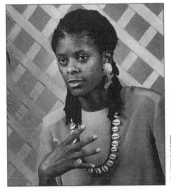

Denise Manning

But be sure they are things the patient wants to do. It can be a temptation to try new things because you think they would be "good" for the patient, or in order to give him something he "always wanted." Find out what the patient wants to do *now*. "Don't assume for them," says Denise Manning. "Don't assume that they want to go parachute because they've never done it before. 'Cause I told my sister, I said, 'We should have took Mama on a trip.' And that's not what she wanted, you know. That wasn't my mother. She needed to be there, to be with the family, to do the things she really enjoyed. She wanted to go to bingo, to play cards with her girlfriends, to take my niece, her granddaughter, back and forth to school. That was her way of saying, 'Okay, this is happening to me, but I'm going to go on.' She needed bingo, and we sent Mama to bingo."

Often it's the little things that matter most. Preparing a simple meal for a patient who usually does her own cooking can turn her bad day around. Sometimes the most helpful thing you can do is to make the patient's meals a pleasant experience. How? "With good food, good conversation, music, relaxation," says Robert Fuhr. "The same way you would make anybody else's meal a pleasant experience." So put candles on the table, serve the patient's favorite dessert, put on that Beatles tape you bought her for a surprise.

There are all kinds of other little things you can do. Rent a movie from a list of the patient's favorites. Offer

"She needed to be there, to be with the family, to do the things she really enjoyed.... She needed bingo, and we sent Mama to bingo."

–Denise Manning

265

"If I think she's depressed, I'll say, 'Let's go somewhere. Let's do something. Let's go out to dinner, do some shopping.' Something to get her mind off what's bothering her."

–June Heitz

a manicure or a pedicure. Make a cassette tape of the patient's favorite psalms and prayers. Carol Landt sent her mother cards or little gifts on the days when she had her radiation treatments. And before her mother had surgery, she says, "I took my scissors in and gave her a real short cropped little haircut in the hospital. Oh, she liked that, because she had a new look that did something for her." Fred Swain made it his job to collect information for his wife. "Going out and looking up all the different types of programs, what doctors are the best doctors to see, where to go to seek help, nutrition, reading material. I would present some options, and then she would pick out the ones that she felt were good for her."

When the patient becomes depressed, family members can help. June Heitz told us how she handled this problem with her daughter. "If I think she's depressed, I'll say, 'Let's go somewhere. Let's do something. Let's go out to dinner, do some shopping.' Something to get her mind off what's bothering her." You might want to ask the patient to help you to think up things to do. ("Let's work on this together. Let's come up with some fun ideas.") Make a list of activities that you can fall back on when the patient needs cheering up.

Other family members told us that they simply waited the depression out and then made themselves available if the patient wanted to talk about it. Still others gently brought up the depression as soon as they noticed it, before, as one of them put it, "it had a chance to run out of control."

The professionals whom we consulted liked these suggestions and made others. They all agreed that it sometimes helps simply to ask the patient what he or she is depressed about. When he tells you, express empathy and support. Talking about it can make the patient feel better. You might even offer to attend support group meetings with him. In short, you want to convey the message "I'm here with you. And I intend to be with you through this."

It's easy to get impatient with someone who is depressed. Sometimes you may even get angry. It's wise to

266

seek professional help, either for yourself or for the patient, before you reach this point. (You should turn the problem over to a professional in any case if the patient's depression is severe.) Above all, if the patient is depressed, talk to his or her doctor. Depression can be a side effect of many medications. It can also be caused by nutritional deficiencies. A change in medicine or in diet is sometimes all it takes to make a patient who is depressed feel better.

There will be times, of course, when you just don't know what to do. The patient may be acting unusual, showing changes in personality, even yelling at you. First ask yourself whether you might have done something to cause the problem. Have you been nagging at the patient to take her pills? Have you been letting your teenager play his guitar after the patient has asked for quiet? But if you can honestly answer no, there may be other reasons. Sometimes this behavior is caused by the medication or by the cancer itself. Sometimes it is the patient's reaction to being seriously ill. Try not to take it personally; try not to get irritated. Sometimes it's best just to choose to do nothing. (This is certainly better than acting hastily just for the sake of doing something, which can often make the problem worse.) Acknowledging your own fear or uncertainty, at least to yourself, can make you feel better. And sometimes a reassuring "We'll get through this together" is really all the patient needs. Or a short visit from a friend or relative—a fresh face on the scene—may be enough to relieve the pressure on both of you.

Some patients, however, may develop severe emotional problems. These can include clinical depression, paranoia, and extreme hostility. One patient we know of accused his wife, who was impeccably honest and to whom he had been married for forty years, of stealing money out of his bank account. We know of another patient who, when her cancer advanced to the dangerous stage, reacted by divorcing her husband and spreading lies about him. In her eyes the cancer was all his fault. These patients felt normal emotions intensified abnormally, and they dealt with these emotions by projecting them onto others.

When the patient has problems as severe as this, it's essential to recognize that they are caused by the cancer experience, not by anything you did. Keep reminding yourself that you are not to blame. In such cases we strongly urge you to give the patient as much love as you can and get him or her into therapy if at all possible.

It's all very well to suggest that the patient may benefit from therapy. But what if the patient refuses to see a therapist? This, after all, is his choice. At worst you may simply have to accept it (and like Art, quoted earlier in this chapter, see a therapist yourself). Before you give up, however, you might like to try the following approach. Focus on one specific problem that the patient has. Give an example of somebody who has seen a therapist for that problem. Explain how the person benefited from the therapy. Encourage the patient to seek therapy just for this one problem. Once he has done so, he can move on to explore other issues if it seems appropriate.

A big part of caring for the patient is dealing with medical professionals. Often you will do this in the patient's presence. But you can also develop your own relationship with the professionals, and the closer that relationship, the more helpful you will be to all concerned.

For instance, you can provide useful information. You know the family's history and its present circumstances. You know the patient's habits. You know how the patient reacts under stress—that she stops talking when she gets depressed, that he jokes constantly when he is nervous. For a doctor or nurse trying to individualize a plan of treatment, insights like these can be extremely valuable.

Asking questions is a good way to show that you want to help. No question is too trivial; if you don't understand something, don't be afraid to ask. Medical jargon can be baffling; for a discussion of common terms, see Chapter 1.

For more on meetings with doctors, see Chapter 1 and Chapter 3.

Try to have a family member present when the patient meets with the doctor. One of you should bring a list of questions and a tape recorder. (If you don't have a tape recorder, take notes.) After the meeting, talk over the doctor's answers to make sure that you both understand what he or she said. In this way you can provide support and relieve the patient of some responsibility. You might also want to make out a medication chart, showing which pills are to be taken when.

A close, supportive relationship with the health care team encourages mutual cooperation. This can be useful. If, for example, you need time off to rest and restore your energy, you can ask the nurse or social worker to help you. Perhaps he or she can arrange in-home care or change an appointment—whatever it takes to keep you functioning at your best. You are likely to get more complete information from the other members of the team if they know that you want to cooperate with them. You and they can consult with one another and back one another up. In short, if you work closely with the health care team, they are likelier to see both the patient and you as real people. This can mean better care for the patient and better support for you.

In dealing with professionals, be wary of overstepping boundaries. Bear in mind that the patient is the one who makes the decisions (unless he or she has specifically asked you to do it). This means that the patient chooses the doctor. It means that the patient chooses the treatment. It means that the patient chooses whether to follow the doctor's orders and the treatment that he or she has chosen. This is important. In fact, you will probably agree with the patient's decisions. But if you do not, try to remember that patients must be free to choose as they see fit. The patient may need your input in order to make informed decisions. But you are there to help, not to take over.

In short, try to serve as a bridge between the patient and the health care professionals. Your goal is to promote a kind of cooperative give-and-take among yourself, the patient, and the doctors and nurses. This is the best way to help the patient. It is also the best way to make your own life easier.

How Friends Can Help

Most of the suggestions we have made so far apply to friends as well as to family members. However, unlike most

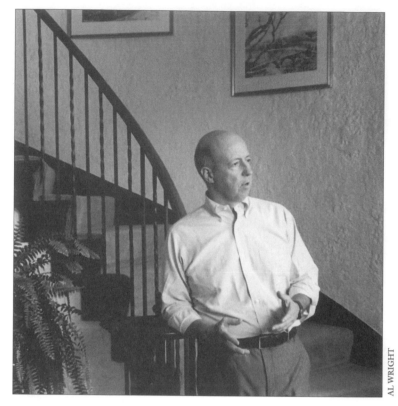

Jay Fritz

"Some people are so frightened that you find yourself putting out more energy trying to make them feel better than you do to make yourself feel better."

–Jay Fritz

family members, friends can choose to avoid the patient. This raises some painful issues that need to be dealt with.

Some friends do choose to avoid the patient. They may do this because they are frightened by people who have cancer. They may do it because they are embarrassed. They may do it because they don't know what to say or do. Then they feel guilty for not having visited and so they continue to stay away. In short, some people cannot deal with a friend's illness. This is a fact of life, as we explained in Chapter 6.

If you can't deal with people who have cancer, it may be best if you do stay away. Your presence probably won't cheer the patient up. As Jay Fritz notes, some people "are so frightened that you find yourself putting out more energy trying to make them feel better than you do to make yourself feel better." On the other hand, if you stay away, you risk hurting the patient. When some of Nancy Heitz's friends stopped visiting, she says she was "left to wonder what I did to drive them away." And on an angrier note, Paul Ryder once asked a close friend who had stayed away, "If I can stand this damned disease, why can't you at least see me with it?"

But let's say you want to overcome your resistance. Let's say you'd really like to support your friend. How do you go about it? How do you prime yourself to make that first visit?

You might start by trying to identify your feelings. Ask yourself what it is exactly that bothers you. What is the worst thing that can happen if you visit your friend? Are you afraid of sick people? Does seeing them remind you that you will die someday? Are you afraid that somehow you could catch your friend's cancer? Do you feel guilty simply because you are well? Once you have identified your feelings, you can begin to put them into perspective. Are they realistic? Are they more important to you than your friend is?

Or if introspection isn't your way, here's another option. "Just do it," suggests Robert Fuhr. Just go and visit; don't try to analyze or change your feelings first. You can make it easier by telling yourself that this first time you'll stay only ten minutes.

If you do choose to support your friend, you are giving a real gift to a person you care about—in some cases a gift that nobody else can give. "Sometimes I feel I have stronger support from friends than family," Sharlynn Crutcher told us, "because I can speak more openly without seeing as much hurt and pain." And you are showing the patient that life can go on, that people still care and want to continue the relationship. Dennis Brown remembered "a close friend who was in the emergency room waiting for me after both my major surgeries, even though I hadn't even told him that I was having them. Somehow he found out and he was there. And since my second surgery, which has been six months now, there hasn't been a day that has passed that he hasn't at least called me to see how I'm doing and whether I'm having a good day or just what's happening. I find that a tremendous source of strength, just to know that there's someone outside of my direct family who cares that much."

The first visit—the one that some friends are never able to make—will probably be the hardest. Once you make it, however, you are very likely to find that worrying about the visit was the hard part. So if you want to get back in touch, remember: it's never too late. Start with a telephone call. If that feels too difficult, phone the patient's family or write a short note or a card. It's sometimes easier to write things than it is to say them (and sometimes easier to read things than it is to hear them face-to-face). You don't need to apologize for having stayed away—just write a friendly note to break the ice. Most patients understand the situation and will look forward to seeing you again.

Getting back in touch is one thing; staying involved is another. It's easy to drift away after a while. The patient who is in long-term treatment or in remission needs your support too. Leslie Haines put it like this:

"I was struck, when recovering from cancer surgery, with the fact that I had never had so many flowers, cards, and good sentiments sent my way before in my life. It was wonderful, and I felt loved and appreciated fully. It made me extremely aware of the fact that we seldom get flowers for keeping ourselves well. One of the best things friends can do is 'reward' wellness efforts with flowers, cards, comments. The flowers seem to say, 'I am so glad you are around and feeling well. You've stayed in remission for a whole year. Congratulations.'"

One good way to stay involved is to form a support team out of a group of friends. Every week one team member contacts the patient with a phone call, a letter, or a card. (You might even buy a stack of cards and address them in advance.) The continuous contact reassures the patient that he or she is being thought of. This approach can be used to provide support to the patient's family, too, especially in cases where the family is overworked. "I had many wonderful friends who reached out to me during the course

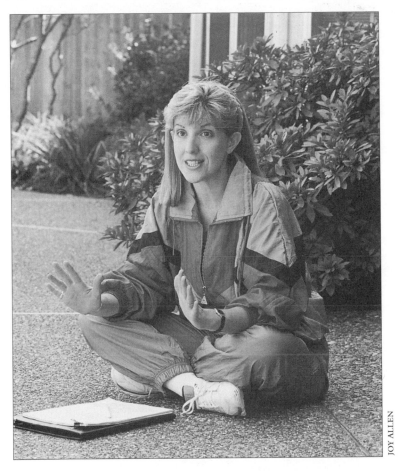

Carol Landt

> *"I had many wonderful friends who reached out to me during the course of my mother's illness. And that was so important, and it was so helpful. And I won't forget those people who reached out to me."*
>
> –Carol Landt

JOY ALLEN

of my mother's illness," says Carol Landt, "and sent me cards and notes and called and chatted, or called and left messages on my answering machine, just to say, you know, 'I'm thinking about you and I'd love to have an update, but I understand if you're busy, and I just want you to know that I care about you and I share your concern.' And that was *so* important, and it was *so* helpful. And I won't forget those people who reached out to me."

When you visit the patient, don't worry about what to say. Being there is what matters. As Paula Carroll points out, "you don't have to have something great to say every time you open your mouth." A cancer patient (not one of

So keep it natural, but keep it positive. Share the latest neighborhood gossip....Share that joke that's going around the office. Just talk about whatever is going on.

our interviewees) who published an article on her experience adds that you don't need to be "reverent" all the time, either. A friend telephoned this patient to ask how she was feeling:

"'Terrible,' I replied; 'I'm depressed.' 'Good,' she said. 'I thought you were going to avoid this part.' I burst out laughing. For me, irreverent stories and fumbling attempts to connect were far better than never responding for fear of doing the 'wrong thing.'"[8]

Don't worry about what to say, but do try to keep your conversation positive. Above all, don't talk about your own operation. Some people do this when they can't think of anything else to say. Others do it out of misplaced kindness; they want to tell the patient, "I know how you feel." In fact, you probably don't know how the patient feels. It is kinder and more helpful to allow the patient to talk about his operation–if he wants to.

This isn't the time to complain about your other problems, either. Friends who do this, says Arnold Schraer, "are just draining. They want me to give to them, rather than give to me. Because of how I'm fighting this battle, they come to me and they want to let down their hair. And they want me to pick them up. And I can't." "One of my friends came over," says Gayle Bartolomei. "And she told me–she had to move from one apartment to another, and a few minor things–that she wished she was dead! And she started crying. Well, I actually wanted to give her a swift kick and then push her out the door and say, 'I really don't need this. You know, I'm fighting. I'm working my tail end off to stay alive, and you want to be dead. Would you mind going home and get your head right?' But I didn't." Cancer patients have enough problems of their own. They don't have the energy to deal with yours.

So keep it natural, but keep it positive. Share the latest neighborhood gossip. Share the news from the patient's church or club. Share that joke that's going around the office. Just talk about whatever is going on.

What if it's the patient who has difficulty making conversation? Try asking questions about the past. This is especially effective if the patient is elderly. Many old people, even those whose short-term memory is impaired, can remember vividly things that they did when they were young. We know of friends who have tape-recorded these stories to give to the patient's children.

When it's too hard for one or both of you to talk, find something else to do. Play board games or cards or checkers or chess. Rent a video and watch it together. Read aloud. Take the patient for a drive or a walk or out to a movie. If the patient has been prayed for in church, share the prayers, and perhaps bring flowers from the altar. If you have a special talent, use it. "One friend of ours draws cartoons," says Fred Swain. "He sends us one or two cartoons a week, just on anything. We look forward to these cartoons, and we have them on the wall." If you can draw or play an instrument or sing, find ways to use your skills to entertain the patient.

And if you simply can't think what to do, you can mow the lawn or feed the dog or offer to watch the house while the patient is in the hospital or recuperating in Hawaii. These are ways of showing both the patient and the family that you care.

Promises mean a great deal to cancer patients, and disappointments are especially hard for them to handle. If you promise to visit, be sure to keep your promise. Being stood up makes the patient feel hurt and abandoned. Bear in mind too that your visit may well be the only thing that the patient has to look forward to that day. "I have never failed to show up when I've promised I would be there," says Paula Carroll. "And I'm right there on the dot at the time. Because with a lot of cancer patients, that's all they've got is time. And they're saying, 'Two o'clock she's going to be here.' They're looking for me at ten to two."

Don't visit when you have a cold or any other illness, even a minor one. Patients who are battling cancer have all they can handle; many patients' resistance is low and they pick up infections easily. Even if you are not contagious, they may feel uneasy having you around. Wait until you are completely well before you visit them.

"I don't want no big outshowing of sympathy. Save that. I don't want no weeping, wailing, gnashing teeth."

–Joe Dodig

Try not to be hurt if the patient doesn't want to see you. Sometimes patients just don't want to see anyone. When this happens, let it be known that you will be available whenever the patient is ready to see you again.

Above all, try not to show pity for the patient. Most patients don't want pity; they just want you to care. Or as Joe Dodig puts it:

"I don't want no big outshowing of sympathy. Save that. I don't want no weeping, wailing, gnashing teeth. Just, 'How you doing, I'm glad to see you, just dropped in to see you. I know you're screwed up there, I know it's hot and heavy on you, but I dropped in to see you and see how everything is.' That's all I want to hear. I don't want to hear no big, long issue."

Expressions of pity, however well meant, are offensive. Cancer patients, like everybody else, deserve respect.

We firmly believe that, like the patients quoted throughout this book, family members and friends can actually benefit from the cancer experience. Friendships and family relationships can grow stronger through cooperative effort in difficult times. When you learn to communicate and pull together, to function together as part of the health care team, to take care of yourselves and of one another, the rewards can be unprecedented.

No one ever wants it to happen. But since it has happened, we urge you to view the cancer experience as an opportunity to focus on what matters most to everyone. Loving one another, caring for one another, sharing one another's feelings–in short, connecting with one another as human beings.

In order of their first appearance, the patients who contributed to this chapter are: Paul Ryder, Jay Fritz, Nancy Heitz, Annette Pont-Gwire, Sharlynn Crutcher, Dennis Brown, Ruth Swain, Julie Benbow, Paula Carroll, Joe Dodig, John Chapman, Leslie Haines, Arnold Schraer, and Gayle Bartolomei. The family members who contributed to this chapter are: Lois Ryder, Vickie Ryder, Brent Ryder, Carol Landt, Denise Manning, June Heitz, Lily Kravcisin, Fred Swain, and Johana Garrison.

Recommended Reading

General

Harwell, Amy. *When Your Friend Gets Cancer.*
Wheaton, IL: Harold Shaw Publishers, 1987.

This short, highly readable book, written by a cancer survivor, explains how you can offer your friend both practical and emotional support. Written from a strongly Christian perspective, it will appeal especially to readers who are Christians, but much of the advice it contains will be valuable for anyone who has a friend with cancer.

Hermann, Joan F., et al. *Helping People Cope: A Guide for Families Facing Cancer.* **Harrisburg, PA: Pennsylvania Cancer Control Program, Pennsylvania Department of Health, 1988. (To obtain a copy of this book, call 1-800-537-4063.)**

This invaluable guide describes all of the services that the patient and the family may need and explains in detail how to find them. The outline format is exceptionally clear and easy to use. The book includes basic information about cancer and cancer treatments, a glossary, and a patient's bill of rights.

Murcia, Andy, and Bob Stewart. *Man to Man: When the Woman You Love Has Breast Cancer.* **New York: St. Martin's Press, 1989.**

The husbands of two breast cancer patients explain to other husbands how they coped with the practical and emotional issues surrounding cancer, and how they helped their wives to cope. The authors take turns speaking directly to the reader, describing their experiences and their feelings. The style is lively and informal.

Peabody, Kathleen L., and Margaret L. Mooney. *The Lonely Pain of Cancer: Home Care for the Terminally Ill.* **Carlsbad, CA: Sharp Publishing, 1991.**

Written for the family caregiver, this book explains in

clear language and in detail how to set up the patient's room, how to provide personal care, how to take vital signs, how to give medication, and how to manage pain. It also tells how to talk to the patient and how to deal with visitors. An indispensable resource for anyone who must care for a chronically or terminally ill patient.

Pomeroy, Dana Rae. *When Someone You Love Has Cancer.* **Santa Monica, CA: IBS Press, 1991.**

Highly personal as well as highly practical, this book describes how the author nursed her husband through terminal lung cancer. It contains a wealth of how-to information, presented in a clear, conversational style, in a series of short but useful chapters. Emotions, home care, and issues surrounding death are emphasized. The author is a nationally known lecturer in hospice work.

Simonton, Stephanie Matthews. *The Healing Family: The Simonton Approach for Families Facing Illness.* **New York: Bantam Books, 1984.**

The author believes that stress and other emotional factors contribute heavily to the development of cancer, and that by helping patients to change their response to stress, the family can help them to recover, or at least to improve their quality of life. The use of visualization is discussed in detail. Although some of the author's assumptions are controversial, this book is well organized, thoughtful, and well written.

Children

Bernstein, Joanne E. *Books to Help Children Cope with Separation and Loss.* **3d ed. New York: R.R. Bowker Co., 1989.**

A bibliographic guide to fiction and nonfiction books for children aged three to sixteen. Part I tells how to use books to help children to cope. Part II describes 606 children's books; topics include death, serious illness (there are five books on cancer specifically), and problems of adjusting to new caregivers. Part III is a reading list for adults.

Bracken, Jeanne Munn. *Children with Cancer: A Comprehensive Reference Guide for Parents.* **New York: Oxford University Press, 1986.**

An easy-to-use, well-researched, down-to-earth book, written by a reference librarian whose daughter survived cancer. It discusses the various childhood cancers, treatments, and coping issues in detail and includes annotated reading lists, a list of pediatric cancer clinics, and an appendix on medical tests. This is the most complete guide we have found for the parents of children with cancer.

Gaes, Geralyn, Craig Gaes, and Philip Bashe. *You Don't Have to Die: A Family's Guide to Surviving Childhood Cancer.* **New York: Villard Books, 1992.**

Written by the parents of a young cancer patient, this comprehensive guidebook is full of concrete practical advice. It describes the various forms of treatment, tells parents how to work with doctors, and discusses life at home for the child with cancer. Anecdotal; inspiring without being unrealistic. Jason Gaes, the young patient, survived to write *My Book for Kids with Cansur: A Child's Autobiography of Hope* (Aberdeen, SD: Melius Publishing, 1991).

McCollum, Audrey T. *The Chronically Ill Child: A Guide for Parents and Professionals.* **New Haven: Yale University Press, 1981.**

This well-organized reference book deals with the physical and emotional problems that the chronically ill child faces at each stage of development from infancy to young adulthood. Emotional reactions of parents and siblings are also discussed. The author is a psychotherapist and a research assistant at the Yale University School of Medicine. Her writing style reflects her professional background, but the book is clear and reasonably readable.

...and Living

Part 1: Gaining Control

"Cancer" is a terrifying word. Most people don't want to hear it, read it, or say it. Some people's fear of cancer borders on superstition–they refuse even to think about it, as if thinking about it could make them get it. They avoid cancer patients who were once their friends; their fear is stronger than their love. They ignore blatant symptoms until it is too late. Other people are oblivious to the threat of cancer. "Who, me worry?" they say, in effect. These people want to believe that cancer will never–can never–happen to them.

Most people fall somewhere between these two extremes. They go to the doctor if they have symptoms; they don't bury their heads in the sand. But the word "cancer" fills them too with dread.

Cancer is a uniquely terrifying disease. It is not one disease but many. Its growth is insidious, its causes not well understood; it may not be discovered until it is too late. It can take over every aspect of your life–time, physical well-being, work, self-image, relationships, your hopes for tomorrow and your enjoyment of today. Finally, of course, it can be fatal; to many people, "cancer" means "pain and death." For all of these reasons, cancer can signify loss of control. Many people's fear of cancer is largely the fear of losing control over their own lives.

This chapter is written for four different groups of readers. Each group fears cancer for a different reason.

If you have never had cancer, you may imagine in horrifying detail exactly what having it would do to you. You may envision the changes it would make: you see yourself as defective, as an invalid; you see yourself in

"Even if you backslide it doesn't matter....
The only thing that would really be a
failure would be to stop trying."

–Charles Fuhrman

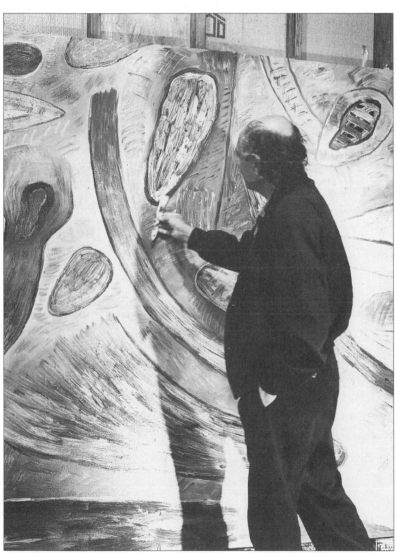

MICHAEL FAHEY

Charles Fuhrman

pain. Once cancer touches you (you may think), you will instantly and permanently lose control over all of the things that make life worth living.

If you have cancer now, you may be terrified for a different reason. Now the thing you feared has happened; now you may fear that the cancer is in control. That the cancer—and the cancer treatment—will determine what happens to you from now on. Will the treatment work? If it does work, what will your life be like? And if it doesn't work? What then?

Perhaps you are in remission; your doctors have told you that the cancer is under control. "But," you ask yourself, "how do they know? Is the cancer still in my body? Could it come back? If it does, can I beat it again?" Worst of all, you may have read that fear causes stress, and that stress itself could trigger a recurrence. How much control *do* you have? Are you really in control at all?

Finally, *you may have a terminal prognosis.* Your doctor has given you six months to live, but you may feel that those six months are not worth living. You feel as if you have no control, over your disease or over the quality of the life you have left. Some people with a terminal prognosis die sooner than they might have. They die of cancer—and despair. In a very real sense, they die because they believe that nothing they can do will make any difference.

But the fact is that *you can make a difference.* There are things you can do to give yourself some control no matter what your situation is. Whether you are in perfect health or facing a terminal prognosis, you don't have to let the fear of cancer rule your life.

Why Is Control Important?

No matter what your state of health, it is possible to gain a measure of control over your life. But before we suggest some ways to do it, we'd like to say a little about control itself. What is control? And why is it so important?

When we talk about control, we *don't* mean the rigid,

authoritarian control that people sometimes impose on themselves ("I must *never* get angry") or on others ("You *must* drink your juice"). This kind of control is limiting, uncreative, inflexible. It doesn't allow for growth; it leads to stagnation, not to change. The other kind of control—the kind we talk about in this book—is just the opposite. It is imaginative, liberating, constructive. It is achieved by identifying your problems, brainstorming possible solutions, choosing the best one, and taking action to implement it. This kind of control is a tool for making life the way you want it to be.

Having a sense of control is good for you psychologically. In people who have cancer, it is associated with an increased sense of well-being.[1] This is true even when these people have been diagnosed as terminal by their physicians.[2] More specifically, there is evidence that a sense of control may reduce anxiety and depression,[3] increase sense of purpose,[4] and even improve the patient's social life.[5]

Having a sense of control is good for you physically as well. If you are a cancer patient, it may improve your actual control over such physical symptoms as nausea and fatigue.[6] One study has shown that people who have a sense of control get sick less often. (The researchers point out that this could be because they tend to take better care of their health in the first place.)[7] Most importantly, a sense of control has been shown to improve the functioning of the immune system.[8] This fact alone makes a sense of control a valuable weapon in fighting cancer.

In this chapter we will be talking about changes that you can make in your life. All of these changes are designed to increase your sense of control. We believe that they can help to reduce your fear of cancer, and that they can help you to fight cancer as well. This is true not just of the changes that involve avoiding risk factors—of avoiding exposure to carcinogens, for example. It is true of all of the changes that we discuss.

Losing control over your life is terrifying. Gaining control over your life can be the healthiest, most rewarding thing you've ever done.

Most importantly, a sense of control has been shown to improve the functioning of the immune system. This fact alone makes a sense of control a valuable weapon in fighting cancer.

Control Means Change

To gain control, you will probably have to make changes. You might have to change your eating habits or your job. You might have to learn how to let go of grudges. And the idea of change may make you very uncomfortable.

But I Don't Want to Change!

It's only natural to resist change. Change means letting go, leaving things behind. If they are pleasant things, such as Mom's batter-fried chicken, of course you don't want to give them up. But even unpleasant things, such as a job you hate, can have the virtue of familiarity, and giving them up can be painful too.

Then there's the question of what you'll replace them with. This can be a real deterrent when you're trying to change pleasant but unhealthy habits. Many people will cling to pleasures that are literally deadly rather than submit to what they imagine will be a lifelong regimen of unrelenting "goodness." Until you learn that change needn't mean making sacrifices, it's natural to resist the whole idea of changing.

Finally, there's the problem of procrastination. This time you want to change. Your mind's made up; you're all prepared; you're really going to do it...but not just yet. Tomorrow, maybe. Or next week? You're procrastinating. Why?

It could be because you're a discomfort dodger or a self-doubter or both, says Dr. William Knaus, author of *Do It Now: How to Stop Procrastinating*.[9] Discomfort dodgers have a vivid imagination; they painfully anticipate every bump in the road of change. They also tend to exaggerate the bumps and to ignore the smooth spots. Every change—even something as minor as shifting your watch to the other wrist—produces some discomfort. Acknowledge that this is going to happen; tell yourself that you can endure it; and think about the benefits of changing.

Self-doubters are preoccupied with their own real and imagined faults. They anticipate failure at every turn, so they put off changing (and doing a lot of other things, for that matter). Why bother? They know they're going to fail. The prescription for eliminating self-doubt is to start working steadily on one small change that is easy to achieve. Achieving it will help give you confidence to try another. Keep the changes small and attack them one by one; in time, you'll have succeeded often enough that you'll have gained control over your self-doubt.

For more on ways of dealing with self-doubt, see the discussion of the Inner Critic on page 178.

How to Do It

So you're ready to make changes. What's the best way to do it? In this section we offer a few pointers.

For further suggestions on problem solving see Chapter 6.

It's important to be willing

If you've accepted the fact that you need to change, you've already taken the first big step. But are you willing—or are you just resigned? It's important to be willing, even excited. Acceptance is important, but a grudging acceptance won't get you far.

Being willing means focusing on the positive. As we have pointed out, it's hard to want to change when change means loss, discomfort, failure. Try not to think about what you're giving up. Think instead about what you are adding to your life. Let's say you decide to stop smoking. Try not to think about the things you are going to miss: the first cigarette of the day; the camaraderie of lighting up with fellow smokers; the relaxed, comforting feeling as you inhale. Think instead about being able to exercise without getting winded; about the respect you'll get from friends who have quit; about the self-confidence and self-esteem you're going to gain from knowing that you've kicked the habit. Another way to think positive is to compare the benefits of the new behavior with the disadvantages of the old one. Think about the money you wasted; the morning cough; the person who wouldn't date you because you smoked. In either case, the idea is to concentrate on what you are gaining, not on what you are losing.

Willingness is followed by commitment. No program will succeed if you are not seriously committed to it. When you make a major life-style change, such as starting an exercise program or quitting smoking, try to make an initial commitment of at least three weeks. Tell yourself that you'll stick to it that long no matter what. This will give you a chance to get the new habit well established, and that will improve your prospects for long-term success.

Commitment has many sources. One of these, oddly enough, is anger. Constructive anger at your own bad habits can be a powerful motivator for change. Notice we said "constructive anger." We aren't talking here about blaming yourself. Nor are we talking about the destructive anger that's often behind the rigid kind of control.

What else might inspire your commitment? An ideal of how you want your life to be? Your determination to succeed? Your love for someone else? Or might it be a good scare—a heart attack or a warning from your doctor? Whatever its source, your commitment gives you drive. You might say that it's the energy that leads to change.

Have a plan of action

In implementing changes, as in any other project, you need a plan of action. That is, you need to decide exactly what you are going to do and exactly how you are going to do it. It's best to put your plan in writing; that way you'll have it to refer to later.

Beware of the New Year's resolution approach to change: resolving on January 1 to transform your life utterly and discovering by March 1 that you're back to your old bad habits because you tried to do too much too soon. Go slow and take it one step at a time. "I always tell my clients, 'You can't move a mountain, but you can move a rock,'" says weight reduction counselor George Somogyi. "'If you move one rock at a time, you can then move the mountain.'"[10]

First list the changes you want to make. If there are a lot of them, rank them in order of priority (see the following

> *"You can't move a mountain, but you can move a rock. If you move one rock at a time, you can then move the mountain."*
>
> **–George Somogyi**

section). Next set a starting date for the first change. Write it down in your plan of action and mark it on your calendar. Now, using the step process, list the small tasks you need to complete to make this first change. Write the small tasks down on your plan of action. You may want to mark them in your calendar as well. List the benefits of making the change that the small tasks lead up to. Keep the list handy (perhaps in your purse or pocket), so you can read it if you get discouraged.

We explain the step process on page 190.

Now it's time to take that first step. Maybe you'd rather not tell anybody; after all, it's your own private business. Or maybe you'd like to start out with a burst of fanfare. Go into your office, announce that you have big news, and tell everybody that today's the day you quit drinking. Some people do best with this approach; telling others reinforces their resolve. Do whatever it takes to get you off to a strong start.

Your plan of action should be well thought-out, but it shouldn't be cast in concrete. Not every change will turn out the way you expect it to; the reality may not be as attractive – or as feasible – as the ideal. In that case you may have to make adjustments.

Let's say you're a grade school teacher. It's a stressful job and you've never really liked it; the kids are wild and you're sick of dealing with the bureaucracy. A year ago you were treated for lymphoma. Your cancer is in remission now, but you're tired and tense; the job is getting to you. You decide that it's time to change careers.

You've always liked carpentry; you built your own house and designed and built most of the furniture. You decide to quit teaching and go to work for yourself remodeling houses.

Six months later you're too tired to get out of bed. You love your new career, but you're just not strong enough to do heavy labor. You alter your plan and start making custom wood furniture. This takes less muscle, and you can concentrate on the detail. Your designs are original; your craftsmanship is superb; you find a ready market, and your business takes off.

Your plan of action should be well thought-out, but it shouldn't be cast in concrete.

Part of being flexible is realizing that change is not a matter of all or nothing.

By all means strive to achieve your dreams, but don't be afraid to modify them. Be flexible. And guard against the idea that you have to do everything. Part of being flexible is realizing that change is not a matter of all or nothing. Out of ten possible changes you can choose to make one, five, or all ten. This is true whether you are making changes in one area—such as diet—or in several areas—such as diet, exercise, stress control, and smoking. If you want to improve your eating habits, say, you can start by eating one piece of fruit a day. Next you can cut out butter. Next you can change to low-fat milk. Or you can commit yourself totally to a healthy diet. Any change, even one, is a step in the right direction. The choice—like every choice—is up to you.

Build support

When it's time to make changes in your life, the more help you can enlist, the better. Family members can provide emotional and practical support. They can support your decision to give up smoking, for example, and can offer you daily encouragement. Bear in mind that building support does not mean shifting responsibility—asking your mate to slap your wrist when you reach for a cigarette. But you can ask her (or him) to be understanding if you're a little more irritable than usual, and to join you in activities that will help you to stick to your plan. If your mate smokes, don't expect him (or her) to quit just because you're quitting. That's not realistic; it's his decision, not yours. But you can ask him to support your attempts to quit, or at least not to undermine your efforts.

It is interesting to note that while women tend to make life-style changes on their own, men tend to make them with the encouragement of their wives.[11] If you're a woman, remember: it's good to support your husband—but it's good to ask your husband to support you too.

Friends can also help. Telling a friend about your plans for change can strengthen your determination to implement them. So can hearing your friend's encouragement. Confide in friends who have already done whatever it is you want to do–in the friend who has already lost fifty pounds, who practices yoga to handle stress, who does her breast self-exam every month. It helps to make mutual-support agreements with friends who have goals like yours–agreements to exercise together, to go to religious services together, or simply to call each other up when one of you is longing for a big slice of pie.

Some people find certain habits easier to break when they can do it in a group, using proven methods. Substance abuse, smoking, and overeating all respond well to this approach. Some people like to start off strong by booking into a health resort. Some of the other guests will be making life-style changes too, and this can provide powerful motivation and support. Being away from your usual pressures and temptations keeps you from slipping up. Health resorts run the gamut from spartan to luxurious; prices start at around $400 a week. If that would strain your budget, let it be your vacation. Enjoy your stay at the resort and do something really good for yourself at the same time.

To find a health resort that suits your pocketbook, your preference, and your needs, call 1-800-ALLSPAS.

What if a health resort is beyond your means? In that case, consider a self-help group. In many states these are available at little or no cost. We discuss some of the better-known groups in the sections on weight control, smoking, and alcohol. For a complete list of groups in your area, telephone the American Self-Help Clearinghouse (1-201-625-7101) or the National Self-Help Clearinghouse (1-212-642-2944). The latter organization publishes a newsletter and can even tell you how to start a group of your own.

Whether you turn to family, friends, or groups, the support is out there. So when it's time to make changes, remember: you don't have to do it alone unless you want to.

Treat yourself kindly

For many people, the hardest part of changing is overcoming perfectionistic tendencies. Go easy on yourself. Try not to ask more of yourself than you can comfortably accomplish. Don't be so ambitious that you

We tell Dennis Brown's story on page 206.

set yourself up to fail (by going on an impossibly strict diet, for example). Remember the story of Dennis Brown.

Many perfectionists are kind to others; they are unreasonable only with themselves. Show yourself the same consideration that you would show a friend. Imagine how you might support a loved one who was trying hard to change. Then try to give yourself that same support.

And if you do slip up? That's part of the process. Accept your setback, pick yourself up, and keep going. Or as Charles Fuhrman put it, "Even if you backslide, it doesn't matter. It's admitting you're off the track that's really important. I'm always backsliding. But I come back. The only thing that would really be a failure would be to stop trying."

The other side of treating yourself kindly is to reward yourself often. Congratulate yourself for every change you make; build as many rewards as you can into your plan of action. Look back at intervals; measure the progress you have made; give yourself full credit for having made it—and then do something special for yourself. Reward yourself whenever you achieve a specific goal—losing ten pounds, making that difficult phone call, getting your blood pressure down into the safe range. Reward yourself for having stayed on your new program for a specific period of time. When you have gone a week without a cigarette, treat yourself to a night at a comedy club or buy a new baseball card to add to your collection. When you have gone a month without yelling at your son, treat yourself to a day off from work or dinner at your favorite restaurant. When you have gone a year without taking a drink, give yourself a vacation in Hawaii or adopt a puppy from the pound.

In choosing rewards, go for things *you* enjoy. You might choose physical pleasures—healthy ones, of course. Massage, saunas, hot tubs—or how about perfume? Or breakfast in bed? Or just sleeping in? Or you might prefer social or emotional pleasures—bowling, acting classes, new cowboy boots, an evening watching the game with friends. Here as elsewhere, do what works best for you.

The Joys of Change

Setting up an effective program for change is like setting up an effective treatment program or coping program. It can take time, patience, research, flexibility, and perseverance. It can take courage too. The prospect of change can be frightening, as we have explained. But undertaken gradually and in the right spirit, change can be challenging, rewarding, and even fun. Change brings the joy of achievement, as you learn to control things that once controlled you.

Change opens up new horizons and brings the joy of discovery. It can teach you things about yourself you never would have known—whether it's the fact that you enjoy being alone or the fact that you feel better when you help other people. Change can lead you to learn new things about the world around you—whether it's how a computer works, how a mayor is elected, or how guppies breed. When you resist change, you limit your potential; when you embrace it, you discover just how great that potential is.

For this book we interviewed hundreds of cancer patients—some who were undergoing treatment, some who were in remission, some who were terminal. These people told us how they learned to make life-style changes that gave them a new sense of control. They told us how this sense of control contributed to their health and peace of mind. They told us how it brought them joy. In Part 2 and Part 3 of this chapter, we describe some of the changes that you can make to gain a sense of control.

Having cancer forced them to set priorities, to reevaluate their lives, and doing this gave them a sense of direction.

Setting Priorities

What is *really* important in your life?

Many of the patients we spoke to said that they actually benefited from having cancer simply because it obliged them to answer this question. It forced them to set priorities, to reevaluate their lives, and doing this gave them a

You can eat a healthy diet and still enjoy a pizza now and then. You can get yourself in shape without training for the Boston Marathon.

sense of direction. They felt—often for the first time—that they were on course at last, that they were no longer just taking life for granted.

What is really important in *your* life? If you are a cancer patient, you will probably say, "Just getting through it. Just making sure that the cancer doesn't come back." But more thought may lead to other answers. What other things are important to you? Why?

Keep asking yourself that question as you read the next few pages. Gradually you will begin to see what you need to focus on. This will help you to develop a strategy for living life to the fullest, in the way that is most appropriate for you.

Your Health

You might want to give your health top priority. Health is the foundation on which the rest of your life is built. This is obvious if you have cancer, but it is also true if you are well. As we shall explain, you can make changes that will give you the best health that is possible for you. And this will help you to enjoy your other priorities.

There's another good reason why you might want to put health first. If you have cancer, this will give you your best chance of recovery. Even patients with a terminal prognosis are justified in caring for their health. Patients diagnosed as terminal do occasionally surprise their doctors, and you are entitled to retain this hope and to give yourself every chance of attaining it. Even if you don't expect a miracle recovery, you may want to give your health a high priority. This helps some people to make the most of the time they have left.

The idea of putting your health first may sound dull, especially if you are healthy now. It conjures up images of sweating at the gym, of solemn talk about organic tofu. "Who needs it?" you think; "who wants to be a health nut?" But change is not a matter of all or nothing. You can eat a healthy diet and still enjoy a pizza now and then. You can get yourself in shape without training for

294

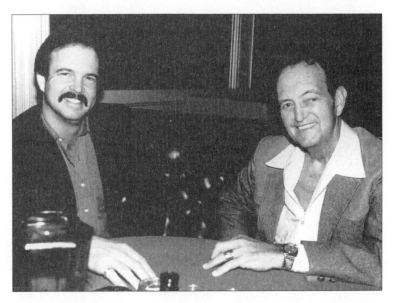

Brent and Paul Ryder

"It took the cancer to make him see that our relationship meant more to him than work-work-work."

–Brent Ryder

the Boston Marathon. So when you think about your health, remember: you don't need to be a fanatic. You can choose what to change, and the number of changes that are right for you.

Your Family and Friends

You may very well wind up making your loved ones a top priority. Most patients realized, when they came to reevaluate their lives, that their close relationships meant more to them than anything else. Many of them added that the biggest changes they made were changes that involved their families and friends.

Sometimes this meant mending fences. This was especially true when the cancer experience had caused rifts in the family. But patients who reexamined the role that other people played in their lives often gained insight into deeper, more basic issues that they had avoided facing before they got cancer. They came to see especially how important it was to let go of petty grudges. As you consider family and friends, you may want to think about your own grudges and grievances—against the son who didn't follow in your footsteps; against the mother who never understood your goals; against the friend who talked behind your back. Are those things *really* important to you now?

Other patients found that even when there were no fences to mend, the demands of work had cut into family time. Solving this problem wasn't always easy; it took thought, planning, and decisive action. This was especially true when the patient had run up big medical bills that had to be paid. If you decide to give more time to family and friends, be open to innovative solutions.

Reordering your priorities to make more time for others can be unexpectedly rewarding. Paul Ryder, who before his cancer was a classic workaholic, took several weeks off from his job to travel through Oregon, to show his son the areas where he had grown up. "It was a great trip for the two of us," says Brent, "but he never would have done it before. It took the cancer to make him see that our relationship meant more to him than work-work-work."

For more on mending fences, see page 197.

Your Work

Most people give a high priority to work. They do so partly from necessity—most people have to work to earn their living—but also from choice; for many people, work is the most satisfying thing in life. And for some people work is the *only* satisfying thing.

What role does work play in your life? Ask yourself the following questions:

- Do I enjoy my work? Does it challenge me? Am I satisfied with the amount of time that I spend working?
- If not, why not? What is the problem? Is there a solution?
- Where does work rank right now on my list of priorities? Is that where I want it to rank?

If you are currently putting work first, ask yourself why. Is your work more important than your health? Your family? Being good to yourself? Workaholics especially tend

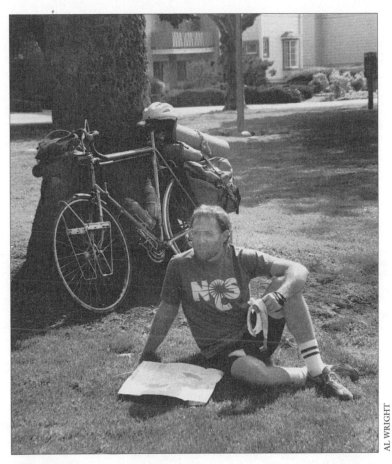

Brad Zebrack

"If I'm going to live, say, seventy-five years, and I'm going to work for forty years, if I take a year off for cancer and a year off for a bike ride around the country,... What's two years in the long run?"

–Brad Zebrack

to rationalize their answers. "The business can't get along without me." "I'm doing it for my family." "I've got bills to pay." Probe a little; are you telling yourself the truth? Is this *really* what's most important to you?

Many of the people we interviewed said that having had cancer made them reevaluate their attitudes toward work. Some of them discovered that they had buried themselves in their jobs and hadn't developed any deep relationships. Others discovered that they had spent years in the wrong line of work altogether.

If this is beginning to sound like you, it's important to remember that you have options. You will need to look at your work in a different light if you want to have time and

297

*Creativity
is a way of
making your
own personal
mark on life.
For some people,
it's a top
priority. It gives
them a sense
of fulfillment,
a sense of who
they are.*

energy to spend on other things. You will need to learn to be flexible—even if you have medical bills, a mortgage, and three kids to raise. Look at *all* your options. Where can you compromise? Can you gain time for other things by working at home? Consulting? Working part-time at several jobs? Can you cut expenses by selling the house and renting an apartment? Getting a roommate? Helping the kids to get a part-time job? Can you pay off your credit cards by selling your motorcycle? If not, why not? What *is* most important to you?

Some people make dramatic changes. Brad Zebrack decided that if he could take a year off work to undergo treatment for Hodgkin's disease, he could take another year off to realize his dream of a cross-country bicycle trip. "If I'm going to live, say, seventy-five years, and I'm going to work for forty years, if I take a year off for cancer and a year off for a bike ride around the country, I'll work thirty-eight years instead. What's the difference? What's two years in the long run?"

A break like this would be impossible for most people. But what changes *can* you make in your own life?

We are not trying to persuade you to work less. We are simply saying that you have choices. The priority you assign to work is your choice and your responsibility. That is part of what it means to be in control.

Your Creative Side

Creativity is a way of making your own personal mark on life. For some people, it's a top priority. It gives them a sense of fulfillment, a sense of who they are.

Look to see *where* (not *whether*) you are creative. Look for the things you do in your own special way. The way you plant your garden, choose your clothes, write a letter, remodel a room, run your business, communicate an idea—all these may indicate your creativity.

Making more time for creativity can involve trying new things as well—learning to play bongo drums, taking a class in flower arranging, learning to restore old furniture or an old house, making a dress, writing about your life when you were young. And take a creative approach to your other priorities. Is exercise one of them? Take up square dancing. Do you want to spend more time with your family? Get them together and shoot home videos. Is work important to you? Find a better way to do one part of your job. No matter what your top priorities are, add creativity to the list and add zest to your life.

Pleasant Events

It can take something as serious as cancer to make you think about setting pleasure as a priority. Along with a new relaxed attitude toward work, many of the patients we interviewed experienced a new urge to seek out and enjoy pleasant events; to savor the moment; to have fun.

And what are pleasant events? They're the little things that add spice to your everyday life. Things you do alone– daydreaming, reminiscing, listening to music, watching your favorite TV show. Things you do with others–calling an old friend, going out for lunch. In a study that examined the relationship between mood and pleasant events, examples given included "read Sunday paper," "party," "sunny day," "letter from Adrienne," and "complimented by Mrs. F."[12] Pleasant events also include play, by which we mean active ways of having fun–whether it's shooting baskets or singing in the shower, playing croquet or just horsing around.

Pleasant events are good for you both physically and psychologically. Studies have shown a strong correlation between pleasant events and daily mood. In other words, they have shown that you feel better on days when you do things that you enjoy.[13] One study found that pleasant events most strongly related to mood were the ones that involved family and leisure activities.[14] Having fun with the children is a good way to make yourself feel good.

Other studies have shown that pleasant events help to counteract both the psychological and the physical effects of stress. One study showed that people who do things

Having fun with the children is a good way to make yourself feel good.

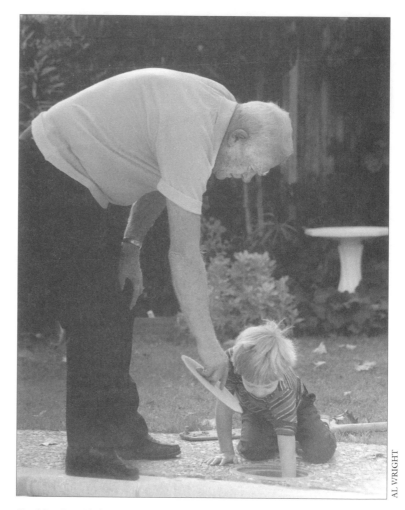

AL WRIGHT

Fred Swain with his grandson Byron

they enjoy are less likely to become depressed than others, even when their lives are stressful.[15] And one interesting study specifically links high positive daily mood with increased functioning of the immune system.[16]

All of which suggests that setting pleasure as a priority isn't nearly as frivolous as it sounds.

If pleasure has been a low priority for you, you may need to learn how to have fun again. Watch a toddler banging on a pan or a puppy racing around the yard. That's the pure essence of fun. Learn to loosen the rigid demands that we adults put upon ourselves.

"But what" (you ask) "can I *do*?" You can do anything that's fun–for you. Fly a kite. Throw sticks for the dog. Go to the park and swing. Take your grandchildren to the circus. Go to the beach and build a castle in the sand. Call up a friend and tell him that new joke you just heard. Make up an option list of things that you think you would enjoy. Try them out; keep trying until you find ones that work for you. Remember: we're talking about fun here. Nothing is fun if you don't enjoy it, no matter how much "fun" it's supposed to be. And nothing is fun if you're trying too hard to excel. The golfer who flies into a rage because he hooks a shot isn't having fun, no matter what he tells himself. He needs to find something else to do– something that he can immerse himself in for the pure pleasure of it. That's what we mean by seeking out pleasant events. That's a priority worth making room for.

Nurturing Yourself

Some people go through their whole lives putting themselves first. Some people go through their whole lives putting themselves last. We don't recommend either extreme. Instead, we recommend being good to yourself.

"But," some people would say, "that's selfish." No; not really.

Being selfish means thinking of your own needs to the exclusion of other people's needs. It means sacrificing other people, and perhaps your own ideals, for the sake of immediate self-gratification.

Nurturing yourself means giving to yourself without depriving others. It means accepting yourself, not being hard on yourself, valuing yourself, treating yourself well. It means living your life in the way that you feel is best for you.

Seeking out pleasant events is one way to nurture yourself. But there are other ways as well.

Nurturing yourself means doing things to promote your own mental and emotional well-being. For some people this could mean meditating. For others it could mean

> *Nothing is fun if you don't enjoy it, no matter how much "fun" it's supposed to be. And nothing is fun if you're trying too hard to excel.*

finishing a task just because finishing it will make you feel good. For others still it could mean seeing a therapist when you're not in crisis, just to get a better perspective on an issue that's always been uncomfortable for you. These ways of nurturing yourself help you to enjoy life more.

Nurturing yourself means thinking, "What can I do this day to give myself pleasure?" Ask yourself this question as you consider each of your priorities. "How can I give myself pleasure as I do my job? As I care for my family? As I look after my health?"

Are you thinking about setting priorities? If so, you have already started to nurture yourself. You are putting your life into the order that is right for you.

We strongly urge you to make nurturing yourself one of the top priorities in your life.

Part 2:
The Body's Way

There are two approaches you can take to gain control over your life. One approach leads to control by way of the body. The other leads to control by way of the mind. Setting priorities helps you to map out your route.

We have stressed throughout this book that everyone is an individual. Gaining control over your life is thus a highly individual matter. Here as elsewhere, choose the way that works best for you. For some people this will be the body's way. For others it will be the mind's way. For most people it will be some combination of the two.

In making changes, there are several points to keep in mind. First, tailor your program to your specific needs. In this section we discuss the body's way and list eight areas where making changes can give you more control. Decide which areas are the most important for you. Then choose the one you need to work on first. If you smoke two packs of cigarettes a day, for example, and also need to lose twenty pounds, you would be wise to concentrate first on the smoking.

Second, try not to fall prey to the all-or-nothing way of thinking. It's usually easier to make changes one at a time. Congratulate yourself for any small improvement. Making any constructive change will give you some control. Don't tell yourself that if you can't do it perfectly there's no point in doing it at all. This is a guaranteed formula for failure.

Third, try to be patient with yourself. Don't expect instant results. As you add healthy habits to your daily routine, unhealthy habits tend to drop away. But it's probably going to take a while, so hang in there.

Choose the way that works best for you. For some people this will be the body's way. For others it will be the mind's way.

Finally, beware of telling yourself, "I don't have time"–to exercise, to eat right, to get that mammogram. It's easy to fall into this trap. The fact is, you can make the time to do what's good for you. In the following pages we'll show you why this is worthwhile.

Reducing Your Risk

There is no way to guarantee that you will not get cancer. However, you can reduce your risk of getting it. And the things that you do to reduce that risk will improve your chances of fighting it if you do get it.

How much the risk can be reduced, and how you can reduce it, depends a lot on which authorities you ask. But even the most conservative sources agree that what you choose to do makes a big difference. It has been estimated that 33 percent to 70 percent of all cancers are preventable.[17] For some types of cancer, the odds are even better. It has been estimated, for example, that 90 percent of all lung cancers among men could be prevented simply by not smoking.[18]

Why does choice play such a large role in the reduction of risk? Simply because most of the known causes of cancer are things that you can choose to avoid. The authors of a recent article in *Science* state: "The majority of the causes of cancer (such as tobacco, alcohol, animal fat, obesity, ultraviolet light) are associated with life-style, that is, with personal choices and not with the environment in general. The widespread public perception that environmental pollution is a major cancer hazard is incorrect."[19]

It is well worthwhile, then, to learn how to reduce

The known causes of cancer are summarized in figure 6 on page 55.

Reducing your risk factors can make a difference no matter what your present state of health.

your risk factors for cancer. In the pages that follow, we will describe many specific ways of doing just that.

We repeat: you will be *reducing* your risk, not *eliminating* it. No one behavior is guaranteed to give you cancer or to protect you from it. Everyone has heard about the three-pack-a-day smoker who lived to be ninety, and the athlete who contracted cancer at twenty-six. Nor can you change your past behavior; and some causes of cancer (such as heredity) are not based on behavior anyway. But there is a lot that you *can* do, and the more good choices you make, the better your odds.

Imagine a big jar full of jellybeans. Most of the jellybeans are white, but a few of them are red. You shut your eyes, stick your hand in the jar, and pull out one jellybean at random. The fewer red beans there are in the jar, the less chance there is that the one you pull out will be red.

It's the same with cancer. The more you reduce the risk factors, the less chance you have of developing the disease. You can't reduce the risk factors to zero, so there will always be a few red beans in the jar. But the fewer risk factors there are in your life, the better your odds will be.

Reducing your risk factors can make a difference no matter what your present state of health. If you are well, it will lessen your chance of developing cancer at all. If you have cancer already, reducing your risk factors can help you to fight it. If you are in remission, the cancer will be less likely to recur. Even if you have a terminal prognosis, you can gain some sense of control by reducing your risk factors. This can help you both physically and psychologically, as we explained earlier.

Reducing your risk factors for cancer will lessen your chance of developing other illnesses, such as heart disease, respiratory disorders, alcoholic hepatitis, and diabetes. It will help you to feel better physically and emotionally. In short, no matter what your situation, reducing your risk factors is very well worthwhile.

In each of the following sections we deal with one area in which you can make changes. First we provide an overview of the area and explain why it may be important for you to change. Next we discuss in detail one provocative fact or explain how to make one critical change. Finally we tell you where you can get all your other questions answered.

Diet

Changing to a healthier diet can give you more control over your life. It can help you to fight cancer and decrease your chance of developing it in the first place. It decreases your chance of developing other diseases as well. What's more, a healthy diet can be delicious.

Facts about Diet

Science has established a definite link between cancer and diet. According to the American Cancer Society (ACS), "it is estimated that about one-third of the annual 500,000 deaths from cancer in the United States...may be attributed to undesirable dietary practices."[20] Though no one diet has been proven to prevent cancer, health author- ities agree that a properly chosen diet can reduce the risk of developing certain cancers. There is also evidence that a properly chosen diet can help you to fight cancer once you have developed it.

This figure includes deaths associated with obesity. We discuss obesity separately on page 323.

The most important risk factor is fat, which we discuss below. But there are other issues to consider as well. First, of course, you should avoid foods that increase the risk of cancer. Which foods are those? You might think first of foods that contain additives and pesticides. In fact, according to the ACS, food additives pose only a small risk.[21] And according to Dr. Bruce Ames, director of the National Institute of Environmental Health Sciences at the University of California, Berkeley, "the number of cases of cancer...caused by man-made pesticide residues in food...is close to zero."[22]

The risk from salt-cured and pickled foods is much higher. These foods contain natural carcinogens that may increase the risk of developing stomach and esophageal cancers. Nitrates and nitrites, used to preserve meat, can enhance the formation of nitrosamine, another carcinogen. Smoked foods can absorb carcinogens out of the smoke. The ACS recommends that you limit consumption of salt-cured, smoked, and nitrate-preserved foods.

Of course, this is only one side of the story. The other side is that certain foods decrease the risk of cancer. These "good" foods are whole grains, legumes, fruits, and vegetables. All of them contain dietary fiber, which is thought to protect against colon cancer. A diet high in fruits and vegetables is also believed to protect against bladder, prostate, stomach, esophageal, and lung cancer.[23]

It is not known exactly how fruits and vegetables protect against cancer. Vitamins, minerals, fiber, and certain nonnutrients, acting alone or together, may all play a role.[24] Many studies have shown that foods rich in Vitamin C can protect against cancers of the mouth, esophagus, pancreas, and stomach, and perhaps also against cancers of the breast, rectum, and cervix.[25] There is also evidence that Vitamins A and E may help to protect against certain cancers by acting as antioxidants, and in the case of vitamin E, by inhibiting the conversion of nitrites into nitrosamines.[26] Finally, there is evidence that eating cruciferous vegetables (brussels sprouts, cabbage, broccoli) may reduce cancer risk.

A diet that reduces your risk of developing cancer can also reduce your risk of developing heart disease, which is linked to a high intake of saturated fat. Furthermore, it can reduce your risk of developing diverticulitis and irritable bowel syndrome, both of which have been linked to a diet low in fiber.[27]

One way to gain control over your life, then, is to eat plenty of whole grains, vegetables, and fruits and to save the salami, the pickles, and the whipped cream for special occasions.

Fat

If you make only one change in your diet, cut down on fat. There are more studies on fat than on any other

> *One way to gain control over your life, then, is to eat plenty of whole grains, vegetables, and fruits and to save the salami, the pickles, and the whipped cream for special occasions.*

dietary risk factor, and there is strong evidence that a high-fat diet increases your risk of developing cancer, especially cancers of the prostate, colon, and breast. A high-fat diet is also associated with cancers of the endometrium, ovary, and pancreas.[28] Although some studies implicate animal fat, most studies suggest that the risk comes from total fat intake, not from any specific kind of fat.[29]

How does a high-fat diet increase cancer risk? This is a controversial subject, and the safest answer is that nobody seems to know for sure. One study suggests that while a high-fat diet may actually help to cause tumors, it is more likely that it simply speeds their growth.[30] Other studies suggest that, especially in breast cancer, hormones may play an important role. Many of the fat-related cancers (breast, endometrium, ovary, prostate) are also hormone related cancers. Since obesity is a risk factor for some of these cancers, it is not clear whether the fat itself or the obesity caused by eating the fat creates the risk.[31]

In short, it appears that a high-fat diet increases the risk of developing several kinds of cancer. If you want to reduce cancer risk, it is safe to say that you should cut down on fat.

Most Americans eat far more fat than is good for them. And fat consumption is rising steadily. In 1910, 24 percent of our average daily caloric consumption was fat; today it is 35 percent to 40 percent.[32] In other words, fat consumption has increased by almost two-thirds in the last eighty years. Much of this increase is due to the growing popularity of fast foods and convenience foods. Between 1978 and 1989, for example, consumption of pizza (loaded with high-fat cheese) went up a whopping 77 percent.[33]

Which foods contain fat? You might be surprised. You probably know that there's fat in french fries and in whipped cream. But do you eat chicken? Dark meat, broiled (*not* fried), with skin, is over 50 percent fat. So are turkey hot dogs. So are eggs. Do you snack on granola bars? They contain 30 percent to 50 percent fat—as much as candy bars or doughnuts. Even vegetarians need to think twice. Tofu—like spareribs and sausage—contains

If you want to reduce cancer risk, it is safe to say that you should cut down on fat.

over 50 percent fat. So do most nuts and seeds. So do most cheeses. And soybeans contain over 30 percent fat—just like most pies.[34]

"Well, at least" (you think) "if I'm a vegetarian I'm getting 'good' fat. Animal fat is 'bad'; vegetable fat is 'good.'" Wrong again. It is true that animal (or saturated) fat is the kind that puts you at risk for heart disease. However, from a cancer prevention standpoint, most studies suggest that all fat is equally "bad."

How much fat is too much? If you eat the average American diet, as we have just explained, up to 40 percent of the calories you consume are fat calories. The National Cancer Institute (NCI) and the American Cancer Society both recommend that this amount be reduced to 30 percent or less.[35]

How, then, can you cut down on fat? The easiest way is simply to cut down on fatty foods—butter, cheese, fried foods, fatty meats, whole-milk ice cream. This is what the ACS recommends, and we shall explain how to do it presently. But for detail-minded people who enjoy a good challenge, there's another way.

First, find out how much fat you should be eating. Start by determining your daily caloric needs. If you are neither under- nor overweight, multiply your current body weight by 13. This will give you the number of calories you need to maintain basal metabolic rate and normal daily activities. Add more calories if you are very active, the amount depending on the type and duration of the activity (see table 1). Finally adjust for your age by subtracting 2 percent for each decade over age thirty.[36]

Once you know your daily caloric needs, multiply this number by your target percentage of fat. This target should be not more than 30 percent and not less than 10 percent to 20 percent of your total. (You need a certain amount of fat to maintain good health. The 10 percent figure, however, is controversial as of this writing.)[37] For example, if you need 1,800 calories a day and your target is 20 percent fat, multiply 1,800 by .20 to arrive at 360.

Divide this number by 9 (the number of calories in a

If you are under- or overweight, consult a registered dietitian to determine your daily caloric needs.

gram of fat). This gives you the number of grams of fat allowed in your diet. In our example, you are allowed 40 grams of fat a day.

Now you know how much fat you should be getting. The next step is to find out how much fat you *are* getting. When you're dealing with packaged food, it's easy: just look at the label. Fat content is usually expressed in grams per serving. But what about other kinds of food (meats, eggs, deli sandwiches, dinner at your mother-in-law's)? For these, registered dietitian Nancy Bennett suggests using a book that lists the fat content of foods.[38] (See the Recommended Reading at the end of this chapter.) Once you know what you should be getting and what you are getting, adjust your diet to bring the two figures into balance.

How can you cut down on fat? In all kinds of ways. Sometimes you can just remove the fatty parts of a piece of meat or buy extra-lean hamburger instead of regular. If you had skinned the chicken in the example cited earlier, you would have reduced the fat content from 51 percent to 35 percent. Four ounces of regular cooked hamburger contains 58 percent fat; four ounces of lean contains 22 percent. Other options are to replace meat with beans or low-fat fish; to replace whole milk with nonfat or 1 percent milk; to replace butter with jam; to replace ice cream with water sherbet or frozen yogurt; to broil meat in a nonstick skillet; and to buy (or make your own) low-fat salad dressing. Nancy Bennett adds that you can replace those croissants and breakfast bars with bagels, English muffins, pita breads, corn tortillas, or matzoh crackers.

Finally, remember that your target daily percentage is an *average*. You don't have to deprive yourself forever of foods you love. Setting your daily average at 30 percent doesn't mean you can't ever enjoy another sausage. It simply means that when you do enjoy a sausage, you need to go easy on fat for the next few meals. If your fat intake is 50 percent today and 20 percent tomorrow and the next day, it will average 30 percent for all three days.

In short, you can reduce the fat in your diet and still enjoy all kinds of tasty food. Not only will this make you

Finally, remember that your target daily percentage is an **average**. *You don't have to deprive yourself forever of foods you love.*

healthier, it will make you feel better as well. "It takes about three hours for fat to clear your stomach," says Nancy Bennett. "Until then you tend to feel tired and full. Most people who go on a low-fat diet find they have more energy. They don't feel so weighted down and groggy. Most people will tell you that they feel great."

As you change over to a low-fat diet, it's best to follow the guidelines we recommend throughout this book. Take it slowly, one step at a time. Don't take an all-or-nothing approach. Don't just give up old pleasures – look for new ones. Explore your options. Do what works best for you.

Finally, to prove our point, we present two sample menus on page 313 and page 314. These menus show you how to cut the fat out of restaurant meals as well as home-cooked ones. Look them over. We think they prove that a low-fat diet doesn't have to taste like straw.

For More Information...

It is widely agreed that diet affects health, but its exact effect is highly controversial. This is especially true when the issue is cancer. We want to make our own position clear. We view diet as *one* positive factor in maintaining good health. We also believe that a diet program can be an appropriate supplement to a standard cancer treatment program. At the same time, we recognize that many alternative practitioners view diet as a form of treatment in itself. We recommend that you evaluate any diet-based cancer treatment using the guidelines given in Chapter 5. Keep your mind open to the various possibilities. But balance what you believe against what you discover to be the facts. Get the best information available – and then make up your mind.

For general information on cancer and diet, call the American Cancer Society (1-800-ACS-2345). Or write to the ACS Public Education Department, 1599 Clifton Road NE, Atlanta, GA 30329-4251.

To choose a diet that is right for you, you may want to consult a registered dietitian. Contact the American

---

Sample Menu

High-Fat Choices	Low-Fat Choices

Breakfast

High-Fat Choices	Low-Fat Choices
1 cup Granola	*1 cup Wheat Flakes*
1 cup Whole Milk	*1 cup 1% Milk*
2 slices Buttered Toast	*2 slices Toast with*
	2 tsp Jam
4 oz Orange Juice	*4 oz Orange Juice*
Coffee with	*Coffee with 1% Milk*
1 tbsp Half-and-Half	
1,050 calories	*462 calories*
42 grams fat	*2 grams fat*
(36% calories are from fat)	*(4% calories are from fat)*
Cheese Omelet	*Mushroom Omelet*
Hashed Browns	*Fresh Fruit*
Bagel with 2 tbsp	*Bagel with 2 tsp Jam*
Cream Cheese	
4 oz Grapefruit Juice	*4 oz Grapefruit Juice*
Coffee with 1 tbsp	*Coffee with 1% Milk*
Half-and-Half	
879 calories	*592 calories*
48 grams fat	*15 grams fat*
(49% calories are from fat)	*(23% calories are from fat)*

Source: Nancy Bennett, MS, RD.

Dietetic Association (1-800-877-1600) for the names of registered dietitians in your area. If you are in the hospital, you can consult the dietitian on the hospital staff.

For information on other specific issues, such as

Sample Menu

High-Fat Choices	Low-Fat Choices

Lunch

At a Carl's Jr. Restaurant

Western Bacon Cheeseburger French Fries Whole Milk	Charbroiled Chicken Sandwich Tossed Green Salad with 1 tbsp Low-Calorie Dressing 1% Milk
1,330 calories 69 grams fat (47% calories are from fat)	480 calories 10 grams fat (19% calories are from fat)

At a Deli

Salami and Swiss on Rye Mustard, 2 tbsp Mayonnaise 1 oz Chips Cola	Turkey on French Mustard 1 oz Pretzels Cola
930 calories 60 grams fat (58% calories are from fat)	500 calories 3 grams fat (5% calories are from fat)

Source: Nancy Bennett, MS, RD.

pesticides in food, call or write the Center for Science in the Public Interest, 1501 16th Street NW, Washington, DC 20036-1499 (1-202-332-9910).

For good books on diet, see the Recommended Reading at the end of this chapter.

Exercise

Most people know that exercise makes you feel better. It helps to quiet the mental chatter; it gets you more in touch with your body; it increases your self-confidence. And it's healthy, too.

Facts about Exercise

Aerobic exercise is exercise that increases respiratory and circulatory function by increasing oxygen consumption. An example would be jogging. Aerobic exercise speeds up metabolism, which burns more calories (table 1) and continues to burn them even after you have stopped exercising. It increases blood volume and lung capacity; it strengthens the heart; and it lowers the level of blood cholesterol. Aerobic exercise increases endurance and reduces the risk of cardiovascular disease. It also helps to strengthen the bones.[39]

Table 1: Calories Burned in Various Forms of Exercise

Activity	Calories Burned		
	Per 1 lb body weight per min	Per 150 lb body weight per min	per hr
Knitting	0.010	1.5	90
Writing	0.013	1.9	114
Cooking	0.022	3.3	198
Volleyball	0.023	3.4	204
Ballroom dancing	0.023	3.4	204
Food shopping	0.028	4.2	252
Fishing	0.028	4.2	252
Weeding	0.033	4.9	294
Walking (normal pace, asphalt road)	0.036	5.5	330
Weight lifting (free weights)	0.039	5.9	354
Cycling (9.5 mph)	0.045	6.8	408
Aerobic dance	0.046	7.0	420
Lawn mowing	0.051	7.6	456
Swimming (slow crawl)	0.058	8.7	522
Running (11.5-minute mile)	0.061	9.1	546
Basketball	0.063	9.4	564
Running (6-minute mile)	0.115	17.2	1,032

Source: Editors of the *University of California at Berkeley Wellness Letter, The Wellness Encyclopedia* (Boston: Houghton Mifflin, 1991), 36-37.

Anaerobic exercise is intense exercise that lasts only a short time. An example would be weight lifting. Because it is not sustained over a long period, anaerobic exercise does not increase oxygen consumption or speed up metabolism. It builds muscle, however, and this helps to burn more calories in the long run, since the more muscles (lean body mass) you have, the more calories it takes just to maintain them.[40]

Slow, gentle *stretching* promotes flexibility; it relieves muscle tension, and it keeps the muscles from tightening up in the first place. (This is why we suggest below that you stretch before you exercise.) Stretching is also good exercise in itself for people who cannot engage in more strenuous activities.

Regular exercise is good for you. It increases physical fitness, and this in turn increases your chance of living longer.[41] It is beneficial in other ways as well. There is evidence that people who exercise regularly are less likely to develop cancer than people who don't.[42] Studies suggest that exercise can decrease the risk of colon cancer in men [43] and of cancers of the breast and reproductive system in women.[44] And a study of 13,344 men and women conducted over eight years found a strong relationship between physical fitness in general and deaths due to cancer. People in the least-fit category of this study were *sixteen times* more likely to die of cancer than people in the most-fit category.[45]

Even patients with a terminal prognosis can benefit from some form of exercise. It can help them to feel that they have some control over their bodies, to feel that they are still in the fight. "I think that one of the basics is to try and keep your body in shape so that you can feel good about yourself. So that you don't think of yourself as a sick person," is how Dennis Brown put it. This attitude can actually improve the patient's chances, as we explained in Chapter 6. It can also improve his quality of life.

Older people especially need regular exercise. Studies have shown that regular weight-bearing exercise (such as walking and stair climbing) can increase bone mass and

> *People in the least-fit category of this study were sixteen times more likely to die of cancer than people in the most-fit category*

prevent osteoporosis in elderly subjects. Exercise also increases metabolism, which makes it easier for the body to take in essential nutrients.[46] If you are over sixty, moderate aerobic exercise can strengthen your heart and lungs. It can also make you feel better mentally and emotionally.[47] Anaerobic and flexibility exercises (such as those taught in slow-stretch classes) can make you stronger and more flexible, and they can improve your range of motion.[48]

...and How to Do It

Yes, you know that exercise is good for you. So why don't you do more of it?

Perhaps you just basically don't like to exercise. "It's hard work" (you think); "I'll sweat; I'm too old; I'll feel like a fool in the gym (swimming pool, aerobics class), where everyone except me has a perfect body. And I don't know how to use the equipment, and I'm flabby, and I'm fat. And I can't walk a block without panting. And people will laugh."

If you don't like to exercise, your first step is to acknowledge that you don't like it. Your second step is to decide that you're going to do it anyway. And your third step is to make it as much fun as possible by cutting out as many negatives as you can. If you don't want to learn to use the equipment, walk. If you don't want anyone to see you, ride a stationary bike at home. If the thought of wearing baggy sweatpants depresses you, buy yourself a snappy leotard.

You may want to consult a doctor before you start your exercise program. This is advisable if you are over forty; if you smoke; if you are overweight; if you have diabetes, high blood pressure, high blood cholesterol, or heart disease; or if there is a history of early heart disease in your family.

The ideal program combines aerobic and anaerobic exercise. Aerobic exercise includes cycling, running, walking, swimming, and water aerobics; the last three are especially appropriate for older people. Anaerobic exercise includes isometrics and light to heavy resistance training

Keep at it. Be persistent; work up gradually to a level that is comfortable but challenging.

with weights. Twenty to thirty minutes of aerobic exercise combined with at least ten minutes of anaerobic exercise three to five times a week constitutes an excellent program.[49] But any exercise is good for you; the important thing is to do it willingly and regularly. So choose whatever appeals to you–but follow two simple rules.

The first rule is: *Use moderation.* Start slowly with something easy. Warm up thoroughly; don't push yourself too hard. In exercise, more is not necessarily better. If it hurts, you're overdoing it or doing it wrong. And while moderate exercise may stimulate the immune system, there is evidence that overdoing it can have just the opposite effect.[50]

It's a good idea to start with a little stretching. Stretch all the major muscle groups; then stretch the muscles used in your particular activity. (If you run, for example, stretch the stomach muscles, the calf muscles, the hamstrings, and the muscles in the backs of your legs.) Stretch each muscle or group of muscles gradually until you reach maximum extension; hold for up to thirty seconds; relax and repeat. Move slowly and gently; bouncing can cause strains and tears.

The second rule is: *Keep at it.* Be persistent; work up gradually to a level that is comfortable but challenging. If staying on an exercise program comes hard, make at least a three-week commitment. At the end of those first three weeks, see how you feel. We think you'll find that you enjoy exercise more than you ever thought you would.

Exercise Makes Other Changes Easier

Not only is exercise valuable in itself, it is valuable because it complements other life-style changes. It can make it easier to initiate those changes and it can also make it easier to maintain them.

There is evidence to suggest that exercise can help you to stop smoking. One study on women enrolled in a smoking cessation program found that of the ones who exercised regularly, 70 percent stayed off cigarettes after they completed the program for periods ranging from seven days to one year. None of the women who didn't exercise made it past twenty-four hours.[51]

Exercise helps you to stay on a healthy diet by reaffirming your commitment to take care of your body. And exercise helps you to control your weight. It burns calories, and it doesn't necessarily make you more hungry. This is an old wives' tale. Studies show that mildly obese women do not eat more when they exercise than when they don't,[52] and in fact they may actually eat less.[53]

Exercise can help you to control stress by relaxing both your body and your mind. Its physical effects on stress are well documented.[54] People who engage in aerobic exercise especially cope better with stress than people who do not.[55]

Other studies have documented the psychological benefits of exercise. Aerobic exercise has been shown to decrease depression.[56] This may be because it helps people to develop self-confidence and a sense of patience; because it shows them that they really can improve their health and looks; because it distracts them from their physical and emotional symptoms; or even because it has some biochemical effect on the causes of depression itself.[57]

Finally and most interestingly, exercise can increase your sense of control. Specifically, it increases self-efficacy, the belief that one can do what is necessary in a given situation. One group of researchers studied the effects on 103 sedentary middle-aged men and women of doing sit-ups, bicycling, walking, and jogging. They found that people who had not originally believed that they could do a certain amount of exercise actually came to believe it during the course of a twenty-week exercise program. This belief in turn affected both their actual performance and their physical responses to exercise. The change was especially dramatic for women, who started out with much lower self-perceptions than men but caught up with them, or even surpassed them, by the end of the program.[58] What this means for you is that exercise can teach you to gain control *in general*–not just over stress and not just over your body, but over your life as a whole.

The ideal is a program of sustained exercise, as we have

For more on how to stop smoking, see page 331.

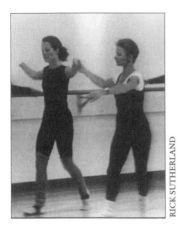

RICK SUTHERLAND

This breast cancer survivor is learning to dance.

Are you trying to be more creative? Take up samba or modern dance.

For more on walking, see page 212.

just explained. But the important thing is to do something that gets you out and moving. You will gain some benefit from *any* activity you undertake. So match your exercise to your own interests and your own abilities, and to your top priorities as well.

Is work a high priority for you? Walk upstairs to your office instead of taking the elevator. Walk on your lunch hour; walk the last mile (or five blocks, or even one block) to your job. If you work on your feet, do stretching exercises on your break. If you drive for a living, do isometric exercises at the stoplights.

Do your family and friends come first? Play games with them—volleyball, softball, basketball, Frisbee, soccer. Too strenuous? Take your mom fishing. Play hide-and-seek with the children. Throw tennis balls for the dog (he's family too). Help a friend to move. If *making* friends is one of your priorities, take a slow-stretch class, an aerobics class, a windsurfing class. Join a gym. Go where the people are and exercise with them.

Are you trying to be more creative? Take up samba or modern dance. There are dance groups designed specifically for people with cancer. Redesign your garden; put in a fish pond. Build a bookcase or a deck. Remember: it's all exercise, whether you're swinging a dumbbell or a hammer. Use your imagination. Do what you enjoy.

Do you want to learn how to have fun? See our suggestions in Part 1 under Pleasant Events. Then ask yourself what's fun for *you*. Rollerskating? Bird watching? Flamenco dancing? Learning to ride a horse? Pushing your granddaughter on a swing? Walking down to the lake to feed the ducks?

We've used a lot of "walking" examples in this chapter. That's because almost everybody can walk. If you're athletic, try a challenging, fast-paced aerobic walk. If you're in average shape, walk a mile to the grocery store. If you're recovering from surgery, walk around your yard. Walk the baby, walk the dog, walk with your wife to the corner for a frozen yogurt. To receive the greatest benefits, work up to thirty minutes three times a week, at a clip fast

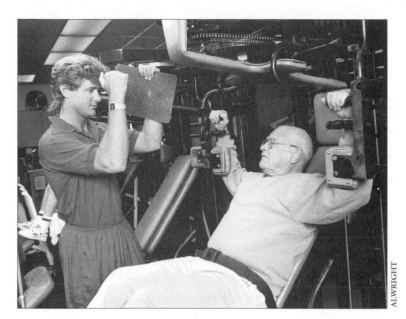

ALWRIGHT

You may want to work with a personal fitness trainer.

enough to speed up your breathing and your heart.

"But," you may be thinking, "I can't walk. I'm in a wheelchair. What about me? How am I supposed to get any exercise?"

Start by looking into the special exercise programs offered by your local Center for Independent Living or Center for Persons with Disabilities. These programs include basketball, swimming, weight lifting, and general body conditioning, among other things. The people who run the programs can also give you good advice on how to exercise as you go about your daily life. For more information, check with your local college or university; with the disabled health clinic of your hospital; and with the local branch of the Visiting Nurse Association. Or talk to a physical therapist. He or she can design a program to meet your specific needs.

In short, no matter what other life-style changes you wish to make, no matter whether you have cancer or not, no matter what your priorities and your interests are, exercise can help you to gain control over your body and help you to get more pleasure out of your life.

If there is no Center for Independent Living in your area, contact the National Council for Independent Living, 1-518-274-1979.

For More Information...

There are many sources of information on exercise. Your library, bookstore, and local newsstand carry books and magazines on a wide variety of sports. Local clubs devoted to a particular activity (hiking clubs, bowling leagues, gardening societies) can introduce you to people who share your interests and can give you the information you need to get started.

If you like to work with experts for direction and motivation, you may be a good candidate for a supervised exercise program. Qualified instructors teach swimming, weight lifting, toning and stretching, and cardiac health programs. They can be found through hospitals, physicians, health clubs, adult schools, and the YMCA and YWCA. (Some Y's offer special water pool programs for people with cancer.) Many employers offer health and wellness programs. You can also arrange to get private instruction with a personal fitness trainer.

If you prefer to set up your own program, there are books available to tell you how. Look in your bookstore under Health for books on self-guided personal wellness training.

For good books on exercise, see the Recommended Reading at the end of this chapter.

Weight Control

Keeping your weight within healthy bounds is another way to gain control over your life. This can mean putting weight on, but it usually means taking it off. If you are fighting cancer now, you may need to focus on gaining weight, and that can be a challenge. If you need to gain weight, you should consult your doctor. (He or she will probably also refer you to a registered dietitian.) On the other hand, some cancer patients need to lose weight; this will help them to improve their overall health. Finally, if you want to reduce your risk of getting cancer in the first place, you may need to lose ten or twenty (or fifty or a hundred) pounds. Losing weight can be a challenge too. In this section, we will talk about losing weight.

Facts about Being Overweight

Being even 10 percent overweight puts you at risk of developing cancer. And the risk increases as your weight goes up. A twelve-year study run by the American Cancer Society on 750,000 people found that men who were 40 percent or more over the average weight for their height were 33 percent likelier to die of cancer than men of average weight. For women the increased risk was 55 percent. For certain cancers the risk was much higher—73 percent for colorectal cancer in men and *542 percent* for endometrial cancer in women. Women were also at greatly increased risk for cancers of the uterus, gallbladder, cervix, ovary, and breast. Nor was the risk confined to people who were grossly overweight. Men who were only 20 percent over average weight were at 37 percent increased risk for prostate cancer. And women even 10 percent overweight were at 36 percent increased risk for endometrial cancer and 59 percent increased risk for cancer of the gallbladder.[59]

Obesity is associated with other diseases as well. These include adult onset diabetes, high blood pressure, gallstones, osteoarthritis, cerebral vascular lesions, and heart disease. The ACS study found that men in their forties who were 10 percent to 19 percent overweight were at 264 percent increased risk for diabetes; for women the figure was 355 percent. Women in their forties who were at least 40 percent overweight were *twenty-four and a half times* as likely to die of diabetes as they would have been if their weight had been average.[60]

So it's important to control your weight. The question is: How are you going to do it?

No, not by going on a "diet." As millions of Americans who are yo-yo dieters can attest, short-term diets don't really work. They may take the pounds off temporarily, but the weight comes right back in 90 percent of

Women in their forties who were at least 40 percent overweight were twenty-four and a half times as likely to die of diabetes as they would have been if their weight had been average.

cases,[61] usually with an added pound or two.

So forget about going on a "diet." To lose weight and to keep it off, you need to develop eating habits that you can maintain comfortably for the rest of your life.

The ideal combination for weight management is to change your eating habits permanently and to exercise regularly several times a week. If you lose the weight slowly–about one pound a week–you should lose fat, not muscle. So set realistic goals; don't be in too much of a hurry. Remember: the more slowly the weight comes off, the longer it stays off.

And how should you change your eating habits? That's easy–theoretically. Just cut your fat intake to between 10 percent and 30 percent, following the guidelines in the section on diet. (Don't try to go below 10 percent. You need that much fat in order to stay healthy.) Why cut fat and not, say, carbohydrates? First, because fat contains more calories per gram. And second, because your body tends to store the fat you eat rather than burn it. Fat, in other words, makes you fat. If you eat carbohydrates, on the other hand, your body uses 23 percent of the calories they contain just to process them. That leaves only 77 percent of those calories to be stored.[62] Weight loss is a complicated issue, and nobody knows exactly how it works. But experts agree that cutting fat and following a moderate exercise program is the best way to lose weight and keep it off for good.[63]

It sounds simple. But in practice it can be extremely difficult.

> Fat contains 9 calories per gram. Carbohydrates contain only 4 calories per gram.

It's All in How You Think

Chronic or compulsive overeating is an emotional issue, and emotional issues are not simple. There is more involved here than calories, or fat. If you want to lose weight and keep it off, you will need to change your attitudes toward food. In fact, how you think and feel about food is as critical to changing your eating habits as knowing what foods will help you to lose weight.

Why do people overeat? There are innumerable reasons. Some people overeat as a way of expressing negative emotions. They're mad at their spouse; they can't talk about it; so they overeat. Some people overeat to punish themselves, or because they're feeling self-destructive. And of course there are people who use food as a reward. This is natural and harmless up to a point; almost everyone likes a treat after a hard day's work; but some people reward themselves for *everything* with food. "It's a way of self-nurturing," says Robert Fuhr, a clinical psychologist who specializes in issues of weight control and smoking cessation. "But for these people it's the only method that they know."[64]

To break the pattern of compulsive overeating, you must first understand why you do it. If you feel able to do so, you might then try solving the problem yourself. The challenge will be to notice when and why you overeat. Identify the negative emotion that is making you do it and then address the issue directly. If you find this difficult, very painful, or impossible, we suggest that you seek professional counseling with a therapist who specializes in this field.

To break the pattern of compulsive overeating, it's important to have support. If you're comfortable with a group approach, you might want to investigate Overeaters Anonymous (OA). This friendly, low-pressure group describes itself as a "fellowship of individuals for compulsive overeating." It is not political or religious, and it charges no fees or dues of any kind. OA does not offer specific diets, calorie reduction techniques, or eating plans. It is a self-help group for people who want to stop overeating. To find the chapter nearest you, look in the white pages of your telephone book under Overeaters Anonymous.

Social support is important too. "Some people who want to lose weight tell me that all their friends do is go out to restaurants and eat a lot, and how can they do anything different?" says Robert Fuhr. If this sound like you, you may need to add to your circle of friends. Look for people who enjoy the things that you enjoy—other than eating.

"Some people who want to lose weight tell me that all their friends do is go out to restaurants and eat a lot, and how can they do anything different?"

–Robert Fuhr

Look for people you can jog with, square dance with, do aerobics with. Look for people who support your efforts to lose weight, not people who urge you to take a second helping. Above all, look for people whose company you enjoy, even when you aren't eating a thing.

If you use food to nurture or reward yourself, you need to learn to do this in other ways. The key is to become aware that you're eating when you're not hungry. Each time you reach for the cookie jar, ask yourself, "Am I really hungry?" If you aren't, try to figure out why you *are* eating. Are you lonely (frightened, angry, proud of yourself, bored)? If you're using food as a coping mechanism, ask yourself what you could do instead to reward yourself or make yourself feel better. Eating is a sensual pleasure. Try to do things that use your other senses—vision, hearing, touch, and smell. Put on your favorite country-and-western tape, play with the cat, take a bubble bath. Choose things that make *you* feel good, things that are truly nurturing and that have no negative long-term consequences. (Don't take up smoking; don't go out and buy $400 worth of new clothes if all of your credit cards are overcharged.) Make a list of nonfood rewards and comforts and keep it handy for those moments when you think you just have to have a chocolate éclair.

For more on nurturing yourself, see page 301.

Finally, remember our suggestions for initiating any kind of change. These are good rules for anybody who is trying to develop new eating habits. Take it one step at a time: this week put jelly instead of butter on your toast; next week put milk in your coffee instead of cream. Small changes won't seem like big sacrifices. Use the step approach to set weight loss goals as well. Say you want to lose thirty pounds. Set yourself the goal of losing five. Reward yourself when you achieve that goal. Then lose another five, and so on until all thirty pounds are gone.

We explain the step approach on page 190.

Suppose you feel the urge to binge. One good technique is simply to wait a while. Walk around the block. Call up a friend and chat. Tell yourself that if you really want to binge, you can binge two hours from now. By that time, the urge may very well have passed.

Try to treat yourself kindly; don't blame yourself if you occasionally eat something you shouldn't. Stick with your program, but go easy on yourself. Berating yourself because you ate that piece of fudge probably does you more harm than the fudge did. Besides, if you convince yourself that you've "failed," you might eat six more pieces out of pure self-disgust. Or you might decide that since you've blown it for today, you'll eat everything in sight and start fresh tomorrow.

Have a plan of action, not only for every day but also—especially—for when you eat out. Bring your own snacks on the plane and avoid the salted nuts. Choose restaurants that you know serve appropriate food; don't wait until the waiter brings you the menu to discover that everything on it is deep-fried. If you're going to a party, eat a snack at home before you leave. This will help you to avoid the liver paté and the chips and dip.

In short, take control of the details if you want to control your eating habits. And rethink your attitudes toward food.

For More Information...

The cancer prevention diet recommended by the ACS is also a good, safe diet for losing weight. Call the ACS at 1-800-ACS-2345 to obtain a copy.

If you are very overweight, or if you think you need guidance in changing your eating habits, you may find a weight management program helpful. Look for one that is led by a registered dietitian with experience in the field. Choose a program with a proven long-term success rate. Avoid short-term programs, programs that feature crash diets or special foods, and any program that makes extraordinary claims. Remember: if it sounds too good to be true, it's probably not true.

To find a qualified dietitian in your area, contact the American Dietetic Association (1-800-877-1600), the American Institute of Nutrition (1-301-530-7050), or

Stick with your program, but go easy on yourself. Berating yourself because you ate that piece of fudge probably does you more harm than the fudge did.

Smoking is responsible for one out of six deaths in the United States. Over 400,000 Americans die each year from the effects of smoking.

the American College of Nutrition (1-919-452-1222). Choose a dietitian who belongs to one of these organizations, who has a degree from an accredited college or university, and who has several years of proven success working with patients in weight management.

For information on weight loss programs in your area, look in the yellow pages of your telephone book under Weight Control Services.

For good books on weight control, see the Recommended Reading at the end of this chapter.

Smoking

Are you a smoker? If so, you probably won't be able to read this. It would be easier to skip over the next few pages and continue to do what's "comfortable" for you. But if you feel adventurous, read on.

Smoking is responsible for one out of six deaths in the United States.[65] Over 400,000 Americans die *each year* from the effects of smoking.[66] This is almost four times as many Americans as died in combat during the entire Vietnam War, a war that lasted over eleven years. It is more Americans than died in combat in World War I, Korea, and Vietnam combined.

Facts about Smoking

Smoking is responsible for 30 percent of all deaths from cancer.[67] It causes almost all deaths from lung cancer, the commonest cancer deaths in both men and women.[68] Smoking is also associated with cancers of the mouth, throat, esophagus, pancreas, kidney, bladder, and cervix.[69] (Smokeless tobacco–snuff–is just as dangerous; it can increase the risk of oral cancer by almost 5,000 percent.)[70]

Even if you escape cancer, you aren't safe. If you smoke, you are two to four times likelier to die of coronary artery disease. You are at increased risk for stroke, respiratory infection, and peptic ulcer. Smoking causes 81.5 percent of deaths from chronic obstructive pulmonary (lung) disease.[71] It is estimated that each cigarette you smoke reduces your life expectancy by five and a half minutes.[72]

You don't even have to smoke to die of smoking. An estimated 53,000 deaths a year are caused by passive smoking–inhaling smoke from other people's cigarettes.[73] Babies and children are especially at risk. The American Academy of Pediatrics estimates that 9 million American children under age five are exposed to secondary smoke, most of it probably from their parents' cigarettes.[74] This is a serious health hazard. One large study showed that the children of mothers who smoked were 70 percent more likely to be hospitalized for respiratory illness than children of mothers who did not smoke.[75] Passive smoking is also a risk factor for Sudden Infant Death Syndrome.[76] Finally, mothers who smoke are at increased risk of complications from pregnancy, and their infants are 35 percent more likely to die at birth than they would have been if their mothers had not smoked at all. About 5,000 babies die each year in the United States simply because their mothers smoked.[77]

Even if it doesn't kill you (or your children), smoking spoils some of the pleasure in life. It can spoil your looks; smoking stains your teeth and it causes wrinkles. One study showed that heavy smokers are almost five times more likely to be wrinkled than nonsmokers.[78]

Finally, studies suggest that men who smoke risk becoming impotent, perhaps because nicotine constricts the blood vessels in the penis. In one study, three-quarters of the men who were tested failed to achieve an erection after smoking only two cigarettes.[79]

Given these hair-raising statistics, why do people smoke? First of all, because they're addicted. Nicotine, the active agent in tobacco, is every bit as addictive as heroin, and it reaches the brain even faster–in seven seconds, to be exact.[80] And since nicotine is an addictive drug, you will experience withdrawal symptoms if you stop taking it. These may include nausea, diarrhea, headache, insomnia, irritability, anxiety, depression, and fatigue. Some people experience only one symptom; others experience several.

Heavy smokers are almost five times more likely to be wrinkled than nonsmokers.

But you can satisfy these needs without smoking. In the next section we'll show you how to do it.

The physical symptoms diminish after a week or two, but the desire to smoke may last much longer.

In fact, the psychological addiction to smoking can be more enslaving than the physical addiction. Many people see smoking as a way to relax, as a stress reducer, or simply as a habit. But it can hook you in other ways as well. Do you use smoking as a way to reward yourself? Something to look forward to? Something to do with your hands? Or just as a familiar and nurturing ritual—grabbing a cigarette, lighting it, and taking that first puff? These psychological needs can be as strong as, and more insidious than, the physical craving for nicotine.

It kills you; it kills your children; it's addictive. How can a cigarette do so much damage?

First of all, cigarette smoke contains tar. As you smoke, this tar condenses in your mouth, esophagus, throat, and lungs. The smoke also damages the cilia—tiny hairs—that help to clear foreign substances out of the airways. This allows the condensed tar to build up in the lungs. The tar in cigarette smoke contains forty-three carcinogens.[81] Over time, as the tar builds up, these carcinogens cause the cells to mutate, and the smoker develops lung cancer. The same general mechanism also causes cancers of the mouth, esophagus, and throat.

The oxygen-carbon dioxide exchange is explained on page 224.

When the cilia are damaged or destroyed, mucus builds up in the lungs. This leads to infection and then to chronic bronchitis. Cigarette smoke also destroys the tiny air sacs in the lungs, which are vital to the exchange of oxygen and carbon dioxide. This leads to emphysema. These two conditions are known collectively as chronic obstructive pulmonary disease. People with advanced COPD die of infection, heart failure, suffocation, or all three.

Cigarette smoke contains nicotine and carbon monoxide. Nicotine constricts the blood vessels and makes the heart beat faster. When this happens, the heart requires more oxygen, but it gets less. Carbon monoxide replaces the oxygen in the blood. When this happens, even less oxygen goes to the heart (and to the rest of the body). All of this overworks the heart. The end result may be death from heart failure.

Nicotine and carbon monoxide also promote the deposit of plaque in the arteries. This leads to atherosclerosis (hardening of the arteries). If the arteries in question are the ones that carry blood to the brain, the result is stroke. Smoking also causes blood clots; these too can obstruct circulation to the brain. Again, the result is stroke.

All of this serves to explain why smoking is such a deadly habit. But…

You Can Quit

It's never too late to quit. One year after you smoke your last cigarette, your risk of disease from smoking is reduced by half. And the longer you go without smoking, the lower your risk.[82]

Ninety percent of people who stop smoking do it on their own.[83] Here as elsewhere, it's important to have a plan of action. Robert Fuhr, who counsels many smokers, suggests using the step approach.

First, list all the reasons why you want to quit—you'll be healthier, you'll be more attractive, you can taste your food, you'll respect yourself, and so on. This gives you a positive incentive.

Second, try to figure out why you smoke. What needs are you meeting by smoking? If, for example, you smoke to relax, recognize that, for you, relaxation is a need. You're going to have to meet that need some other way.

Third, become aware of your smoking pattern—of the times and places where you usually smoke during the day. Do you smoke when you first get up? After phone calls? After work in the evening? These are your high-risk times. Imagine your whole day in detail and make a list of the times when you are at the highest risk of smoking.

Fourth, figure out how you can meet your needs in other ways. For example, if you smoke to relax, decide how you're going to relax after you stop smoking. In this particular case, it might help to remember that smoking doesn't really relax you at all. "The level of anxiety drops

It's never too late to quit. One year after you smoke your last cigarette, your risk of disease from smoking is reduced by half.

Table 2. Cues and High-Risk Situations for Smoking and Suggested Interventions for Patients Trying to Quit

Cues and High-Risk Situations	Suggested Interventions
Awakening in the morning	Brush your teeth as soon as you awake. Start an activity right away; don't sit around thinking about smoking.
Drinking coffee	Have your coffee while doing something with your hands so that smoking is difficult. Have tea or another beverage instead.
Eating meals	Eat lunch in a different location. Sit in nonsmoking sections at restaurants. Get up from the table right away after eating and start another activity (e.g., take a walk). Brush your teeth right after eating.
Watching television	Have an activity ready to keep your hands busy. Play a game, do a puzzle, sew, build a model, give yourself a manicure, write a letter. Keep low-calorie snacks readily available. Watch television with a nonsmoker, either a friend or a family member. Have carpets and upholstery cleaned when you quit smoking and make the television room a no-smoking area.
Driving a car	Have car cleaned and deodorized when you quit smoking. Keep low-calorie snacks on hand or keep toothpicks or a fake cigarette with you. Chew sugarless gum. Try public transportation, which prohibits smoking.
Taking a break with coworkers	Brush your teeth or start chewing a piece of sugarless gum at the beginning of breaks. Take several slow, deep breaths and visualize a peaceful scene to help you relax. Take breaks with nonsmoking associates until you feel more confident about not smoking.
Having a drink at a bar, restaurant, or party	Try to take a nonsmoker with you or associate with nonsmokers. Let friends know that you have just quit. Moderate your intake of alcohol (it can weaken your resolve).
Socializing with friends or family members who smoke	Suggest frequenting no-smoking events (movies, theater, shopping in department stores) until you are more confident. Let these people know you're trying to quit and ask for their support. Ask them not to smoke around you, offer you cigarettes, or give you cigarettes if you ask for them. Consider quitting with someone else (especially a family member). You can offer each other support and avoid extra temptation.
Encountering stressful occasions (feeling lonely or under pressure, arguments with family or friends)	Review your reasons for quitting. Relax by taking several deep breaths and thinking of a peaceful scene. Then congratulate yourself for relaxing without smoking. Get out of the house. Take a walk or go to a no-smoking establishment. Take a shower. Reward yourself for having quit smoking (e.g., buy something with the money you've saved on cigarettes).
Have a lapse (smoking one or two cigarettes)	Recognize the lapse as a small setback, *not* a failure. Don't give up! Resolve to remain a nonsmoker. Get rid of any cigarettes you may have bought. Identify the reason for the lapse and plan how to avoid or cope with the situation the next time.

Source: Sarah E. Kraner and Kathryn E. Graham, "Helping Your Patients Who Smoke to Quit for Good," *Postgraduate Medicine* 90, no. 1 (July 1991): 242-43.

right after you've had a cigarette. But your overall level of anxiety is higher," says Fuhr. "Most people say they're more relaxed once they've stopped smoking."

Fifth, plan ahead for your high-risk times. If you always have a cigarette first thing in the morning, decide exactly what you're doing to do first thing in the morning to avoid having a cigarette. "Set up a plan ahead of time, so that when you're in that situation you already know what to do." Table 2 lists various high-risk situations and offers suggestions for handling them.

Sixth, reward yourself for quitting. You may find that being free of cigarettes is its own reward. But if external rewards work well for you, by all means use them. Earlier in this chapter we discussed the use of rewards. Refer back to page 292 and see what appeals to you. One cancer patient whose diagnosis prompted him to give up smoking put into a glass jar every morning the money he would have spent that day on cigarettes. Seeing the pile of dollar bills grow higher was a reward in itself. (It also served to remind the patient how much money he had been wasting on cigarettes.) And at the end of one smoke-free year, he had enough money to take himself on a trip to Hawaii.

Seventh, build support. We discussed support earlier in this chapter too. When you quit smoking, you can use the buddy system to prevent relapse. Arrange in advance to call a friend when you think you can't go another minute without a cigarette.

Here are some more useful suggestions to supplement your seven-step plan. Start by setting a quit date–preferably within three weeks, but the sooner the better. Be specific, and don't put it off too long. Next throw out all your cigarettes. This is essential if you really want to stop smoking.

Some people find visualization helpful. "I have my clients picture themselves having more energy, being more relaxed, with clean lungs and a healthy heart," says Fuhr. "Enjoying life more. Being happier. Then I have them visualize rejecting a cigarette and all the poisons in it. As they come to value better health and see that it is

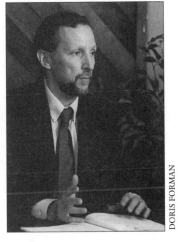

DORIS FORMAN

Robert Fuhr

"As they come to value better health and see that it is attainable, they learn to choose to reject cigarettes as they would reject a glass of poison."

–Robert Fuhr

For more on visualization, see page 220.

attainable, they learn to choose to reject cigarettes as they would reject a glass of poison."

Some people keep a log of the things that trigger the urge to smoke. There are feeling triggers, social triggers, and thought triggers. A feeling trigger might be the anxiety that you feel when you have to make a difficult phone call. The anxiety triggers the urge to have a cigarette. A thought trigger might be thinking you need a cigarette in order to work faster. A social trigger might be seeing somebody smoking. In each case you need to find a different way of responding to the trigger. If you see somebody smoking, for example, "it is vital to change the way you interpret what you see," says Robert Fuhr. "If you say to yourself, 'Boy, I bet that person really wants to quit,' you'll be much less likely to want to smoke yourself than if you say, 'Boy, I bet that person must really be enjoying that cigarette!'"

Of the 90 percent of people who stop smoking on their own, most quit "cold turkey" – that is, abruptly, completely, and without aids.[84] However, there are all kinds of aids for people who find them helpful. Nicotine gum, a prescription drug, is one of the most effective. It has a 40 percent one-year success rate, provided it is used in conjunction with counseling.[85] Because it helps to satisfy the craving for nicotine, it works best for smokers who are heavily addicted. It is expensive, however; a three months' supply can cost over $500. It can have side effects too, including dizziness, mouth sores, ulcers, and possible addiction. Nicotine patches are also sold on prescription, but they must be used under a doctor's supervision. It is important not to smoke while wearing the patch. Correctly used, the nicotine patch has a one-year success rate of up to 29 percent; this figure rises to 35 percent when the patch is used together with behavior modification.[86]

Antidepressant and antianxiety drugs have been used in trial studies to help people to stop smoking. As of this writing, it is too soon to tell how effective they are.[87] Two other popular techniques are hypnosis and acupuncture. Although the proponents of hypnosis claim success rates of up to 88 percent, these claims have not been scientifically validated; most studies suggest that 15 percent to 20 percent is more like it. The same holds true for acupuncture.[88]

One last word of warning. When you've gone a couple of months without smoking, you're through the most difficult period. At this point, you may consider that you've quit. You need to be prepared for the fact that at times you may still experience a strong urge to smoke. Be ready with your own relapse prevention strategy. Make a list of things that work for you–things that will get your mind off cigarettes.

It's not easy to quit smoking, but over 40 million Americans have done it.[89] Most of them didn't succeed on their first attempt. So if you've tried and failed, try again. And again. Don't give up. If there's one change that's really worth making, this is it.

It's not easy to quit smoking, but over 40 million Americans have done it.

For More Information...

If you are one of the 10 percent who prefer to join an organized program, you can choose among a variety of clinics and groups. The ACS, the American Lung Association, and the Seventh-Day Adventist Church all sponsor clinics that employ education and behavior modification. There are also many commercial smoking cessation programs. One of the oldest and largest is SmokEnders, which uses behavior modification techniques, that is, techniques that reward desired behavior. Smokers Anonymous takes a different approach. Modeled after Alcoholics Anonymous, this is a support group–not a clinic–for people who want to stop smoking. To find a smoking cessation program, contact your local office of the ACS or the American Lung Association, get a reference from your hospital, or look in the yellow pages of your telephone directory under Smokers' Information and Treatment Centers. Keep looking until you find a program that appeals to you. Choose one with a success rate of at least 30 percent. That is, ask for data indicating that one year after they quit, at least 30 percent of the program participants haven't started smoking again.

The American Lung Association publishes Freedom from Smoking® self-help manuals and a home video. To obtain them, contact the office nearest you, or telephone 1-212-315-8700. The American Cancer Society (1-800-ACS-2345) and the National Cancer Institute (1-800-4-CANCER) also provide self-help materials.

For good books on quitting smoking, see the Recommended Reading at the end of this chapter.

Alcohol

Alcohol is a poison. However, most people's bodies can handle alcohol in small amounts. A glass or two of wine with your dinner probably won't hurt you. But add two sherries or two beers before dinner and you put your drinking into the heavy class. There is good evidence that heavy drinking (defined as twenty-one or more drinks a week) increases your risk of developing cancer, to say nothing of a variety of other diseases.

Facts about Alcohol

Although the link between alcohol and cancer is not as well established as the link between smoking and cancer, it is widely accepted that heavy drinking is a factor in the development of certain cancers. One of these is cancer of the liver, for which alcoholics are at a 50 percent increased risk.[90] But the evidence against alcohol is strongest in the case of mouth and throat cancer. Heavy drinkers are fifteen times more likely than nondrinkers to develop oral cancer and eleven times more likely to develop cancers of the throat and larynx.[91] And the risk is very much greater for drinkers who smoke. This group accounts for about three-quarters of oropharyngeal cancers in the United States. One study showed that men who take more than four drinks and smoke two or more packs of cigarettes a day are 38 times as likely to develop these cancers of the mouth and throat as they would be if they neither smoked nor drank—and women are 108 times more likely.[92]

The more you drink, the more you are likely to sabotage your eating habits. Studies suggest that heavy drinkers eat fewer fruits and vegetables, and that this too increases the risk of oropharyngeal cancer. There is also strong evidence that people who don't eat well because they drink instead are at increased risk of developing cancer of the esophagus.[93] In short, alcohol is a risk factor in itself, and the combination of alcohol and smoking, or alcohol and poor nutrition, constitutes an even greater risk factor.

Alcohol causes other diseases and disabilities. These include osteoporosis, stroke, hypoglycemia, impotence, and nerve damage. Drinking is believed to be the leading cause of hypertension (high blood pressure) in the United States.[94] Alcohol is especially hard on the heart. It weakens the heart muscle, and the heart compensates by enlarging. Alcohol also weakens the contractions of the heart muscle by interfering with the hormones that regulate these contractions. All this can lead to congestive heart failure. Unfortunately, by the time you first start to feel fatigued, or notice that your heart is beating abnormally, your health may be severely damaged.[95]

Alcohol is hardest of all on the liver. Heavy drinking causes this organ to become swollen with fats, protein, and water. In time the liver will become inflamed and parts of it may die. You will then become jaundiced, run a fever, and experience abdominal pain. These are the symptoms of alcoholic hepatitis. If you stop drinking now, the damage may correct itself, but your liver will remain scarred for the rest of your life. If, on the other hand, you continue to drink, the liver will become even more scarred. At this point the damage cannot be corrected, and if you continue to drink, you may very well die of liver failure. Or you might die of cancer. As we noted above, 50 percent of liver cancer patients are alcoholics.[96]

Finally, of course, heavy drinking can kill you in other ways. Between 1982 and 1989, it was estimated that almost half of all traffic fatalities involved alcohol. During

Alcohol is especially hard on the heart. It weakens the heart muscle, and the heart compensates by enlarging.

your lifetime, you stand about a 40 percent chance of being in a traffic accident in which someone was drinking.[97] In 1990 in California alone, alcohol was a factor in 13,465 deaths. Of these, 1,613 were murders and another 1,041 were suicides.[98]

Alcohol is a liar. It makes you think you've got your stress under control. But you don't.

But It Helps Me to Relax!

If you are more than a casual drinker, the chances are that you drink because it makes you feel good. Experts disagree as to how alcohol achieves its pleasant effect. Some say that it generates euphoria; some say that it reduces anxiety; some say that you enjoy drinking because you associate it with pleasant situations—with parties, for example.[99] Whatever the reason, the fact remains that alcohol can make you feel good. It makes you feel relaxed, and it reduces stress.

"What's wrong with that?" you ask. "All through this book you've been saying how important it is to reduce stress. If alcohol is all it takes, terrific!"

What's wrong with that is that alcohol is a liar. It makes you think you've got your stress under control. But you don't. It's important to learn to manage stress if you want to stay healthy. The trouble with alcohol is that it doesn't teach you to manage stress. It just masks the symptoms temporarily. And heavy drinking makes it much, much harder to maintain healthy habits—habits that would improve your quality of life. In short, alcohol doesn't really make your life better. In fact, it can make your life a great deal worse.

When you drink, the alcohol enters the bloodstream and is carried throughout the body. Once inside the brain cells, it "shorts out the wiring" in the brain. That is, it disrupts your ability to move, think, speak, sense, and feel.[100] When you drink, then, you feel more relaxed because your brain has been disrupted. That relaxed feeling is caused by the alcohol—by an agent outside yourself. In effect, the alcohol acts as a crutch.

Furthermore, alcohol is addictive. This means that if

you keep drinking, it takes more and more alcohol to relax you. Worse yet, once your brain becomes adapted to alcohol, it will function normally only if you keep drinking. If you stop, you will suffer withdrawal symptoms. In the early stages, these include restlessness, anxiety, insomnia, and tremors. In the later stages, they include hyperactivity, disorientation, confusion, and hallucinations. You may crave alcohol to such an extent that you will give up everything else just to get it. In short, if you habitually drink to relax, you run a real risk of becoming both physically and psychologically hooked.

"Not me," you say. "*I* haven't got a problem. I can stop any time I want to." That's characteristic. That's the standard response made by people who have lost control to an addictive substance—whether it's alcohol, nicotine, or cocaine.

Finally, although drinking masks the symptoms of stress, it doesn't do this in a way that makes it easier for you to function. The reason we encourage you to learn to reduce stress is that by doing so you can improve your health and accomplish other useful life-style changes. Far from improving your health, alcohol can destroy it, as we have just explained. And it doesn't help you to make useful changes, either. On the contrary, it makes these changes more difficult. The more you drink, the harder it will be for you to maintain good eating habits, to go for that jog, to stay off cigarettes. And the harder it will be for you to make a commitment to the other priorities in your life—to stick with that new business you've just started, to find time to play with the children, to get that RN degree, to have that heart-to-heart conversation with your wife. You'll be compromising all that just to feel good for a few hours.

But when the effects of the alcohol wear off, you'll be right back where you started from. And next time it will be just a little bit harder to go for that jog, to have that heart-to-heart conversation. And it might take two drinks instead of one to make you feel better.

Why not drink to manage stress? Because it doesn't work.

"Not me," you say. "I haven't got a problem. I can stop any time I want to."

For More Information...

If you have a serious drinking problem, you will probably need help to overcome it. Alcoholics Anonymous (AA) offers excellent support; to contact the chapter nearest you, look in the white pages of your telephone book. Alcoholics Anonymous takes the approach that in order to overcome addiction, you must admit that you can't control it yourself and must give yourself over to a higher power. AA usually defines a "higher power" as God, but participants may define the term however they choose. If you prefer a group with a completely nonspiritual orientation, try Secular Organizations for Sobriety (SOS) or Rational Recovery (RR) or Women for Sobriety (WFS), all listed in the yellow pages under Alcoholism. These groups reject the AA emphasis on your own powerlessness; they stress the importance of personal responsibility and choice.

There are a number of special resources for members of specific ethnic groups. If you are African American, contact the National Black Alcoholism Council (NBAC) at 1-312-663-5780. If you are Hispanic, contact the National Coalition of Hispanic Health and Human Services Organizations (COSSMHO) at 1-202-371-2100. If you are Native American, contact the alcoholism/substance abuse coordinator at the Indian Health Service Office nearest you.

If you are unable or reluctant to attend a group, and if you own a computer, you might want to investigate computer recovery meetings. Compuserve, a national computer service, offers twelve-step (AA-style) meetings on line. You can log on using any name you like; anonymity is guaranteed. Or check out an electronic recovery bulletin board (BBS). Recovery BBS (1-415-223-1119), located in San Francisco, can provide you with a list of these boards. They let you access information from all over the country; some of them list group meetings in your area.

For good books on alcohol addiction, see the Recommended Reading at the end of this chapter.

Environmental Hazards

You can't open the newspaper nowadays without reading about carcinogens in the environment. There's pollution. There are food additives. There are chemical pesticides, such as 2,4-D. There are naturally occurring carcinogens, such as radon gas. Carcinogens are everywhere. Sometimes it's enough to make you think you should be living in an isolation chamber.

In fact, the risk of actually developing cancer from environmental sources is quite small–with one major exception. (We'll discuss that exception in a minute.) If you want to avoid *any* exposure to carcinogens, either because you have cancer now or simply because you dislike the idea of any exposure, then you may want to investigate this issue more fully. Learn all you can, and remove as many suspected carcinogens from your own environment as possible. To protect his environment, Charles Fuhrman got rid of the carcinogenic chemicals that he used in his graphic art. Now he uses gloves when he paints with oils; he uses a nontoxic thinner; and he makes sure to keep his studio well ventilated. Charles feels more in control now; he is doing all he can to give himself the best possible health.

The risk of actually developing cancer from environmental sources is quite small–with one major exception.

Facts about Environmental Hazards

If you live in today's society, you are going to be exposed to carcinogens. Here are examples of a few common substances that you may find in your environment.

Old insulation and old furnaces may contain *asbestos*. So, of course, do asbestos vinyl floors. The risk of contamination from asbestos is greatest when it is broken up (as during remodeling). If possible, asbestos should be left alone. If it must be removed, the work should be done by a specially licensed professional. Asbestos causes lung cancer, chest cancer, and abdominal cancer.

Radon gas is odorless, colorless, and radioactive. It is found in some building materials and in some well water. It may also be in the ground under your house. Radon causes lung cancer.

Benzene is found in lead-free gasoline. Benzene has been linked to leukemia. *Carbon tetrachloride*, another carcinogen, is found in some cleaning fluids.

Particleboard and fiberboard contain *formaldehyde*. So do some permanent-press fabrics. So do some glues. Formaldehyde gives off a strong-smelling, colorless, carcinogenic gas.

Indoor insect sprays contain many cancer-causing chemicals. So do many garden pesticides. Two of the best-known examples are *DDT* (now banned from sale) and *2,4-D*.

Vinyl chloride, found in PVC pipe, increases the risk of various cancers, especially liver cancer.[101]

All of these common substances are known or suspected carcinogens. Most of them can cause other diseases as well. Pesticides can cause damage to the central nervous system; formaldehyde can cause severe allergic reactions; and asbestos can cause asbestosis, an occupational lung disease.[102]

You don't have to isolate yourself in order to avoid exposure to carcinogens. You can reduce the risk they pose by making a few simple life-style changes. Even one change helps, and a few changes can make a big difference. But there is one carcinogen that everyone should avoid.

The Deadly Sun

> *Most people know that sunlight causes cancer. But most people still act as if sunlight were good for them.*

Most people know that sunlight causes cancer. But most people still act as if sunlight were good for them. If they're well, they work and play in the sun; if they're ill, they look forward to getting back out in the sunshine. And how many people think that they look healthier with a tan?

But sunlight kills.

Sunlight is responsible for almost all basal and squamous cell skin cancers, and it is a major risk factor for melanoma, the deadliest form of skin cancer. (The cure rate for advanced melanoma is just 14 percent.)[103]

Sunlight causes cancer because some of those golden

> ## Self-Exam for Skin Cancer
>
> Every two months check your body for lesions or moles, using the ABCD method:
> - Is the mark **A**symmetrical?
> - Does it have an irregular or jagged **B**order?
> - Is the **C**olor uneven?
> - Is it larger than a pencil eraser in **D**iameter?
>
> If the answer to any of these questions is yes, have the mark checked by a dermatologist.

rays are ultraviolet (UV) rays. Sit unprotected in the sun for a few hours and the UV rays start to kill your skin cells and destroy the connective tissue in the skin. UV radiation also distorts the DNA in skin cells. Over time this damage accumulates, causing the cells to grow abnormally. Eventually a cancer develops. Sometimes sunlight causes the formation of actinic keratoses. These rough, scaly patches are not cancers but they can develop into cancers.[104] Finally, UV radiation is thought to suppress immune function in the skin cells. This increases the risk of cancer even more.[105]

It's important to remember that the danger of sunlight is cumulative. Regular exposure over the years is what causes the damage. In fact, according to Dr. Sidney Hurwitz, professor of dermatology at Yale's School of Medicine, "most skin cancers begin in childhood."[106] On the other hand, ten minutes of exposure here and there also has a cumulative effect. That walk on your lunch hour, that fifteen minutes you spend mowing the lawn, that trip to the outpatient clinic in your wheelchair—it all adds up.

So how are you going to protect yourself?

In three ways. First, use a sunscreen whenever you go outside (and remember that "outside" includes riding in the car). Choose one with an SPF value of 15 or higher if you burn easily; of 8 to 15 if your skin is less sensitive; and be sure that it blocks both UVA and UVB rays. Don't

It's a good idea to make sure that your children wear sunscreen whenever they go out.

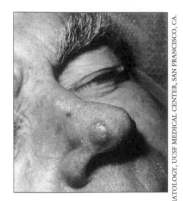

Basal cell carcinoma

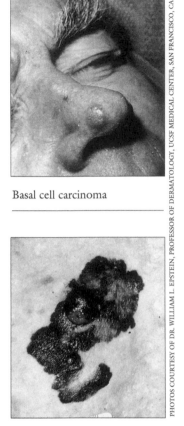

Melanoma

PHOTOS COURTESY OF DR. WILLIAM L. EPSTEIN, PROFESSOR OF DERMATOLOGY, UCSF MEDICAL CENTER, SAN FRANCISCO, CA.

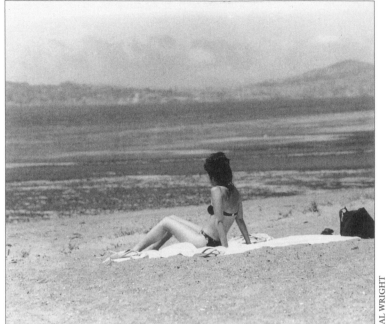

AL WRIGHT

Tanning is a suicidal practice.

forget that these rules apply if you are dark-skinned, too, especially if you'll be out in the sun for hours.

Second, wear loose clothing and a sun visor or a hat. And third, try to stay out of direct sunlight altogether between 10:00 A.M. and 3:00 P.M. That's when the sun's rays are the strongest.

"But," you say, "I want to get a tan."

For some people, getting a good tan is a major goal in life. They lie out in the sun, soaking up the warmth, imagining how great they're going to look. A little color may make you look healthier, and that warm glow may make you feel more alive. But that warm glow is already evidence of skin damage. Tanning is a suicidal practice, as we have just explained. "Think of the sun as a giant nuclear reactor," says one expert. "How much time would [you] want to risk in the glow of a nuclear power plant?"[107]

Besides, the beauty doesn't last. Tanning causes wrinkles, especially if you smoke. The tan is temporary, but the wrinkles are permanent. Tanning ages the skin prematurely.

It makes it dry, yellow, blotchy, inelastic, and baggy.[108] Do you really want to look like an alligator handbag and risk getting cancer at the same time? Think about that the next time you're lying out in the sun.

And don't think tanning with a sunlamp or in a tanning booth is any safer. Artificial sunlight is just as deadly as natural sunlight.

Sunlight is probably the single most dangerous carcinogen in your environment. Luckily, it is also one of the easiest to avoid. Not many life-style changes pay such big dividends with so little effort on your part.

For More Information...

In an emergency involving an environmental hazard, contact your local fire department. If poisons are involved, contact the nearest poison control center; look in the white pages under Emergency Crisis Hotlines.

If you suspect that there has been a toxic spill in your area, contact the National Response Center (NRC) at 1-800-424-8802. If you suspect long-term contamination of the air, soil, or water, you may want to have your house tested for toxic pollutants by a private independent testing lab. Look in the yellow pages under Laboratories, Testing, or Environmental Services. If the situation poses a threat to the public health, contact the nearest regional Environmental Protection Agency (EPA) office. These offices are listed in *Environmental Enforcement: A Citizen's Guide*, which also tells you how to see that the laws are enforced. To obtain a copy of this booklet, or of other EPA documents on enforcement, write to EPA, Office of Enforcement and Compliance Monitoring (LE-133), 401 M Street SW, Washington, DC 20460. If you suspect that a law is being violated, you can also contact the environmental health division of your city or county health department, listed in the white pages of the telephone book.

If your job brings you in contact with hazardous

"Think of the sun as a giant nuclear reactor," says one expert. "How much time would you want to risk in the glow of a nuclear power plant?"

substances, first make sure that safety regulations are stringently enforced. Next, learn all you can about the hazards of your workplace. In addition to the sources cited above, call the State Industrial Relations Department, Division of Occupational Safety and Health (OSHA), listed in the white pages under State Government. (In some states, this is a federal office.) Cal/OSHA publishes *A Guide to Developing Your Workplace Injury and Illness Prevention Program*; to obtain a copy, contact Cal/OSHA, 395 Oyster Point Blvd., Room 325, South San Francisco, CA 94080 (1-415-737-2843). If safety regulations are not being enforced, or if they do not cover known hazards, let management know. If this doesn't solve the problem, contact OSHA or the other sources cited above.

For help in assessing the safety of consumer products, call the Consumer Product Safety Commission at 1-800-638-2772.

For good books on environmental hazards and on ways of dealing with them, see the Recommended Reading at the end of this chapter.

Stress Reduction

In Chapter 6 we discussed stress reduction as a coping strategy. But stress reduction is more than just a tactic for coping with cancer (or with any other problem for that matter). Reducing stress is an important part of making any life-style change. It's an essential part of your long-range plan.

When you reduce the stress in your life, it's easier to focus on other priorities. It's easier to make changes. Above all, with stress under control, it's easier to stick to those changes once they are made. All this improves your quality of life.

Our position here is based upon our interviews with hundreds of cancer patients. It is also consistent with the findings of current research. One study of men and women who took a nine-hour course in stress control showed that the people who reduced their stress levels the most made the most life-style changes in subsequent years. These changes included taking up new hobbies ("pleasant events"), spending more time with other people ("family and friends"), and taking better care of their health.[109] Other studies suggest that stress management training helps cardiac patients to lose weight and to stop smoking,[110] and that it helps healthy people to eat less.[111]

Suppose you use stress control strategies to cope with the cancer experience and drop them when the cancer goes into remission. As you resume your previous life-style, the stresses of that life-style will return. They may even be worse as a result of the cancer experience. And you may deal with them by overeating, smoking, drinking, getting depressed, holding it all in–whatever mechanisms you used before. All this undermines the goal of your new program, which is to increase your control and so to achieve the highest possible quality of life.

That's why you need to make stress control part of any new program of change. Refer back to Chapter 6 for a discussion of stress control strategies and a list of Recommended Reading.

Screening

If you're a woman, do you give yourself a monthly breast exam? Most women know they should, but not all women do it. And yet, if breast cancer is caught in situ (before it has had a chance to spread), the cure rate is almost 100 percent.[112] That's just one example of the importance of screening.

If you don't do anything else we recommend, *get yourself screened regularly for cancer*. Screening can mean the difference between life and death. Unlike the other changes that we discuss, screening does not reduce your risk of developing cancer. However, *it greatly reduces the risk that any cancer you develop will have reached the incurable stage before you discover it.*

If you don't do anything else we recommend, get yourself screened regularly for cancer. Screening can mean the difference between life and death.

Breast Self-Examination

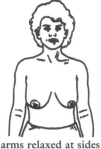

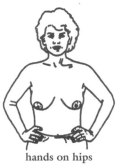

arms relaxed at sides

hands on hips

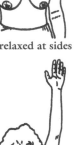

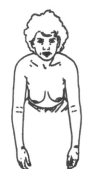

arms raised above head

bending forward

1. Positions

Visual Inspection: Standing

In each position, look for changes in contour and shape of the breasts, color and texture of the skin and nipple, and evidence of discharge from the nipples.

Palpation:

Use your left hand to palpate the right breast, while holding your right arm at a right angle to the rib cage, with the elbow bent. Repeat the procedure on the other side.

Side-Lying Position:

Lie on the opposite side of the breast to be examined. Rotate the shoulder (on the same side as the breast to be examined) back to the flat surface.

2. Perimeter

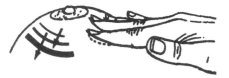

The examination a bounded by a line extends down fror middle of the arm to just beneath the breast, continues across along the underside of the b_ _ _ _ _ the middle of the breast bone, then moves up to and along the collarbone and back to the middle of the armpit. Most breast cancers occur in the upper outer area of the breast (shaded area).

light
medium
deep

3. Pressure

Use varying levels of pressure for *each palpation,* from light to deep, to examine the full thickness of your breast tissue. Using pressure will not injure the breast.

4. Pattern of Search

Vertical Strip:

Start in the armpit, proceed downward to the lower boundary. Move a finger's width toward the middle and continue palpating upward until you reach the collarbone. Repeat this until you have covered all breast tissue. Make at least six strips before the nipple and four strips

start in armpit

after the nipple. You may need between 10 and 16 strips. Palpate carefully beneath the nipple. Any incision should also be carefully examined from end to end. Women who have had any breast surgery should still examine the entire area and the incision.

Source: American Cancer Society, California Division, *Breast Self Examination: A New Approach,* Publication no. 6438.39, revised May 1992. Printed with permission of the American Cancer Society, California Division.

Facts about Screening

The American Cancer Society states that regular screening can detect cancers of the breast, tongue, mouth, colon, rectum, cervix, prostate, and testis. Regular screening can also detect early melanoma. These nine sites represent half of all new cases. With early detection about 89 percent of these cancers can be cured.[113]

So it's critically important to catch cancer early. There are two ways of doing this. First, the ACS lists seven warning signs that may indicate cancer. Memorize these warning signs. See a doctor immediately if you spot any one of them:

- A change in bowel or bladder habits
- A sore that does not heal
- Unusual bleeding or discharge from the genital, urinary, or digestive tract
- A thickening or lump in the breast or elsewhere
- Indigestion or difficulty in swallowing
- An obvious change in a wart or mole
- A persistent cough or hoarseness

Remember: if you exhibit one or two of these signs, it doesn't necessarily mean that you have cancer. Don't panic. But see the doctor promptly, to make sure.

On the other hand, remember that cancer can start in your body without causing any of these signs. That is why it is important to get regular screenings.

When we say "screenings," here and throughout, we mean *cancer-related screenings*. We do not mean ordinary annual checkups, which are not designed to screen for early cancer. The ACS recommends a cancer-related screening every three years for men and women between twenty and thirty-nine and every year for men and women forty and over. In addition, women between twenty and thirty-nine should have a breast exam done by a doctor every three years; women forty and over should have one every year. Women eighteen or older, and younger women who have been sexually active, should have a Pap smear every year. After three or more consecutive normal annual exams, the Pap smear may be done less often; discuss it

Table 3: Summary of American Cancer Society Recommendations for Early Detection of Cancer in Asymptomatic Persons at Average Risk

Examination	Sex	Age	Periodicity
Sigmoidoscopy	M and F	Age 50 and older	1 exam every 3 to 5 years
Stool Blood Test	M and F	Age 50 and older	Every year
Digital Rectal Examination	M and F	Age 40 and older	Every year
Testicular Self-Examination	M	Age 15 and older	Every month
Pap Test and Pelvic Examination	F	Women who have been sexually active or have reached age 18 or older	Every year. After 3 or more satisfactory, consecutive, normal annual examinations, the Pap test may be performed less frequently at the discretion of the physician.
Endometrial Tissue Sample	F	At menopause; women at high risk*	At menopause
Breast Self-Examination	F	Age 20 and older	Every month
Clinical Breast Examination	F	20-39 Age 40 and older	Every 3 years Every year
Mammography	F	35-39 40-49 50 and over	Baseline Every 1 to 2 years Every year
Health Counseling**	M and F	20-40	Every 3 years
Cancer Checkup***	M and F	Age 40 and older	Every year

*History of infertility, obesity, failure to ovulate, abnormal uterine bleeding, or estrogen therapy.
**To include counseling about tobacco control, sun exposure, diet and nutrition, risk factors, sexual practices, and environmental and other occupational exposures.
***To include examination for cancers of the thyroid, testicles, prostate, ovaries, lymph nodes, oral cavity, and skin.

Source: Diane J. Fink, *Guidelines for the Cancer-Related Checkup* (Atlanta, GA: American Cancer Society, 1991), 4; "For Men Only: Testicular Cancer and How to Do TSE," brochure published by the American Cancer Society, 2093-LE, 1990.

with your doctor. Men and women forty and over should have an annual digital rectal examination, and men and women fifty and over should have an annual stool blood test. The ACS also recommends that they have a sigmoidoscopy every three to five years.

Men should perform a monthly self-examination for testicular cancer. This is important for men of all ages, but especially for those between fifteen and thirty-four, who are at highest risk. If you find an abnormal nodule or lump, consult your doctor. Finally, the ACS recommends that women twenty and older do a breast self-examination every month and that older women have regular mammograms. A baseline mammogram should be done between age thirty-five and thirty-nine; this is used for comparison with mammograms taken later. Starting at age forty, women should have a mammogram every one to two years. Starting at age fifty, they should have mammograms taken yearly. These recommendations are summarized in table 3.

These are the standard recommendations. Your own physician may recommend that you be tested more frequently or at different intervals, particularly if you are at a high risk of cancer. Especially if you fall into the high-risk category, we suggest that you follow your own doctor's recommendations. That way you will get the screening best suited to your individual needs.

Men can get breast cancer too. If you are a man, you should consult a doctor promptly if you find a lump or other noticeable change in the breast area.

Eight Bad Reasons for Not Getting Screened

Fear of cancer

How often have you heard someone say, "If I have cancer, I don't want to know"? This is the first big reason why people don't get screened. As we said at the beginning of this chapter, "cancer" is a terrifying word. Some people are so afraid of cancer that they refuse to think about it. But if you refuse to think about it, you have no control at all; cancer—or the fear of cancer—has control of you. If you want to take control of your life, you must be prepared to face and deal with your anxiety.

For more on mastering emotions, see Chapter 6.

Fatalistic thinking

Some people have an even more fatalistic attitude. These people believe that cancer equals death; their position is "Why bother to get screened? If I have cancer,

The risk you run by getting the X ray is nothing compared to the risk you run by not getting it.

I'm going to die anyway." This is a particularly irrational argument in view of the survival rates cited earlier. Look again at those figures; they show that almost all of the people with nine common cancers can be completely cured *if the cancer is caught early.* But that's *if* the cancer is caught early. You won't catch it early if you don't get screened.

Denial

Then there's the "Why worry?" approach, also known as "If it ain't broke, don't fix it." People who take this approach tell themselves that cancer won't happen to them. As we pointed out at the beginning of this chapter, this is just another form of denial. And denial can be deadly.

Fear of X rays

X rays are often used to screen for cancer. That's enough to keep some people from getting screened. These people have read that X rays give you cancer; to them, getting an X ray is like walking into the lion's den. If this sounds like you, ask your doctor to explain how little risk is actually involved, and why it's important for you to have the test. You will learn that the risk you run by getting the X ray is nothing compared to the risk you run by not getting it.

Fear of embarrassment

One out of eleven American men will develop prostate cancer; it is second only to skin cancer among this population. And prostate cancer is the second leading cause of cancer deaths in men (the first is lung cancer). Scary? Yes; but the cure rate for prostate cancer is 88 percent when it is detected while it is still localized. This can be done during a routine rectal exam. It can also be done from a blood sample drawn during a routine physical (the so-called PSA exam). Getting both exams increases the chance of detecting the cancer by 34 percent.[114] It has been estimated that getting a regular screening for prostate cancer could save the lives of about 116,000 men a year.[115] Yet the majority of American men don't get screened.[116]

Why not? Usually because they are uncomfortable undergoing this examination. Ask yourself: Is it worth a little discomfort to save your life?

Fear of pain

It has been estimated that routine mammograms could reduce breast cancer deaths by up to 50 percent.[117] Yet many women avoid getting mammograms because they are afraid of the pain. It is true that a mammogram is mildly uncomfortable. It is not painful (or "agonizing" or "excruciating"), no matter what your friends may have told you. And the discomfort, if any, lasts only a few seconds. Sigmoidoscopy, used to screen for colon cancer, is another exam with an undeservedly scary reputation. One of the Alpha team of writers underwent her first sigmoidoscopy after working on the chapter you are now reading. In this exam, a long, flexible scope is inserted about twenty inches into the lower colon. The writer had heard many horror stories about this procedure, but she found that in fact the pain was negligible. A little discomfort, or even a little pain, is a small price to pay for catching cancer early.

Expense

Some people avoid getting screened for reasons that have nothing to do with fear. Sometimes they think it's just too expensive. In fact, the cost of screening varies widely. A mammogram that might cost $100 if it was done by a private physician can cost as little as $27 in a community screening program. Some health insurance plans cover screening mammography. A Pap smear can run from $34 to $100, and a digital rectal exam can cost $20 or $30 if it requires a special visit to the doctor's office. If you're seeing the doctor for something else anyway, it will cost less.[118] If money is an issue, remember that screening can save your life, and ask yourself what else you can economize on instead. Can you do without that new coat for a while? Or think of the money you could save if you quit smoking.

If you want to gain control, you must make a commitment to your health and to the quality of your life. This includes making a commitment to getting screened regularly for cancer.

Ignorance

Finally, some people don't get screened because they don't know that there is such a thing as screening. Maybe you can tell them.

We've said it before and we'll say it again: if you want to gain control, you must make a commitment to your health and to the quality of your life. This includes making a commitment to getting screened regularly for cancer.

For More Information...

For more specific information about the hows and whys of screening, contact the American Cancer Society at 1-800-ACS-2345.

For information on where to get screening, contact your local office of the ACS. Be sure to get your mammograms from a center accredited by the American College of Radiology (ACR). Some mammography test units use poor equipment and inadequately trained personnel. To learn whether a center is accredited, call the ACS at 1-800-ACS-2345 or the American College of Radiology at 1-703-648-8900. And ask the center to show you an individual certificate for the mammography machine that will be used to test you. The equipment should be designed specifically for mammography.

Part 3:
The Mind's Way

There are two approaches you can take to gain control over your life. The first one is the body's way; the second one is the mind's way. In the following pages we examine faith and sense of purpose—two areas where you may want to consider making changes. We also examine the role of cancer as teacher.

Faith

Faith plays a vital role in many people's lives, but especially in the lives of many cancer patients. Most cancer patients face the possibility of death, and some must ultimately accept that they are going to die. Coming face-to-face with death can change deeply held beliefs, sometimes dramatically, sometimes in subtle ways. Faith helps these patients to deal with their fear, and so to gain more control over their lives.

In this section we discuss both religious beliefs and nonreligious, or what we call "spiritual," beliefs. We define *religious belief* as belief in the doctrine of an orthodox religion. We define *spiritual belief* as a belief that focuses on a personal relationship with a higher power, but one that is not necessarily dependent on religious doctrine. In the following discussion, we use the word "faith" to refer to both. When we wish to distinguish religious beliefs from spiritual beliefs, we use those terms.

Some of the patients we spoke with engaged in formal religious practices. Others took solace in reading religious or spiritual material. Although these patients felt no need to participate in formal ceremonies, they took time to reflect on ideas that had become important to them. This

"God has given us the opportunity to live each moment. And how we live that is up to us. Our commitment, always, from day one, was a commitment to life."

–John Wienecke

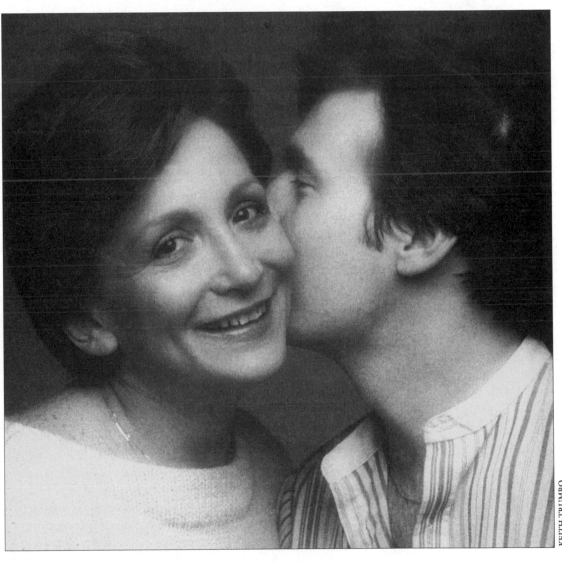

Marcie and John Wienecke

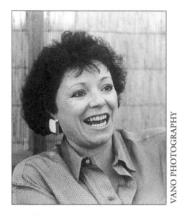

Julie Benbow

VANO PHOTOGRAPHY

"It's faith in a thing other than yourself. A belief that you have to—you want to—go on because it's good to go on."

—Julie Benbow

meditation comforted them and often provided them with insights on how they wanted to live their lives.

Other patients gained inspiration from nontraditional sources. "I'm a New Age kind of person," says Nancy Heitz. "I believe in crystal healing. I meditate. And when I'm really feeling depressed, I go in my room and I turn out the lights and just get into myself." And nature—sunrises, night skies, magnificent storms—can provide many people with deep comfort. That's where they feel closest to their higher being. "When I'm hiking in the mountains or walking by the ocean, I feel the closest to God," one patient told us. "I can really feel His presence there."

In general, patients in whose lives faith played an important role fell into three categories: those for whom faith had always been important; those who had returned to their former faith after having abandoned it; and those who had just discovered, or were in the process of discovering, the value of religious or spiritual beliefs. Patients in this last group came to their faith in a variety of ways. Some spoke of slowly developing a trust in something outside themselves. Others described their faith as a blessing or a gift. A positive experience—having a test come back negative, for example—strengthened some people's belief in the existence of a higher power. And for others faith developed more or less of its own accord, growing directly out of the cancer experience. As Nancy Heitz succinctly put it, "The minute you find out you're dying, you believe in something."

What was that something? What did these patients have faith in? Most of them simply believed in God. Shortly after a massive tumor was discovered in his chest, Jeff Losea, a devout Christian, heard a voice inside his head that said, "Don't worry. I'm with you." Jeff believed that "the Lord spoke to me, and I could relax, because it was in His hands."

The sense of giving in to something higher than themselves was common to all the patients for whom faith was a factor, whether or not they held religious beliefs. "It's not just faith in God," Julie Benbow told us. "It's faith in a thing other than yourself. A belief that you have to—you want to—go on because it's good to go on." And Odile Belladonna described it as "a sense of trust that I never experienced before in my life. Just a sense of very deep trust that it wasn't just me. I didn't have to do it alone."

Faith helped these patients to overcome their fear. But paradoxically, they gained control by giving up control. For many, faith meant a kind of profound surrender, a giving in to a higher power. Odile Belladonna called it "giving up the fearful control and allowing for the greater control to take over. It's like clutching onto something so tightly because you don't know what's on the other side. When you let go of that, something else can take form. There's room for something else." Or as another patient put it, echoing a tenet of Alcoholics Anonymous, it can be a profound relief to "let go and let God."

What did these patients gain from their faith? First, it gave them a sense that there was meaning to their lives, to the experience of having cancer. "You have to believe that because something bad is happening to you now," says Julie Benbow, "that maybe it's a way of becoming a better person." Barbara Fritz, a patient and the wife of a patient, expressed a similar view from the perspective of her own religion. "I've had too many things happen to me, and too many challenges, to be able to not think that there's a God. I mean, there is a reason for me to be here. And I hope to get to a certain point in my life where I can really leave it in the hands of God, instead of trying to fix it myself. And realize that there's a reason that He gives me challenges, and that after I go through them, maybe I will gain more insight into life itself and just why I'm here."

Faith gave our patients a deep sense of security in the face of death. "Faith is a tremendous help," says Barbara Johns. "I don't know if I could ever get through without my faith, really. So many people are just living thinking they're going to die every minute. I don't." Jay Fritz says that his faith allowed him to accept with composure the possibility "that for some reason I was only going to get forty years where others get eighty." When her husband was diagnosed with cancer, Diane Losea's faith enabled her

> *"I've had too many things happen to me, and too many challenges, to be able to not think that there's a God."*
>
> —**Barbara Fritz**

to believe that even if Jeff didn't make it, "it was going to be OK. It was going to be OK." And she adds, "God has given me such peace, where I know before, without God, I was a mess."

And when death did occur, faith helped our patients' families to find meaning in the experience and to accept it. "I had to accept it, and I couldn't have, by myself," says Lois Ryder. "It was through my faith in God. I have said many times, 'Not my will, but God's will.' I think it was God's will that time. I had to believe that to overcome my own sadness."

Faith quiets the mind; it silences the voice of the Inner Critic; it replaces insecurity with calm. A renewed sense of faith enabled Odile Belladonna to find her inner balance for the first time. "I'm not stressed out anymore. I used to explode at the drop of a hat because there was so much I had repressed within myself. Now I have a willingness to accept what is. I don't try to control out of insecurity or fear."

Faith provides social support. Patients who attended church after a long absence were often touched by the concern of others who shared their beliefs. "I just couldn't believe it," says Barbara Johns. "When I was in the hospital, I had just really started getting involved in the church. And care—the people that came, caring! There is not one Sunday goes by that you're not prayed for in church. It's just really very caring."

If faith is your way, we urge you to use it as a complement to—not a substitute for—treatment. Dennis Brown tells a joke about a cancer patient who prayed to God for help "—and he saw a vision of God saying, 'Don't worry, my son. I'm going to cure you.' The oncologist came in and told him they were going to start chemotherapy. And he said, 'Oh, no, I don't need you. God's going to cure me.' The radiation therapist came in and told him, 'You're going to have radiation.' And he said, 'No, I don't need it. God's going to cure me.' He saw a nutritionist and said the same thing. A little while later he died and went to Heaven. And he said, 'God, I just don't

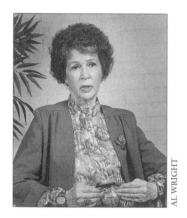

Lois Ryder

AL WRIGHT

"I had to accept it, and I couldn't have, by myself."

–Lois Ryder

360

understand it. How could you let me down?' God said, 'I didn't. I sent you an oncologist and a radiation therapist and a nutritionist. And you sent them all away.'"

Don't make that mistake. Better to be like Jeff Losea. Jeff's faith that he was in God's hands gave him the courage to explore all the medical options.

There are innumerable faiths—Western and Eastern, old and new, traditional and nontraditional—and many ways of developing a spiritual life. Finding the way that is right for you is a highly individual matter. It's a little like finding the right doctor or the right treatment program. You want something that feels right to you, but also something that your mind accepts, something that makes sense to you intellectually and emotionally. To start your search, read up on the faiths that interest you. Go to churches, temples, lectures, and meetings; talk to the people who share the beliefs you are investigating. What do they say? What do they seem to get out of their faith? Do they, and their answers, appeal to you? Listen with your mind and heart. Above all, what is your gut-level reaction? Does it *feel* right for you?

Be patient. It can take time, and sometimes considerable searching, to develop a spiritual life. Then again, you may find your path immediately, with no search at all. But the search itself can start to open your mind and heart to the benefits of having faith.

Sense of Purpose

What is *your* purpose in life?

Some people don't need one. Some people do need one, and they know exactly what it is. Many people need to have a purpose in life but they can't seem to find one; this makes them feel frustrated, anxious, and depressed. If that sounds familiar, this section may be for you. Because a sense of purpose can be developed.

We define *purpose* as the way you want to live, and what you want to be the result of your living. We define *sense of purpose* as your commitment to that ideal.

Your purpose is not the same thing as your priorities. Your purpose is *why;* your priorities are *how.* Your priorities are the things you do in order to achieve your purpose.

To understand the difference between purpose and priorities, consider Stan, a drug addict in recovery. Stan's purpose in life is to help other people to stay clean. His first priority is to stay clean himself. His second priority is to get an honest job. His third priority is to learn how to relate to other people. Helping others to stay clean is Stan's ideal. Stan's priorities are the steps that keep him headed toward that ideal.

Having a sense of purpose gives you more control over your life. It helps you to reach your full potential in one area – the area that is most important to you – and this, in turn, increases your self-esteem. A keen sense of purpose is a powerful motivation to look beyond your current problems, to see them as obstacles to be surmounted. Many of the patients we interviewed told us that having a strong sense of purpose was as helpful in this respect as having faith. (The two can be interrelated, as you will see presently.)

It's important to realize that your purpose in life can change. This is especially true for people who have cancer. When you are actually battling cancer, your purpose in life is usually to win, to get through the illness, to survive. But when you are cured or are in remission, you may ask yourself, "What now? What am I going to do with the rest of my life?" And you may have trouble coming up with an answer.

If you find yourself in this position, try not to worry. Honor the intense battle you have just fought and give yourself time to rest and recuperate. But while you rest, leave yourself open to discovery.

Developing a sense of purpose isn't always easy. To the recovering cancer patient, developing a sense of purpose can seem like having to move yet another mountain. But as patients throughout this book testify, mountains *can* be moved, stone by stone.

"I didn't want to do it," Julie Benbow told us. "I mean,

I left it as long as I could. You can do it fairly superficially, or you can do it from a fundamental point of view. 'What is my life worth? What am I doing with my life? Am I being a good person? How am I relating to other people?' And that takes a lot out of you. But it also gives you the gift of life again. The gift to go forward with a new set of eyes and a new identity."

So don't be discouraged. Do the best you can. Take your time and let the answers come. And have faith that they will come in time.

Meanwhile, try to get the most you can out of your life. You may discover, after you think about it for a while, how good your life really is right now. You may even discover that you had a purpose all along–and that you are already fulfilling that purpose.

What is *your* purpose in life? To save the rain forest? To have your own business? To work for world peace? To have a family? To be happy? To get you started thinking, we discuss one possible answer to this question and illustrate it with examples provided by our patients. For these people, the answer was "Helping others."

Going through the cancer experience often shows patients another side of life, one that they may not have known much about before. This can lead them to find a new purpose in giving to others. "I do feel a strong compulsion that I should help other people," Polly McMahon told us. "I felt it was something I had to learn, that I had missed out on. And so I have gravitated toward helping people who are sick." And she adds, "I feel that my life is expanding into different horizons than it would have done had I remained perfectly healthy."

This last comment was echoed by many of the patients we talked to. As having cancer led them to help others, so the experience of helping others altered their feelings about having cancer. Esther Joyce made this discovery while she was teaching orthopedically handicapped children:

"I had been crying all night. I went to work, and I found by the time I hit the classroom until the time the children left, I didn't have a thought about it. It was the best therapy

> *"I had been crying all night. I went to work, and I found by the time I hit the classroom until the time the children left, I didn't have a thought about it. It was the best therapy I could have had."*
>
> –Esther Joyce

I could have had. Here were these three-year-olds; one was pushing a walker, saying ,'Look at me! I'm standing! I'm walking!' The courage of these babies was something to behold. So it was, from my point of view, very fortunate that I started on this job and that I was in an atmosphere where I could be helping very brave youngsters."

It was their faith that led some patients to help others. Jay Fritz, a practicing Catholic, told us quite simply that his purpose in life was to emulate Christ's Gospel, and he described the satisfaction he got out of doing so:

"I get a really good sense that I am doing what Christ said, 'to help the least of mine.' I know I feel good sharing. It just gives you a sense that you're doing the right thing. You know you've helped people. You go out to the Little Sisters of the Poor, and a couple of months ago we gave them a Christmas party. I'll never forget—I was tending bar, actually, after Mass, and one of the ladies came up and said, 'Do you serve any bourbon?' And I turned around, and I heard a voice saying, 'That's for me!' There was an old, ninety-six-year-old lady in a wheelchair, and saying, 'Boy, I look forward to this day!' You know, you just feel good about it. I mean, somehow I brought happiness into her life."

Jay is a member of the Knights of Malta, a 900-year-old Catholic lay order whose purpose is to help the sick and the poor. Members of the order go on an annual pilgrimage to the Shrine of Lourdes, in southern France:

"We are assigned a [sick] person, usually a different person every day, and we take care of that person. Anything that he or she wants to do for that day. It might mean getting them cleansed in the baths, if they wanted to use the baths…the healing water in the baths. The Lourdes water, that is responsible for sixty or seventy-five or in that range of miracles that have been documented."

Jay described movingly for us what he gets out of these pilgrimages:

"Growing up in America, we really don't see the poor and the sick very much. We're sort of sanitized. Some of us go through life not seeing anything. When I first went to

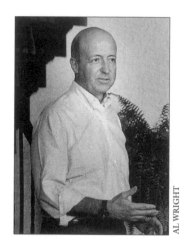

Jay Fritz

"I know I feel good sharing. It just gives you a sense that you're doing the right thing. You know you've helped people."

–Jay Fritz

AL WRIGHT

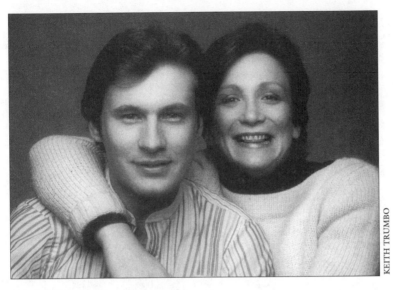

John and Marcie Wienecke

"My purpose was providing quality life for her....The time that we had together in that last thirteen months was one of the richest times I ever had."

–John Wienecke

Lourdes, it was like a shock to me, because there were people all over, and they were all sick. And many of them very ill or deformed. You almost want to shrink away a little bit, because you don't know how to handle it. But it builds up every time you help. I feel better; it's easier for me to do. And I'm doing more of it."

Some family members found their purpose in helping the patient. John Wienecke found it in helping his wife, Marcie:

"My purpose was providing quality life for her. To be with her in a transition that would be nurturing to her. To empower her to face that situation. The time that we had together in that last thirteen months was one of the richest times I ever had. It was exciting, it was joyful, it was living life with all cylinders in gear. And it was just my commitment to another person."

If you want to help others, one good way to start is to work through organizations that can use your skills. Jay Fritz, a successful entrepreneur, put his business skills to good use by serving on hospital and school boards. Esther Joyce, a retired schoolteacher, used her skills to help handicapped children. Take a look at *your* skills. Can you cook? Find a program that provides meals for the

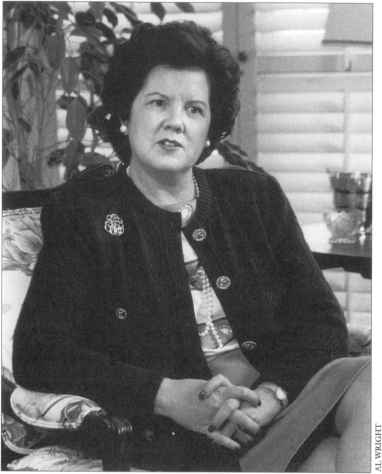

AL WRIGHT

Barbara Fritz

housebound or the homeless. Do you like books? Volunteer to read to the blind or take charge of the library cart in a local hospital. Can you teach? Teach adults to read or help recent immigrants to learn English. Are you good with animals? Volunteer at the local animal shelter or join an organization such as Therapy Dogs, Inc. that takes pets to visit people in nursing homes. Can you drive? Type? Make simple repairs? There are hundreds of organizations that can use your skills. What can you do to help others? As Esther Joyce says, "Look around in the world. A lot of horrible things are going on, but there's also a lot of opportunity for a better world. And it's important to see that. Grab hold of it."

Some people's purpose is to live life to the fullest. Like so much else, what this means depends on whom you ask. For some people, it means having fun–enjoying each moment to the fullest. For some people, it means doing as much as you can as well as you can. For some people, living life to the fullest means being the best person you can be. –Like Barbara Fritz:

"My main purpose is to try to continually improve upon the goodness that has been given me. I mean, to continue to grow, to grow as a stronger person. So I'm basically just trying to be a better person every single day. The best I know how."

But living life to the fullest is really a whole new subject in itself. And it's all tied in with the subject of cancer as teacher.

Cancer as Teacher

At the beginning of this chapter we listed four groups of people who fear cancer, because for each of them cancer can mean loss of control. These were people who have never had cancer, people who have cancer now, people who are in remission, and people who are facing a terminal prognosis. People in all four of these groups told us how they set priorities, made changes based on those priorities, and in this way gained a new sense of control over their lives. Throughout this chapter we have explained how you can do this too.

In this last section, we describe what the patients and family members whom we interviewed learned by going through the cancer experience. We have known many people who have learned these same things without being touched by cancer in any way. We don't mean to suggest, then, that one must get cancer in order to learn how to live. Cancer, however, can be a powerful teacher.

Dealing with cancer taught our patients several important lessons. First and most simply, it taught them to deal with

> *"My main purpose is to try to continually improve upon the goodness that has been given me....to continue to grow."*
>
> –Barbara Fritz

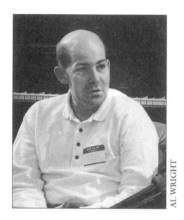

Chris Maggart

"Whether patients want to believe it or not, they will be exposed to all sorts of new ideas and people, and their lives will change for the better."

–Chris Maggart

AL WRIGHT

life. Patients who learned to cope using the skills outlined in Chapter 6, and to gain control using the skills discussed in this chapter, found that they could use these skills to deal with problems and setbacks of any kind. Learning to deal with cancer taught them to deal with their health, their families, and their work in new, creative ways.

Beyond this, cancer taught these patients and their families to see their lives in a new light. It expanded their horizons; it gave them a sense of opportunity; and this, in turn, taught them to see the cancer itself in a new light. Chris Maggart, who was cured of a brain tumor, put it like this:

"Whether patients want to believe it or not, they will be exposed to all sorts of new ideas and people, and their lives will change for the better. Experience is the best form of learning. And this learning expands your horizons– sometimes one-thousandfold."

And Julie Benbow, who underwent radiation treatment for cancer of the thyroid, describes the cancer experience as "gray fog. And you have to get from one side of it to the other. But when you get to the other side, you're standing at the end of Green Street [in San Francisco] going, 'Look at the view!'"

Above all, cancer taught these patients and their families to live life to the fullest. What does this mean?

Living life to the fullest means getting all you can out of every aspect of your life–your whole life, not just your career, say, or your relationships. Living life to the fullest means learning the skills of living. Ultimately, living life to the fullest means developing faith in your own value, in the value of other people, in the value of your goals and of your ability to achieve those goals.

Living life to the fullest means being committed. Committed to doing the best you can with whatever life hands you. Committed to seeking the best possible quality of life, even under difficult circumstances. Committed to your own standards, your own values, your own sense of integrity. John Wienecke, who nursed his wife through breast cancer that had metastasized to the spine, put it like this:

"God has given us the opportunity to live each moment.

And how we live that is up to us. Our commitment, always, from day one, was a commitment to life. And what that means is doing the things that make life work."

It may seem strange to think of cancer as a teacher. But perhaps it is not so strange. Lily Kravcisin, whose mother died of ovarian cancer, comments:

"The existentialists believe that until you get in touch with your own death, you're really not going to live your life fully. You're not going to appreciate what life has to offer. So in many ways, all this ends up being a gift. It's a painful gift, but that's what people grow from."

How did cancer teach these patients to live life fully? In the rest of this section, we're going to let them answer that question for themselves.

Lesson One: Learning to Accept Life as It Is

To live life to the fullest means to accept life as it is. It means accepting the pain along with the pleasure, the trough of the wave along with the crest. Accepting life means using your energy to work with life as it is, not wasting your energy wishing that things were different. Charles Fuhrman puts it like this:

"Before anything happened to me, when I was healthy, I was miserable, because nothing was enough. I wasn't successful enough. I wasn't tall enough. I wasn't good-looking enough. I wasn't smart enough. I wasn't talented enough. You name it. All the way down. I didn't have a Mercedes. I wasn't famous. I wasn't well known. I wasn't selling my work. And now, the big difference, because this happened, is that for the first time in my life I am satisfied with what I have. And you know, it's too bad that I had to learn it this way, but I did. One of the great gifts of having this illness."

Interestingly, learning to accept life as it is gave some patients a new sense of control. "My whole life I felt like I was swimming upstream," says Linda Sumner. "I have always been fighting life and never flowing with it. And I think if there's one thing this illness has taught me, it's

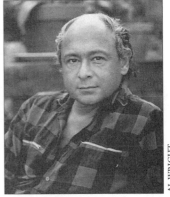

Charles Fuhrman

AL WRIGHT

"The big difference, because this happened, is that for the first time in my life I am satisfied with what I have."

–**Charles Fuhrman**

> *"I learned that you need to let other people live their life path. And everybody has their own life path."*
>
> **– Kris Richardson**

how to flow with life." And she adds, "It helped me to understand that there are certain things that I'm never going to be able to control. And not to waste my energy on those areas. And to really focus in on those areas that I can control, which would be my diet, my exercise, taking care of Linda. And when I do that, I feel empowered."

Learning to accept life as it is means learning to accept the changes that cancer brings. This can be extremely painful, but the pain diminishes with acceptance. "One has to embrace that change," Charles Fuhrman told us. "You can't resist it. You can't fight it. The more one fights it, the more problems it's going to cause. That's the hardest thing in the world–to accept that, that it's really here. It's really happened. Once one accepts it, it loses power over you."

Kris Richardson sums up this lesson in her own way. Kris, who nursed her mother when she was dying of breast cancer, learned that "there are certain things that just seem to be beyond our control. That seem to be our life path. I know that I can't go out there and fix the world. There's a part of me that wants to go out there and fix it. Through this experience with my mother I learned that you need to let other people live their life path. And everybody has their own life path."

Lesson Two: Learning to Deal with Fear

One of the most important lessons that cancer teaches is how to deal with fear–the fear of the unknown, the fear of death, the fear of fear itself. The fear of losing control. For Paula Carroll, who was told after ten years that her breast cancer had recurred, the key was knowing that she had beaten cancer before:

"I could feel this fear just overtaking me. And I thought, 'Now, come on, Paula. You've been through a lot. I mean, this isn't the first time that you've gone through this.' It was, to be honest with you, frightening. But I thought, 'I'm not going to give in to it.' I thought, 'What are my resources? What is my strength?' What was I able to call forth? So by the time my husband came home about an hour later, I was able to say to him, 'This is the call I got.' But I knew I already had a game plan."

Many patients found that learning the facts helped them to deal with fear. Nancy Heitz, who has had incurable bone cancer since childhood, told us:

"The last bone scan I had, I was really scared to go back to the doctor, knowing that it had gone to the kidneys, and different various things like that. I thought, 'Ohh, Nancy, you don't want to do this. You don't want to go to the doctor and hear all this bad news.' And I thought, 'No, I don't want to go and hear bad news; you're right. I want to go and get the facts. The facts I can live with. The being dumb and afraid and scared will kill me.' So I went and found out the facts, and they weren't as bad as I had envisioned."

Sometimes the fear turns out to be *completely* unjustified. Lois Ryder told us about her old friend Tom Watt, who "was scared to death because a lump under one kneecap was getting bigger and bigger. He was so afraid that it was cancer that he waited seven years before he finally went to the doctor. By that time the lump was so huge that it was hard to get any pants to fit. He said he knew now that he was going to die. The doctor told him that it was just a big old benign cyst. He says, 'And to think I wasted seven long years worrying!'"

Cancer can teach family members to deal with fear, sometimes by forcing them to face an issue that they had been avoiding. This is what happened to Kris Richardson when her mother died:

"I started working on my career. I'd always been kind of slaphappy about it, and that's changed. I've really decided to take responsibility for myself. Because a lot of that floundering around and being lackadaisical about it was simply fear. I always had the feeling that if it all went wrong, I could go home and live with my mother. And that was very eye-opening. That I didn't really have her to go home to."

Cancer taught many patients that, when it comes to fear, the thing they had imagined was often worse than the reality. Living with terminal melanoma, said Arnold

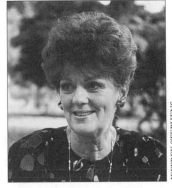

JEFFREY STEPHENS

Paula Carroll

"I could feel this fear just overtaking me. And I thought, 'Now, come on, Paula....I mean, this isn't the first time that you've gone through this.'"

–Paula Carroll

371

"We're really all one. You know, that destroys a lot of the fear of death. Because the fear comes from the separation.... When I don't feel separate from everybody, I don't feel fear."

–Arnold Schraer

Schraer, "you envision scenarios that are frightening–that way down are frightening. But my friend pointed out to me, she says, 'Arnold, you've already faced what everybody is scared of. There's really nothing else to be afraid of.'"

For many, the deepest fear is the fear of death. Everyone who is diagnosed with cancer faces this fear, and our patients dealt with it in a variety of ways. Some of them found that the cancer experience taught them to view death in a more constructive light. Charles Fuhrman put it like this:

"Even if you do get a recurrence, you can look at it in a positive way. I mean, it's frightening. Terribly frightening. But also, the other side of it is that it's another journey. It can be another journey."

Some patients said that cancer taught them other lessons that helped them to face the fear of death. Arnold Schraer, who gave a party for all his friends when he was dying, said that cancer had taught him that he was connected to other people:

"I've been able to learn how to ask for my needs to be met. It's been a great gift that everyone's given me, and I want to be able to share it, give that back in some way to people who feel like their lives are just narrow and isolated. That they're not; they're part of a larger community; that we're really all one. You know, that destroys a lot of the fear of death. Because the fear comes from the separation–that you feel separate. When I don't feel separate from everybody, I don't feel fear."

No matter where you are in the cancer experience, we believe that you can learn to deal with fear. If you are in good health, you can learn from the experiences of the patients we interviewed. If you have cancer now, you can say, like Nancy Heitz, "The facts I can live with. The being dumb and afraid and scared will kill me." If you fear a recurrence, you can say, like Paula Carroll, "It wouldn't be the first time you've gone through this." And if, like Arnold Schraer, you are facing a terminal prognosis, you can learn to say, "We're part of a larger community. We're really all one."

Lesson Three: Learning to Appreciate Yourself

Dealing with cancer can cause a shift, sometimes a radical shift, in the patient's self-image. The fact that you are able to deal with the problems that cancer poses can become more significant than the problems themselves. This can be enormously empowering. And it can teach you things you never knew about yourself.

"You find out that you're made of some really tough stuff," says Carol Landt, who helped to nurse her mother through terminal brain cancer. "I discovered that, no matter what else, we could *both* count on me, and that I was *very* capable."

What taught the cancer patients their own strength? The answer varied with the patient. For Dennis Brown, it was simply discovering how much he could take:

"I think learning that I have very high, if any, upper limits to what I can tolerate has been an advantage. Because if you aren't really put to the test, there's no way you can ever be certain of what your limits of endurance are. So I think you could say that's a positive. It's certainly been of benefit to me to show me how much strength I actually have."

In a dark moment, Charles Fuhrman said it was the realization that he could rely on himself, even when it seemed that there was no one else to rely on:

"When it really comes down to it, we're in the dark. And we crawl. And we make it on our own through that dark tunnel. Somehow we come out the other end. And we've done it on our own."

Some patients learned not only how strong they were, but also how much love they were capable of. Julie Benbow says:

"You know, this thing attacks your body, so you attack it back, but you attack it with love. And then, because you've overcome the worst possible thing in your life, you realize that you have love. I have a lot of love inside me that I want to get rid of, is about the only way to describe it. I just want to give it to you and to give it to you and to give

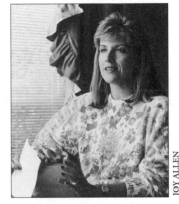

Carol Landt

JOY ALLEN

"I discovered that, no matter what else, we could both *count on me, and that I was very capable."*

–Carol Landt

"When you realize, 'There's a part of me that I didn't even know existed. Wow, I've got a lot more strength than I ever thought I did. That makes me special. Wow! That's great!'"

–Paula Carroll

it to the taxi driver. And I never had that before. So you know, I am always now in the same frame of mind that it used to take me three gin and tonics to get into."

Discovering their own inner resources gave many patients an enormous boost in their self-esteem. "It's a well of strength," Charles Fuhrman told us. "I know I could face anything, you know. Once you face it, you can face anything. So I know it. And I have a lot of respect for myself that I didn't give in, that I didn't fold up. That I had good attitudes. That I was out to take this thing and turn it into a positive experience."

"You love yourself the way you're supposed to love yourself," says Paula Carroll, who beat breast cancer twice. "When you realize, 'There's a part of me that I didn't even know existed. Wow, I've got a lot more strength than I ever thought I did. That makes me special. Wow! That's great!'" And she adds, "I don't mean this in an arrogant way. But I think a lot of times people are arrogant because they don't know their own worth. The more you realize what a special person every one of us is, the more humble you are."

Whether, like Dennis Brown, you have undergone years of cancer therapy, or whether you have never had a sick day in your life, dealing with the issues that cancer raises can teach you to appreciate your own strengths. And this in turn can teach you who you are–in Paula Carroll's words, how special you are.

Lesson Four: Learning to Do What Matters Most to You

Cancer taught our patients to do what mattered the most to them. "I think I benefited from cancer by having to confront these issues," says Brad Zebrack. "What do I want with my life? What do I want my life to become? Given that cancer was a threat in my life, I had to decide how I wanted to live the rest of it without knowing how long it was going to last." Esther Joyce made the same point even more bluntly: "Why not review your life and find out what it is you want to do today? And if you want to do it, by God, do it."

This meant setting priorities. Charles Fuhrman found that what mattered the most to him was "my inner peace. My painting—it's my center; it's who I am. My life, my wife, my family, my friends. That's it. And I decided to just dedicate my life to those things in the most honest, humble way I possibly can. And let go of all the rest."

"Letting go of all the rest" sometimes meant letting go of old emotional needs. For Brad Zebrack, what mattered most turned out to be honoring his principles, and this meant letting go of the need to be liked. "Now if I'm around people who prevent that, I can push them aside, as opposed to worrying that, 'Oh, gosh, if I don't get in with these people then they're not going to like me.' I feel stronger about standing up for what I think and what I believe. Having principles is more important to me now than having people like me."

Kris Richardson made a similar point. She told us that her mother's cancer "made me realize that our time here is short, and it's not to be squandered. And that if I'm hanging out with people who aren't absolutely loving and totally supportive of what I'm doing and who I am, they're not in my life anymore. So I did a major house-cleaning. I hang out with people who are positive, and usually spiritually searching, and who will add something to my life."

What mattered most was different for each patient. For Jeff Losea, it was his relationship with God:

"Before I had cancer, I was happy. And I was just kind of stumbling through life, making ends meet and looking for enjoyment for the flesh—restaurants, fun things to do, vacations, days off. But when I found out I had cancer and was dealing with my mortality, I came closer to God, much closer. I'd rather die now, knowing God, than live to eighty and not know Him. It's enriched my life so much—the people that I've met. The feeling that I get inside knowing that I don't lie, I don't steal. I mean, not that I did before, but I live the life of a Christian. And

> *"Why not review your life and find out what it is you want to do today? And if you want to do it, by God, do it."*
>
> —Esther Joyce

Kris Richardson told us that her mother's cancer "made me realize that our time here is short, and it's not to be squandered."

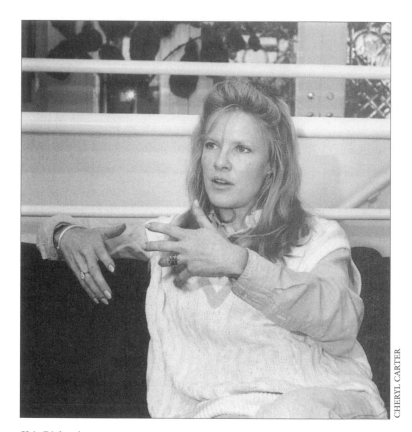

Kris Richardson

believe in God. And He loves me. I thank God for the experience, actually."

Doing what matters most includes living by one's own standards. When Marcie Wienecke was in bed, following a spine operation, John Wienecke told us, "she could not move. And a tooth broke off when she was eating a bagel. She called the dentist. The dentist could not work on her there. She made a request to get taken to his office. We took her by ambulance; he did his work on a stretcher in his office. Now if someone has six weeks to live, who cares whether your teeth are in or not? But that was not her standard. She wanted her teeth taken care of. So she made the request."

For a great many patients, what mattered most turned out to be relationships. "Cancer is a great teacher of the things that are important in life, which gets down to relationships with other people. That's all that's really important," said Dennis Brown. Many of the other patients agreed. Dealing with cancer taught the people we interviewed to look at relationships in a new light. John Wienecke told us how it affected Marcie:

"And what she did is, she started making lists of all her resentments and regrets, and issues she had with people. And she started communicating to people. Her relationship with her mother was transformed out of one of always fighting and being antagonistic with each other to a real partnership, where they shared things they'd never talked about. And there was crying, there was laughter."

This was true for family members as well as for the patients themselves. Diane Losea found that "the things that seemed so significant before–the little habits that somebody may have–just became so insignificant. When something like this hits, you find the real person. It's made me look at things deeply instead of on the surface."

And John Wienecke says, "She was in a wheelchair, she was bald, but it no longer mattered. I started to see that a person isn't what they look like. And what I got out of it was that I love people for who they are."

Finally, cancer taught many patients to think in terms of helping others–especially other people who are facing cancer. Dennis Brown, who owned a large chain of motels, told us:

"I think one of the things to come out of this experience is a stronger desire on my part to be helpful to cancer patients in the future. It opens up an entirely new area of community service for me. So what I intend to do is to set up a counseling service, counseling and research, aimed primarily at people who are in situations that are similar to mine."

And Judy Lakotas, who works behind the counter in a deli, says much the same thing in her own way:

"It's made me aware of other people's problems. My big passion is if I can help other people. This is one thing having cancer has done for me. What can I do

"The things that seemed so significant before–the little habits that somebody may have–just became so insignificant. When something like this hits, you find the real person. It's made me look at things deeply instead of on the surface."

–Diane Losea

"It's kind of sweet out here....Boy, you don't realize how sweet it is being out here."

–Joe Dodig

to help–really help–other people?"

And she adds:

"You know, people hear the word 'cancer' and they see death. I think I can encourage people by telling them there is hope. It's not the end of the world."

To live life to the fullest, do what matters the most to you. Earlier in this chapter, we suggested some ways to do this, whether you have cancer or not. The first step is to set priorities. The second step is to live your life according to those priorities, like the patients and family members quoted above.

Lesson Five: Learning to Enjoy Life

People who have been through the cancer experience know, in Sue Olitt's words, "just how precious life is." Cancer has taught these patients to enjoy life. Or, as Joe Dodig put it, "It's kind of sweet out here. Unless you're in the hospital a couple times in intensive care, boy, you don't realize how sweet it is being out here."

For some patients, enjoying life meant enjoying the little things. For Polly McMahon, who was recovering from colon cancer, it meant "getting up in the morning. Living in one of the prettiest places in the country. I love the fresh air up here. I like my garden, my cat, my house. I love to look at all my beautiful paintings. I've met a lot of nice people in my work. I'm an avid reader. There's just so much to do in life, and I thoroughly enjoy it."

For Jeff Losea, who was dying of metastasized esophageal cancer, it meant "the ability to get up and get out of bed, and have the strength to get up and go to the bathroom, or just take a shower. Just to have a heartbeat, to breathe. Just to appreciate everything. Because people are so caught up in their lives, until something catastrophic hits, they don't take time to smell the roses, so to speak."

For Marcie Wienecke, says John, enjoying life meant participating in everyday activities:

"She did what she wanted to do. When people came over to see her, she would joke, she would talk about it, she would show them her scars from the operation. She planned dinner. Even though she couldn't cook dinner, she would help her mother cook it. She participated fully in everything. I'd moved the bed downstairs to the dining room so she could participate. I picked her up and I would take her to the living room so she could sit in the living room and participate."

Whether you are recovering from cancer, like Polly McMahon, or like Jeff Losea have been diagnosed as terminal, we believe that you can learn to "smell the roses." Even if you have never had cancer, we believe that the experiences of cancer patients can teach you new ways to enjoy life. The cancer experience often brings with it an intense appreciation of little things. What once seemed ordinary is suddenly extraordinary–seeing the crocuses break through the soil, eating a hot-cross bun, watching a squirrel run along a telephone wire. Learn to develop this sense of appreciation. Ask yourself questions that open your awareness. "How can I get the most out of this experience?" "What can I experience today that will be pleasurable for me?" Appreciating things makes you happy with what you have, because you are focusing on what you have and not on what you want. This is an example of thinking positive, a coping skill that we discussed in Chapter 6. Listen to Nancy Heitz:

"I believe that if they don't find a cure for what I have, I'll still be able to be around and enjoy my life. Maybe I might have to make some adaptations, maybe I will have to be in a wheelchair. But being in a wheelchair does not mean I'm in a coffin. I could still be valuable; I can still be a person. I'll just be motorized. Hey, great."

Finally, learn to live in the present. "I think that was the big lesson," says Arnold Schraer. "It's a lesson we hear all the time. But you know, most of us, our minds are in the future with worries and fears. And the present just slips by us. And we never harvest from the moment the beauty of it, and the joy and the wonder of it. And I think that with this disease–it's not that I focus on the disease–it's that I have focused so much on releasing all those things that

> *"Most of us, our minds are in the future with worries and fears....And we never harvest from the moment the beauty of it, and the joy and the wonder of it."*
>
> –**Arnold Schraer**

made me frightened, that all there really is is now. And I feel much more able to tune into that, and it's real. It's a joy and a wonder. I've never had this–I mean, I've had it at times, but I've never had it so consistently. Being able to respond to my environment in a complete way."

To live life to the fullest, learn to live and enjoy one day at a time. Learn to focus on each moment and to live in that moment. Learn to enjoy that moment for itself. The more you do this, the more you become aware of all the things that your life has to offer.

In order of their first appearance, the patients who contributed to this chapter are: Dennis Brown, Charles Fuhrman, Paul Ryder, Brad Zebrack, Nancy Heitz, Jeff Losea, Julie Benbow, Odile Belladonna, Barbara Fritz, Barbara Johns, Jay Fritz, Polly McMahon, Esther Joyce, Chris Maggart, Linda Sumner, Paula Carroll, Arnold Schraer, Marcie Wienecke, Judy Lakotas, Sue Olitt, and Joe Dodig. The family members who contributed to this chapter are: Brent Ryder, Diane Losea, Lois Ryder, John Wienecke, Lily Kravcisin, Kris Richardson, and Carol Landt.

Recommended Reading

Part 1

Benson, Herbert. *Your Maximum Mind.* New York: Times Books, 1987.

This easy-to-read, practical book explains how changes occur in our thought patterns and shows how you can use this information to break old habits or learn new ones. Dr. Benson is chief of the Division of Behavioral Medicine at the New England Deaconess Hospital and president of the Mind-Body Medical Institute.

——————————, and Eileen M. Stuart, eds. *The Wellness Book: A Comprehensive Guide to Maintaining Health and Treating Stress-Related Illness.* New York: Birch Lane Press, 1992.

Exercise, nutrition, stress management, and stress-related illness are discussed in the context of the mind-body connection. This is a self-help book; each discussion, illustrated with case histories, is accompanied by lists of questions, worksheets, and exercises designed to help you to decide what changes you need to make and how to go about making them. There are chapters on problem solving and on living with cancer and an excellent reading list. All of the authors are specialists on the staff of the Mind-Body Medical Institute at the New England Deaconess Hospital and Harvard Medical School.

Bolles, Richard Nelson. *The 1993 What Color Is Your Parachute? A Practical Manual for Job Hunters and Career-Changers.* Berkeley, CA: Ten Speed Press, 1993.

This is the book to buy if you don't know what kind of work you want to do or how to go about finding it. *Parachute* is packed with practical advice, which is updated annually. It is famous for its lively style and its elaborate graphics. The appendix on how to find your mission in life is written from a Christian perspective, but non-Christians may find it helpful too.

Farquhar, John W. *The American Way of Life Need Not Be Hazardous to Your Health*. New York: Addison-Wesley Publishing Co., 1987.

An excellent overall sourcebook on self-directed change, stress management, nutrition and weight control, exercise, and smoking cessation. Clear, readable, and easy to use, it explains how to make changes that will improve your quality of life and reduce your risk of cancer, heart disease, and stroke. There is an extensive resource list of books, magazines, technical articles, and organizations. The author is the director of the Stanford Center for Research on Disease Prevention; he is known internationally for his research and writing.

Robbins, Anthony. *Awaken the Giant Within: How to Take Immediate Control of Your Mental, Emotional, Physical, and Financial Destiny*. New York: Summit Books, 1991.

This popular book shows you how to set goals and how to make the changes necessary to achieve them. It explains in detail how to gain control over your emotions, your health, your relationships, your money, and your time. Written in an upbeat, inspirational style and heavily illustrated with personal anecdotes, it is full of concrete, practical advice.

Yoder, Barbara. *The Recovery Resource Book*. New York: Simon & Schuster, Fireside, 1990.

A comprehensive directory of books, organizations, and other resources, organized by type of dependency. The basics of addiction, recovery, self-help, and treatment are discussed in detail, both in general and with respect to each specific substance. Problems specific to various ethnic groups, women, children, and the elderly are covered as well. There are long chapters on alcohol, nicotine, and food dependencies. There is also a section on addictions to relationships, money, and work. Packed with information and enlivened by first-person recovery stories, this is an excellent resource for readers who feel that they need outside help to make changes in their lives.

Part 2

Bailey, Covert. *The New Fit or Fat.* **Boston: Houghton Mifflin Co., 1991.**

Concise and clearly written, this is an invaluable handbook for readers who want to set up their own exercise program. It is designed especially for readers who want to lose weight, but much of the information in it will be valuable for anyone. The chapters on choosing an aerobic exercise and on how to get started are especially useful. The author conducts the Bailey Seminars on fitness; he holds a degree in nutritional biochemistry from MIT.

Bennett, William I., Stephen E. Goldfinger, and G. Timothy Johnson, eds. *Your Good Health: How to Stay Well and What to Do When You're Not.* **Cambridge, MA: Harvard University Press, 1987.**

An authoritative guide for readers who want to take responsibility for their own health. The chapters on environmental hazards; on tobacco, alcohol, and other drugs; and on dealing with the medical establishment are first-rate. The writing is lively and informal and the contributors' credentials are impeccable; they are all on the staff of the Harvard Medical School Health Letter.

Bohannon, Richard, Terri P. Wuerthner, and Kathy Klett Weinstock. *Food for Life: The Cancer Prevention Cookbook.* **Chicago: Contemporary Books, 1986.**

An oncologist and a caterer have collaborated to produce these recipes, which are based on the nutrition guidelines of the National Research Council and the ACS. This cookbook includes a table listing the nutritive values of many common foods.

Brody, Jane. *Jane Brody's Good Food Book: Living the High-Carbohydrate Way.* **New York: Bantam Books, 1987.**

The first half of this classic cookbook offers detailed guidelines for good nutrition and explains how to follow them. The second half consists of 350 recipes. There is a special section on weight control.

————————. *Jane Brody's Good Food Gourmet: Recipes and Menus for Delicious and Healthful Entertaining.* New York: Bantam Books, 1992.

Nutritious, low-fat recipes by this nationally respected health writer, who is also a gourmet cook.

Dadd, Debra Lynn. *The Nontoxic Home: Protecting Yourself and Your Family from Everyday Toxics and Health Hazards.* Los Angeles: Jeremy P. Tarcher, 1986.

This easy-to-use handbook lists known and suspected toxic chemicals and other health hazards found in the home and suggests nontoxic alternatives. It will appeal especially to readers who want to avoid any exposure to possible carcinogens. The author is the editor of *Everything Natural,* a newsletter on nontoxic and natural consumer products.

Evans, William, and Irwin H. Rosenberg. *Biomarkers: The Ten Determinants of Aging You Can Control.* New York: Simon & Schuster, 1991.

How to use exercise to improve your health and increase your longevity. The authors explain how to choose, set up, and follow the exercise program that is right for you. Their suggestions are based on research conducted at the USDA Human Nutrition Research Program at Tufts University. This book is designed primarily for middle-aged readers, but older readers will also find it helpful. Practical, easy to read, and encouraging.

Farquhar, John W., and Gene A. Spiller. *The Last Puff: Ex-Smokers Share Their Secrets of Success.* New York: W.W. Norton & Co., 1990.

Thirty-three ex-smokers tell how they did it. Dr. Farquhar also discusses physical and psychological addiction; he emphasizes the individual nature of the stopping process. There is a chapter on preventing relapses. Very readable.

Johnson, Vernon E. *I'll Quit Tomorrow: A Practical Guide to Alcoholism Treatment.* Rev. ed. San Francisco: Harper & Row Publishers, 1990.

This book focuses on the psychological aspects of alcohol addiction, treatment, and recovery. It is addressed to treatment providers, but readers who suspect that they or someone they know may have a drinking problem will find it valuable too. The material is clearly presented, and the case histories are riveting. The author is the founder of the Johnson Institute in Minneapolis, which provides training programs for treatment providers.

Lindsay, Anne, and Diane J. Fink. *The American Cancer Society Cookbook.* **New York: Hearst Books, 1988.**

Simple, appealing recipes to help you to reduce your risk of developing cancer. This cookbook will be especially useful for readers who want to cut down on fat.

Milam, James R., and Katherine Ketcham. *Under the Influence: A Guide to the Myths and Realities of Alcoholism.* **New York: Bantam Books, 1983.**

The first half of this book focuses on the physical aspects of alcohol addiction. It covers predisposing factors and traces the development of the disease through the adaptive, dependent, and deteriorative stages. Cancer in alcoholics is discussed briefly. The second half of the book focuses on the psychological and behavioral aspects of alcoholism and on treatment. Easy to read for patients and families alike. Dr. Milam is a clinical psychologist and a nationally known authority on alcoholism.

Natow, Annette B., and Jo-Ann Heslin. *The Fat Counter.* **New York: Simon & Schuster, Pocket Books, 1989.**

This handy paperback gives the fat content of over 10,000 different foods. Part 1 lists brand name and generic foods; Part 2 lists items on the menus of twenty-four restaurant and fast-food chains. The introduction offers practical suggestions for reducing the amount of fat in your diet. The authors have published eight books on nutrition; they are registered dietitians and faculty members of Adelphi University.

Samuels, Mike, and Hal Zina Bennett. *Well Body, Well Earth.* **San Francisco: Sierra Club Books, 1983.**

The first two sections of this book explain how human

health is related to the health of the planet. The third section is a sourcebook of environmental hazards; radiation, chemicals, and air and water pollution are discussed in detail. The last section tells how to reduce your exposure to environmental hazards, and how to reduce the hazards themselves. This book presents a great deal of complex material in language that is easy to understand. Heavily illustrated. There are many charts and tables and a long bibliography.

Schwartz, Bob. *Diets Don't Work!* Houston, TX: Breakthru Publishing, 1984.

Methods for losing weight and keeping it off, based on the author's Diets Don't Work Seminar Programs. This book helps readers to examine the reasons why they overeat and shows them how to develop a thin mentality. The emphasis is on changing attitudes toward food and forming new eating habits based on the new attitudes. Each chapter contains checklists and written exercises. The writing is lively, full of anecdotes, and very easy to read.

Siegel, Mary-Ellen. *Safe in the Sun.* New York: Walker & Co., 1990.

How exposure to the sun affects your skin and eyes, and how to protect yourself. There are chapters on black skin, children's skin, sunscreens, and sunless tanning, and three chapters on skin cancer. Authoritative and easy to read. The author is a senior teaching associate at the Mount Sinai School of Medicine and the author of *The Cancer Patient's Handbook.*

Simone, Charles B. *Cancer and Nutrition: A Ten-Point Plan to Reduce Your Risk of Getting Cancer.* Garden City Park, NY: Avery Publishing Group, 1992.

This book discusses in detail the nutritional factors that increase–or reduce–the risk of cancer. Smoking, alcohol, environmental hazards, and other risk factors are discussed as well. The author provides guidelines for avoiding all of these risk factors, but the emphasis is on learning how to modify your diet. This book is not easy to read; it is packed with technical information, and the style is dry and scientific. However, it is an excellent resource. Dr. Simone is a nationally known expert in cancer prevention and research.

Stuart, Richard B., and Barbara Jacobson. *Weight, Sex and Marriage: A Delicate Balance*. New York: W.W. Norton & Co., 1987.

This book discusses some of the reasons why women may overeat. The relationship between weight problems and marital or sexual issues is examined at length. There is a thought-provoking chapter on the pros and cons of losing weight. Richard B. Stuart is a marriage therapist who specializes in issues of weight control. Barbara Jacobson is a counselor with an interest in obesity.

Yoder, Barbara. *The Recovery Resource Book*. New York: Simon & Schuster, Fireside, 1990.

This book includes material on alcohol, tobacco, and food dependencies. We give a complete description in the Recommended Reading for Part 1.

Editors of the *University of California at Berkeley Wellness Letter. The Wellness Encyclopedia*. Boston: Houghton Mifflin, 1991.

Nutrition, exercise, and environmental safety are thoroughly discussed in this comprehensive, authoritative family health guide. There is a section on common health risk factors and a large section on self-care. Clearly written, well illustrated, and backed by solid research, this book is a pleasure to use.

Part 3

Berman, Phillip L. *The Search for Meaning: Americans Talk about What They Believe and Why.* **New York: Ballantine Books, 1990.**

Over a hundred ordinary Americans tell you in their own words about their religious and philosophical beliefs. The author spent four years taping interviews with people from every walk of life: a contemplative nun, a rodeo clown, a farm laborer, a theoretical physicist, a grand wizard of the Ku Klux Klan, a street person, a Japanese-American Buddhist priest. The questions that these people raise, and the answers that they give, will fascinate readers who are exploring issues of faith and sense of purpose.

Buscaglia, Leo F. *Personhood: The Art of Being Fully Human.* **New York: Ballantine Books, Fawcett Columbine, 1992.**

The first part of this short, readable book describes the five stages of growth toward full humanness, from adolescence through old age. The second part summarizes what the world's major religions have to say about what it means to be fully human. The third part explains how you can learn to apply these same principles to your own life. Leo Buscaglia is a professor of education at the University of Southern California and the author of the best-seller *Love*.

Fields, Rick, et al. *Chop Wood Carry Water: A Guide to Finding Spiritual Fulfillment in Everyday Life.* **Los Angeles: Jeremy P. Tarcher, 1984.**

A collection of advice drawn from a wide range of sources, with heavy emphasis on Eastern and New Age spirituality. Each chapter focuses on one aspect of everyday life; topics include intimate relationships, work, money, healing, technology, and social action. There is an excellent chapter on beginning the spiritual journey and another on the perils of the spiritual path. This lively, popular book includes lists of recommended reading and other resources.

Jampolsky, Gerald G., and Diane V. Cirincione. *Change Your Mind, Change Your Life: Concepts in Attitudinal Healing.* **New York: Bantam Books, 1993.**

The authors show you how to change your life by changing your attitudes—by letting go of fear and recognizing that your true identity is love. There is a chapter on attitudes toward death. This book is highly inspirational; it will appeal especially to readers who believe in God or in a higher power. Dr. Jampolsky is the founder of the Center for Attitudinal Healing in Tiburon, California, which provides support to patients with life-threatening illnesses.

Lash, John. *The Seeker's Handbook: The Complete Guide to Spiritual Pathfinding.* **New York: Harmony Books, 1990.**

A guide to the New Age religions. Essays on thirty themes of the modern spiritual movement, from crystal healing to shamanism. There is a 200-page glossary of terms. A useful sourcebook for readers who want to learn more about alternative spirituality. The author's approach is unbiased; he neither promotes nor disparages any of the religions that he describes.

Peck, M. Scott. *The Road Less Traveled: A New Psychology of Love, Traditional Values, and Spiritual Growth.* **New York: Simon & Schuster, Touchstone, 1978.**

How to achieve mental and spiritual growth by confronting and solving the problems that life poses. Using case histories drawn from his own psychiatric practice, Dr. Peck discusses the role of discipline, love, religion, and the love of God. This book will appeal to readers who seek to develop a spiritual life by combining the insights of modern psychology with those of Christian spirituality.

Rosten, Leo, ed. *Religions of America: Ferment and Faith in an Age of Crisis.* **New York: Simon & Schuster, 1975.**

Part 1 of this comprehensive pocket reference book describes the major Christian denominations, Judaism, agnosticism, and the beliefs of the nonchurchgoer and the scientist. Written in question-and-answer format, it outlines the history of each denomination and summarizes its beliefs, practices, and positions on various social issues. Part 2 is an almanac of facts and figures on various aspects of religion in America. Non-Western religions are not discussed, but the book includes a short section on the Black Muslims.

Smith, Huston. *The World's Religions.* **New York: HarperCollins Publishers, HarperSanFrancisco, 1991.**

This new, revised edition of the classic *Religions of Man* gives the history, basic teachings, and unique insights of each of the world's major religions and discusses the meaning that each religion holds for its followers. There are chapters on Hinduism, Buddhism, Confucianism, Taoism, Islam, Judaism, Christianity, and native traditions. An excellent introductory text, this book is written for the general reader and requires no special knowledge to understand. The author is a visiting professor at the University of California at Berkeley and a nationally recognized authority on the history of religion.

——————————. *Forgotten Truth: The Common Vision of the World's Religions.* **New York: HarperCollins Publishers, HarperSanFrancisco, 1992.**

Smith believes that all religions share a common view of reality, which differs from the modern nonreligious Western view. He argues that the latter view has been shaped by the misapplication of scientific thought. This book is very challenging reading; try it if you are curious about the apparent contradictions between scientific thinking and spiritual belief.

Hope

Hope

Countless people have survived cancer.
Countless more have found that the cancer
experience has transformed their lives,
that cancer has given life new richness and
new meaning.

In the course of writing this book, we have
witnessed this transformation repeatedly. We have
also witnessed the infinite power of hope.

Hope comes naturally to some people. Others may
have to work to achieve it. Acquiring information,
gaining control, developing faith, setting priorities,
finding a sense of purpose—all these are ways of
getting in touch with hope.

When most patients say "hope," they mean the
hope of a cure. To us, hope means much more than
that. We define hope as a positive attitude, not
necessarily related to achieving a cure. Hope means
accepting the reality of any situation but focusing
on the redeeming aspects of that situation. To hope
is to look for the positive in one's circumstances,
whether those circumstances are good or bad.
Hope does not necessarily mean overcoming fear.
It means feeling the presence of life even while
you are afraid.

To hope is to be able to focus on what matters
the most to you. This means that hope is highly
individual. And hope can be an act of renewal—or
discovery. To hope is to discover what gives your life

meaning, to discover your own personal truth.

For one person, hope might be the hope of a cure. For another, it might be the hope of a peaceful death.

For one person, hope might be hope for the highest possible quality of life. For another, it might be the hope of bringing life to a positive completion—by mending old quarrels, by finishing work left undone, by coming to terms with old fears.

For one person, hope might be the hope of living in such a way that one's life has made a difference to others. For another, it might be the hope of dying in such a way that one's death has made a difference to others.

Or hope can simply be a readiness to experience the present moment, a total appreciation of whatever life still has to offer. Some patients never lose this readiness to appreciate life. A few hours before Arnold Schraer died, he came out of a deep sleep and opened his eyes. His nurse offered him a ripe, red strawberry. Arnold's eyes lit up with pleasure. In a moment of complete clarity, he exclaimed: "…To be able to eat strawberries one more time!"

We have seen countless people's lives enriched by hope. We have witnessed its power, its light. Our hope for you is that your life too will be touched by this power.

To hope is to discover what gives your life meaning, to discover your own personal truth.

393

Glossary

Action list A list of specific, immediate goals.

Aerobic exercise Exercise that increases respiratory and circulatory function by increasing oxygen consumption.

Affirmation A simple, positive statement that is repeated over and over to correct negative thinking patterns.

Alternative treatment Treatment that is neither standard nor investigational. Sometimes called "unorthodox treatment," "unconventional treatment."

Anaerobic exercise Intense exercise that lasts only a short time.

Anecdotal evidence Evidence provided by stories, case histories, or testimonials that are not backed by scientific studies.

Antibody A protein secreted by certain lymphocytes. Each antibody attacks a particular antigen.

Antigen A foreign substance that activates the immune system by causing the body to form antibodies.

Benign Not cancerous.

Biopsy Removal of a small piece of tumor tissue for diagnosis by microscopic examination.

Blood count The number of red cells, white cells, and platelets in a given blood sample.

Board-certified Refers to a physician who is certified by the American Board of Internal Medicine and, in the case of an oncologist, who belongs to the American Society of Clinical Oncology.

Body energy In alternative medicine, a life force that is believed to flow through the body, the blockage of which is believed to cause disease.

Brachytherapy Treatment with radioactive material placed in a body cavity, in the tumor, or on the surface of the body. The term is sometimes used to refer to surface placement specifically.

Cachexia   General wasting of the body, often caused by advanced disease.

Cancer   A general term for more than 100 different diseases that involve the uncontrolled increase of abnormal new cells. These cells form tumors that can destroy surrounding tissue and spread throughout the body.

Cancer initiator   An agent that causes cells to mutate.

Cancer promoter   An agent that weakens the body's resistance to carcinogens.

Carcinogen   A substance that initiates or promotes the development of cancer.

Carcinoma   A cancer that originates in epithelial tissue (the glands, the skin, and the lining of the internal organs).

Chemotherapy   The treatment of cancer (or other disease) with drugs.

Clinical trial   A study conducted with cancer (or other) patients, using the scientific method, to evaluate new therapies or procedures.

Cognitive therapy   A form of psychotherapy that is based on the premise that stress is often caused by negative thought patterns.

Colony stimulating factor (CSF) An agent that stimulates the production of disease-fighting cells in the bone marrow, enabling the patient to tolerate higher doses of chemotherapy.

Colorectal surgeon   A physician who specializes in surgery of the lower colon and the rectum.

Complementary therapy Alternative therapy used to support standard treatment. Sometimes called "secondary therapy," "supportive therapy."

Comprehensive Cancer Center An NCI-designated cancer center that takes a multidisciplinary approach to cancer research, patient care, and community outreach.

Control group   In a clinical trial, a group of subjects who receive standard treatment, in order to compare the effects of the therapy being studied with the effects of standard treatment.

Cure   Refers to the elimination of all signs of cancer for a period of at least five years from the end of treatment.

Cure rate   The percentage of patients who have survived a given cancer for five years.

Debulking   A procedure that reduces the size of a tumor so that further treatment may be applied.

Diagnostic radiologist A physician who uses X rays to perform diagnostic tests for cancer.

Dietitian A professional who specializes in planning nutritious diets.

Discharge planner A hospital staff member who helps to arrange for patients' needs after they leave the hospital.

DNA (deoxyribonucleic acid) Acid found in the nucleus of the cell that carries genetic information.

Dosimetrist A specialist who calculates the number and length of the radiation sessions.

Doubling rate The time it takes a tumor to double in size.

Exploratory surgery Surgery that is undertaken to explore an area for diagnostic purposes.

Family illness An illness that makes demands on the patient's whole family.

Gene The biologic unit of heredity; a segment of DNA that controls the transmission of a single trait.

Genetic counselor A counselor who is a specialist on the role of heredity in the development of cancer.

Geneticist A specialist in the study of heredity.

Glioma A cancer that originates in the nervous system.

Grade A term used to describe the extent to which the cells of a tumor resemble ordinary cells.

Gynecologist A physician who specializes in diseases of the female genital tract.

Hereditary cancer A cancer that is associated with risk factors that run in families.

Hodgkin's disease A kind of lymphoma.

Holistic medicine A form of alternative medicine that treats the mind and the body together, as a single unit.

Homeopathic medicine A form of alternative medicine that treats illnesses by administering very small doses of substances that would produce symptoms of the illness if administered in large amounts to a healthy person.

Hormonal therapy The treatment of cancer by administering natural or synthetic hormones, which cause some tumors to stabilize or shrink.

Hormone antagonists Pharmaceutical drugs that inhibit the production of male or female hormones.

Hormones Chemicals produced in the body that regulate the activity of certain cells or organs.

Hyperthermia The use of heat to destroy cancer cells.

Immune system The body mechanisms that fight disease by recognizing and neutralizing foreign cells.

Immunotherapy A form of therapy that stimulates the immune system to kill or control cancer cells.

Informed consent A legal standard that defines how much a patient must know about the potential benefits and risks before he or she agrees to undergo certain procedures or to participate in a clinical trial.

Interferons Natural proteins produced by white blood cells; used in cancer immunotherapy.

Interleukin-2 An agent that stimulates the growth of specific types of white blood cells; used in cancer immunotherapy.

Intracavity radiation Treatment with radioactive material placed in a body cavity.

Intramuscular Into a muscle.

Intrastitial radiation Treatment with radioactive material implanted in the tumor.

Intravenous Into a vein.

Investigational treatment Clinical trials conducted with cancer patients, using the scientific method, to evaluate new therapies or procedures. Formerly called "experimental treatment."

Leukemia A cancer of the blood-forming tissues (such as bone marrow or lymph glands) that causes an overproduction of white blood cells.

Lymph An infection-fighting, plasmalike substance that contains white blood cells and antibodies.

Lymphatic system The system of nodes and vessels that carry lymph throughout the body.

Lymph nodes Glands that produce lymph and that filter out harmful agents (such as bacteria, viruses, and cancer cells).

Lymphocytes Disease-fighting white blood cells.

Lymphoma A cancer that originates in the lymph glands. Unlike leukemia, it forms a tumor.

Macrophages White blood cells that ingest and destroy foreign invader cells.

Malignant Cancerous.

Medical oncologist An oncologist who is not a surgeon.

Megavitamin therapy An alternative therapy that treats cancer with massive doses of vitamins.

Melanoma A highly malignant type of skin cancer.

Metabolic therapy An alternative therapy that is based on the belief that an impaired metabolism causes cancer.

Metastasis The spread of cancer cells from their point of origin to other parts of the body by way of the bloodstream or the lymphatic system.

Monoclonal antibodies Antibodies made in the laboratory that can locate cancer cells.

Multidisciplinary second opinion A second opinion that is provided by a variety of specialists.

Mutation A permanent change in the structure of a cell that may cause it to become cancerous.

Myeloma A cancer of the plasma cells in the bone marrow.

Natural killer (NK) cell A class of white blood cell that attacks cancer cells.

Naturopathic medicine A form of alternative treatment that uses natural substances to treat illness and rid the body of "impurities."

Neoplasm Any new abnormal growth. A neoplasm may be malignant or benign.

Neurosurgeon A physician who specializes in surgery of the nervous system.

Nuclear medicine physician A physician who traces radioactive material introduced into the bloodstream to assess the function of organs.

Nucleus The rounded core of a cell; it contains the genes.

Nurse A professional who is trained to assist the doctor or to provide direct care for the patient under the doctor's supervision. A nurse's responsibilities vary depending on his or her level of training.

Nurse's aide A worker who assists trained nurses in a hospital by performing tasks that do not require extensive training.

Occult tumor A hidden tumor.

Oncogene A particular kind of gene that, when activated by carcinogens, disrupts the nucleus and contributes to the transformation of a normal cell into a cancer cell.

Oncologist A physician who specializes in treating cancer.

Ophthalmologist A physician who specializes in diseases of the eye.

Option list A list of things that you could do to help yourself to solve a problem or to achieve a goal.

Otolaryngologist A physician who specializes in diseases of the ear, nose, and throat.

GLOSSARY

Palliation   Relief from symptoms, especially those which cause discomfort.

Partial response   A 50 percent reduction in the size of the tumor that lasts longer than one month.

Pathologist   A physician who specializes in studying the effects of disease on body tissue.

Photodynamic therapy (PDT)   The use of lasers and light-activated drugs to destroy tumors.

Physical therapist   A professional who helps the patient to regain function and mobility by teaching exercises and new ways to perform tasks such as walking.

Physician's assistant   A professional who performs some of the functions of a doctor under the doctor's super-vision.

Placebo effect   An improvement caused not by the treatment itself but by the patient's belief in the treatment.

Plastic surgeon   A physician who specializes in reconstructive surgery.

Primary caregiver   The person who does most of the work involved in caring for the patient.

Primary (parent) tumor   The site where the tumor first appeared.

Prognosis   A prediction of the probable course of the disease.

Protocols   The guidelines that specify how a clinical trial will be conducted.

Psychoneuroimmunology (PNI)   The study of the interrelationships among stress, the emotions, the central nervous system, and the immune system.

Radiation oncologist   A physician who treats cancer with radiation therapy.

Radiation physicist   A specialist who ensures that the radiation machine delivers the correct amount of radiation.

Radiation technologist   A specialist who runs the equipment that delivers radiation.

Radiation therapist   A radiation oncologist or a radiation technologist.

Radiation therapy   The treatment of cancer with high-energy X rays.

Radiosensitive   Sensitive to X rays or other forms of radiation.

Reconstructive (plastic) surgery   Surgery to remove or restructure tissue after the tumor has been removed.

Recurrence   The reappearance of a cancer after a period of remission.

Religious belief   Belief in the doctrine of an orthodox religion.

Remission   Complete or partial disappearance of a cancer, usually after treatment.

Resection   The removal of a malignant tumor in its entirety.

Risk   The possibility of injury resulting from treatment.

Risk factor   Any agent, substance, condition, or habit that increases a person's chance of developing cancer.

Sarcoma   A cancer that originates in nonepithelial tissue (bone, cartilage, muscle, blood vessels, lymph vessels, or fat).

Scalp hypothermia   The use of a cold cap to reduce or prevent hair loss during chemotherapy.

Secondary tumor   A tumor that has spread from its point of origin to another part of the body.

Second-opinion clinic   A group of specialists who collaborate to diagnose cancers and recommend treatment.

Side effect   A secondary adverse effect of treatment.

Site   The part of the body where a cancer first appears.

Spiritual belief   Belief that focuses on a personal relationship with a higher power but that is not necessarily dependent on religious doctrine.

Spontaneous remission   A remission that occurs without treatment.

Staging   A system for determining how far a tumor has spread from its point of origin.

Standard treatment   Treatment that is currently being used by physicians and that has been proven effective by scientific studies. Sometimes called "orthodox treatment," "conventional treatment," "traditional treatment." The four standard treatments for cancer are surgery, chemotherapy, radiation, and hormonal therapy.

Stress   A physical response to a perceived threat.

Subcutaneous   Under the skin.

Surgeon   A physician who specializes in surgery.

Surgery   The treatment of cancer (or other disease) by removing part of the body.

Survival   Refers to the elimination of all signs of cancer for a period of up to five years from the end of treatment.

Survival rate   The percentage of patients who have survived a given cancer up to a given time.

Thoracic surgeon   A physician who specializes in chest surgery.

Tumor   An abnormal mass of tissue. A tumor may be benign or malignant.

Tumor board   A group of specialists who help doctors to prescribe treatment in unusual cases.

GLOSSARY

Urologist A physician who specializes in diseases of the urinary system in women and diseases of the genitourinary tract in men.

Vaccination The injection of microorganisms associated with a disease to bolster the body's immunity to that disease.

Visualization Focusing on a mental picture. A problem-solving or stress reduction technique.

Appendices

1. The Dying Patient

2. Financial, Legal, Insurance, and Employment

3. Resources

The Dying Patient

We call this the *Alpha Book on Cancer and Living*. Why, then, do we include a section on death? We do so because people do sometimes die of cancer. This is a fact; but it is also a fact that there are things you can do that can make death easier to face, both for the patient and for the family and friends. In this section we tell you about those things.

The information in this section is straightforward and practical. We don't discuss philosophical or religious issues at length. We do suggest places where you can get more information on these issues. In this section we give a brief overview of the practical problems that surround death and dying, and we provide a list of Recommended Reading.

For the Patient

It's natural to be afraid of death. Death is the ultimate unknown—and now you're facing that unknown. If you are dying, you may have trouble dealing with that fear.

One of life's greatest challenges can be simply to acknowledge that you are dying. But doing so has practical benefits. And it can have psychological benefits as well.

If you can acknowledge that you are dying, you can make certain plans. You can plan for your last days; for example, you can tell your family what to do if you get to the point where you can no longer make your own decisions. You can give one member of your family power of attorney—the power to sign legal documents on your behalf. You can make out a Living Will. You can leave instructions concerning your own care. You can specify, for example, that you want to be given enough medication to

Power of attorney and Living Wills are discussed in Appendix 2.

"One of the most important things...was a series of conversations that she and I had....And I realized after she died that she was actually saying goodbye to me."

–James Carse

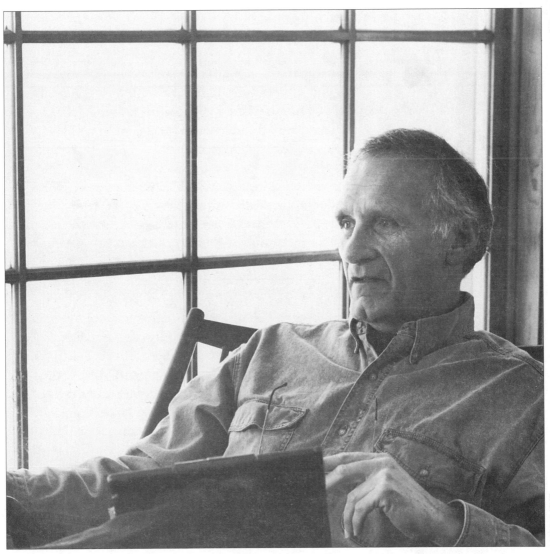

James Carse

keep you free of pain. The fear of death is partly the fear of pain. Knowing that you will not die in pain can greatly reduce this fear.

You can, if you wish, make your own funeral arrangements. One woman we know of wrote her own obituary when she was on her deathbed. After she died, her daughter sent it to the newspaper, which ran the announcement exactly as her mother had written it. "I wish she could have read it," the daughter told us. "It said just exactly what she wanted it to say."

You can make plans for your family's future too. Making out a will, getting your business affairs in order, making it easier for your family to go on without you—when you do this you give your loved ones a tremendous gift. You can give them tangible gifts, as well. Kris Richardson told us how her mother gave mementos to all of her friends and family:

"She had the most wonderful collection of things—art pieces and antiques—and I'll never forget seeing her sitting up in her little bed, with no hair, happy, just delighted: 'Oh, that's what I'm going to give to so-and-so!' and writing out a list that I had to dole out later, all these little things to all of these people. She was like Santa Claus. You've never seen anyone happier giving away all her worldly possessions."

Finally, when you acknowledge that you are dying, you give yourself a chance to say goodbye, to say the things you always wanted to say, to resolve old issues, to ask and offer forgiveness if that seems appropriate. In Chapter 8 we told you how Arnold Schraer gave a party for all of his friends when he was dying, and how Marcie Wienecke transformed her relationship with her mother "out of one of always fighting and being antagonistic with each other to a real partnership, where they shared things they'd never talked about."

Many people die the way they lived. But as this last example shows, it is also possible to die in a way that gives your life new meaning. Now may be the time, if it seems right to you, to look back on your life and resolve old

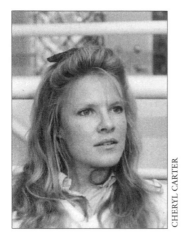

CHERYL CARTER

Kris Richardson

grudges, straighten out old misunderstandings. And now is the time to tell your loved ones how much you love them – to say those things you always wanted to say, but somehow never got around to saying.

Just as there are different ways to cope with life, so there are different ways to cope with death. It's an individual process. Here are some possibilities for you to think about.

It may help to talk it over with other people who are facing the same thing. Your hospital may sponsor a support group for dying patients. If not, check with your doctor, your social worker, or the local office of the American Cancer Society (ACS) to find out what groups are available in your area.

Faith is a traditional weapon against the fear of death. Faith can answer the questions that make you afraid: "What will happen to me when I die?" "Is there life after death?" "What will it be like?" In Chapter 8 we discuss the issue of faith and describe both religious and nonreligious, or what we call "spiritual," beliefs. In that chapter we offer suggestions on finding the way that is right for you.

Some of the orthodox religions – Christianity and Islam in particular – teach that each person has a soul that lives on after death. Others – such as Judaism – don't emphasize life after death very much at all. Members of some orthodox Eastern religions, as well as some adherents of "spiritual" beliefs, believe in reincarnation, or believe that one's life is a kind of energy that continues on after death in another form. The possibility of life after death has also been studied by researchers; to find out what they think, contact the International Association for Near-Death Studies, U-20, University of Connecticut, Storrs, CT 06268. Books that discuss life after death from various perspectives are included in the Recommended Reading on page 418.

Faith can be a source of deep comfort when you are facing death. However, we have known people to resist it for just that reason; their position seems to be that if they didn't need faith when they were well, they aren't going to embrace it now just because they're dying. Faith is an intensely individual matter, but in our view this attitude

"She had the most wonderful collection of things – art pieces and antiques....She was like Santa Claus. You've never seen anyone happier giving away all her worldly possessions."

– Kris Richardson

"People can learn a lot from the way they go through their dying."

–James Carse

is counterproductive. If nurturing your spiritual side could bring you comfort now, we feel that it may be shortsighted to refuse to explore the issue just because you never needed to do so before.

Some people can gain a sense of control over their own death by deciding where they are going to die. Admittedly, this is not always possible. Most people nowadays die in the hospital or in a nursing home. However, if there is a hospice program in your area, you may be able to die at home, surrounded by your friends and family, supported by the members of a hospice care team.

To be eligible for this program, you must be diagnosed as having less than six months to live. Besides a medical director (who acts in collaboration with your doctor) and a registered nurse (who acts as case manager), the hospice team may include a social worker, home health aides, a chaplain, and volunteers. The nurse will make regularly scheduled visits during the day; at night a nurse is available for telephone consultation. Other team members will come to your home on an as-needed basis. Hospice does not provide round-the-clock care until the last few days of the patient's life. Therefore in order to be eligible for this program you must have a friend or family member who can act as your primary caregiver. The hospice team will train this person to look after your physical needs.

The hospice team's job is to help out your family and to provide skilled care for you. This means managing your symptoms, controlling your pain, and providing emotional and psychological support. Hospice can sometimes also arrange for beds, canes, commodes, and other medical equipment.

The cost of hospice care varies depending on the services provided. It is covered under Medicare, Medicaid, and most private insurance plans.

To learn more about hospice, telephone your local Visiting Nurse Association or check with your physician, your hospital, or your State Department of Health. The Hospice Education Institute (1-800-331-1620) supplies referrals to local hospices. The National Hospice

Organization (1-800-658-8898) can also provide information on hospice programs in your area.

Finally, you can decide—at least to some extent—when you are going to die. That is, you can decide when to stop your treatments and let the cancer take its natural course. Some patients feel most in control when they fight to the very end. This helps them to maintain a sense of hope. Others may choose to stop their treatments for a variety of reasons. These reasons may have to do with quality of life, with their personal beliefs, with money issues, with family issues, and so forth. Here we have no specific suggestions to make. We want only to emphasize that stopping treatments is a personal choice. It is your decision and yours alone.

People can learn a lot from the way they go through their dying, says James Carse, who for fifteen years taught courses on death and dying in the religion department of New York University, and whose wife died of cancer in 1991. In Chapter 8, many of the patients we interviewed—including a number of patients who were dying—told you what having cancer had taught them about life. Above all, it taught them the value of relationships—of love. What can you learn as you go through your dying? We hope you will learn how much you love other people. And we hope you will learn how much other people—even those whose feelings you may never have suspected—love you.

Do you want to make sure that your wishes will be followed? See the discussion of Living Wills in Appendix 2.

For Family and Friends

If a member of your family or a friend is dying, that person's death can be very hard on you. How you deal with the stress and the pain will have a profound effect on both you and the patient. You have two tasks: to do what is best for the patient and to do what you need to do for yourself. It can be very difficult to balance these tasks, and your natural tendency may be to overlook your own needs. For a general discussion of how best to nurture yourself, see Chapter 7, page 252. In this section we suggest ways to support the dying patient and ways to deal with your own grief.

Supporting the Patient

The rule is to *support the patient in the way that is best for the patient.* This can sometimes be extremely difficult. But commit yourself to do the best you can, knowing that you won't always do everything right, and that that's OK.

Most patients need to express their feelings – feelings about dying, perhaps, about things left undone, about not being there for the children, about a future that they will not share. Let the patient talk; your job is to listen. Put the patient's need to talk about things that may be painful for both of you above your own need not to talk about those things. Expressing his or her feelings helps the patient to say goodbye. Listen without judgment or debate.

Letting the patient express his feelings can be good for both of you. "One of the most important things that happened during those last few months was a series of conversations that she and I had," James Carse told us. "We thought we should talk about everything that I might later wish we had talked about. So we talked about our children, our lives, our married life together, our friends, our professions, and my future. She had a lot to say about my future. And I realized after she died that she was actually saying goodbye to me. I think it was very important for her to do that."[1]

People who are dying often go through a series of stages. One of these stages may be anger. This can be a natural reaction to impending death. If the patient says things that sound hateful, try to accept it. Above all, don't blame yourself. You may be tempted to avoid the patient or to judge him. Try instead to understand why he might be angry. Can you put yourself in his position and imagine how he would feel? Respect and attention, says Elisabeth Kübler-Ross, help to defuse the patient's anger. Anger is a natural stage that often (not always) precedes acceptance. Don't say things that will invalidate that anger ("It's God's

For more on these stages, see the books by Elisabeth Kübler-Ross in the list of Recommended Reading on page 418.

For more on dealing with the angry patient, see page 267.

will." "You should be grateful for the years you had.") before the patient has had a chance to reach the acceptance stage. –And if you can't defuse the patient's anger? "At least," says Lois Ryder, "try not to lash back. It can be a comfort later to know that you did the best you could for the patient."

The last stage before death is often detachment. The patient who has accepted death may seem cool toward his or her loved ones. Don't see this as a rejection or as a sign of failure on your part. Patients "often die easier if they are allowed and helped to detach themselves slowly from all the meaningful relationships in their life," says Dr. Kübler-Ross.[2] The best thing you can offer the patient in this last stage is sometimes just your silent presence.

No matter what he or she chooses to say, let the patient set the pace and the agenda. Many patients who have not yet reached the last stage do need to express their feelings. However, a few patients need to suppress them. "A lifetime habit of suppressing feelings may be difficult to break, even though you are dying," says clinical psychologist Robert Fuhr.[3] If your husband refuses to tell you how he feels, if your wife wears a cheerful mask no matter what, don't push it. Support these patients in the way that helps them the most, by not discussing what they don't want to discuss. This too can be a gift of love. "I talked about the things he wanted to talk about," says Lois Ryder. "It was my way of showing him that I loved him."

Should you tell the patient that he or she is dying? Here there are no set rules–except, perhaps, the rule that, again, you should do what is best for the patient. "A patient has a right to die in peace and dignity," says Dr. Kübler-Ross. "…He should not be used to fulfill our own needs when his own wishes are in opposition to ours."[4] Ask yourself, then, whose ends would be served by telling him. Would it be in the patient's own best interest? Or would it serve your own emotional needs? Your principles? Your own practical interests? In our opinion, you should never force anyone to confront the fact that he or she is dying. James Carse agrees. "You don't just rush in with

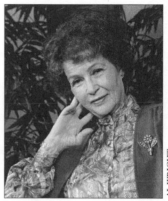

AL WRIGHT

Lois Ryder

"*I talked about the things he wanted to talk about. It was my way of showing him that I loved him.*"

–Lois Ryder

> *"A patient has a right to die in peace and dignity....He should not be used to fulfill our own needs when his own wishes are in opposition to ours."*
>
> **– Dr. Elisabeth Kübler-Ross**

a principle – namely, that everyone's got to know everything about their condition, no matter what. You look at the whole situation with as much humanity as you can and try to determine whether this person is really going to be well served by being told. And that's a very, very hard decision." Look for signs that the patient wants to discuss the subject, says Robert Fuhr. And Carse adds, "I think you could ask, 'Do you know what the disease is?' 'Do you want to know more about it?' Questions like that." In short, open the door – but let the patient decide whether to walk through it.

Finally, remember that if you decide not to tell the patient, everyone has to be in on the decision. If Grandmother believes that she's going to get well, you don't want your four-year-old to tell her, "Daddy says you're dying."

On the other hand, sometimes the patient initiates the questions. James Carse told us that his wife "definitely wanted to know how she was going to die, and she asked the nurse several times to explain how it would happen. Would she go into a coma? What is coma like? And so on." If the patient asks questions like these, answer them tactfully but honestly. If you don't know the answers, get them from someone who does.

Don't force your religious beliefs on the patient, either. We described in Chapter 6 how a well-meaning relative told one of the patients we interviewed that he must convert to her religion if he hoped to save his eternal soul. This advice may have made the relative feel better, but it did the patient no good; he already had his own beliefs.

This is not to say that you shouldn't mention your beliefs at all. You might say, for example, "I really believe in life after death. Shall I tell you why? You might find it comforting. I know I do." But wait for the patient to say yes before you go on.

In short, once again, open the door – but let the patient decide whether to walk through it. And if he chooses not to, respect his choice.

What if the patient doesn't know that he or she is dying,

and yet there are practical decisions that have to be made? What if, for example, you need to make business decisions on the patient's behalf? In cases like this, we suggest that you open the door by saying, "While you're ill (*not* "Since you're dying"), why not let me pay the bills?" or "… it would be a good time to let me learn more about the business." When one of the family members we interviewed was obliged to put her mother into a nursing home, she told her that she was putting her there "until you get better." She never told her mother that she was dying.

In short, there may be times when a little creative truth bending is in order. Use what you know about the patient to get his or her needs met without having to say things that you know the patient doesn't want to hear.

What if the patient wants to talk about death, but you can't handle the topic of death yourself? Again, do what's best for the patient. This doesn't mean forcing yourself to respond; the patient needs someone who can actively listen. Don't feel guilty if you can't be that person. Acknowledge the patient's need to talk. "I know this is important to you, and I wish I could talk about it, but I can't. But don't worry. I'll find someone who can." Perhaps the patient will suggest someone. If not, it's up to you to find a person who can fill this need. If no one in the family can talk about death, ask a nurse, a member of the clergy, or a hospice worker to help out.

Like the patient, you may feel the need to resolve old issues, or new ones. Open the door to see whether the patient is receptive. You might say, for example, "You know, I'd like to discuss this with you. Do you want to talk about it?" But accept that the patient may not want to talk about it, and that you should respect his or her wishes.

You may want to bring up the issue of your own grief. It takes skill here to balance the patient's needs with your own. "I was very much aware of the pain of losing her," says James Carse, "so I started to develop a pattern of private grieving. I would be a little bit upbeat with her and then very sad away from her. But that was a kind of dishonesty that I didn't like living with. So I let her know

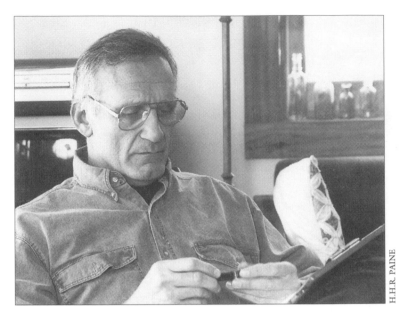

H.H.R. PAINE

James Carse

"I started to develop a pattern of private grieving. I would be a little bit upbeat with her and then very sad away from her."

– James Carse

What's wrong with the cheerleader approach? See page 255.

my feelings. For example, I cried with her on several occasions. But once or twice she asked me not to cry. I think it was hard for her to deal with the full range of emotions, hers and mine. But on the whole, she was very happy to know my feelings."

Sometimes you may need to say things without using words. Suppose, for example, that you need to tell your father how much you love him. But your father has always avoided talking about love, and you know it would make him uncomfortable to talk about it now. Find ways to express your love nonverbally. Offer him a back rub. Ask him which foods would taste good to him. Be there when he needs you. Give his shoulder a squeeze. Show him that you're willing to put him first.

It's possible to express love in the wrong way, or even for the wrong reasons. As John Chapman pointed out in Chapter 7, love can sometimes be overbearing. Expressing your love doesn't mean smothering the patient. It doesn't mean talking to the patient when the patient would rather be quiet. Above all, it doesn't mean always putting a bright face on things. If you're tempted to express your love in any of these ways, try to sense what the patient really needs. Then ask yourself as honestly as you can whether you are serving the patient's needs–or your own.

What you say to the patient can turn out to be extremely important to both of you. Ask yourself, "Three years from now, what will I wish I had said?" What issues will you wish you had resolved? Try to resolve those issues now. If the patient is receptive, and if you feel comfortable doing so, talk about your own life after he or she dies. How do you see your future? How does the patient see it? "–So that anticipating the loss will become part of your relationship with the person," says James Carse. "In that way, you can somehow together face the loss of each other. And I think that's very powerful, very healing."

One final point as we conclude this section. Try not to let the dying process take over your life. If you get too consumed with the dying process, you lose sight of other things–things that you could use to meet your own needs, things that you could share with the patient. If you forget to water the garden, there will be no flowers for you, or for the patient, to enjoy. If you let death take over your life, you run the risk of losing your perspective.

Dealing with Grief

When the patient dies, you will have to deal with your own grief. Don't be surprised if you start to grieve while the patient is still alive. This anticipatory grief is normal. It helps to prepare you for the death. Deal with it by acknowledging it, by realizing that it *is* normal, and by sharing it with others, says Robert Fuhr.

When should you share your grief with the patient? That depends on the patient's own emotional state. Sometimes sharing your grief just makes it that much harder for him or her. This is especially true when the patient is in denial, or is still enjoying living in the moment. This would be the wrong time to tell him how much you are going to miss him. When the patient is actively facing death, when he himself is engaged in anticipatory grieving, you can

Simply say, "I'm sorry for your loss." Express your affection naturally, without overdoing it.

support him by sharing your own grief, says Fuhr.

It can take months, or even years, to work through your grief after the patient dies. Here again there are no rules. Don't judge yourself if you want to start dating after six months–or if you are still mourning the loss of your spouse after five years. Every person and every relationship is different; working through grief is a highly individual process. However long it takes, that's normal–for you.

And even after you've worked through your grief, there may be times when a holiday, or a memory, or a special song triggers a sense of loss. That's normal too.

When the patient dies, you may also have to deal with other people's grief. Here the most important rule is to listen. Give the person who is grieving a chance to say whatever he or she feels like saying. Ask questions ("How do you feel about that?") if it seems appropriate, but don't push. Once again, open the door, but let the other person walk through it. Above all, don't offer advice. Don't offer what Charles Fuhrman calls "healing wisdom." Don't say things like "It's better this way." "You'll get over it." "You'll have another child." This doesn't acknowledge the pain the other person is feeling. It can sound as if you're saying, "Hurry up and stop feeling that way." That hurts the other person when he or she needs to be comforted.

Instead, simply say, "I'm sorry for your loss." Express your affection naturally, without overdoing it ("Are you doing OK?"). Offer specific help ("Would you like me to make up some food for you?" "Would you like me to stay with you for a day or two?" "Would you like me to give you a call tomorrow morning?"). Gestures like these comfort the survivor and show him that you care without putting any emotional demands on him.

What do you tell the children when the patient dies? That too is an individual matter. It depends on the child's age, on the child's relationship to the patient, on the family's religious beliefs. There are excellent books that deal with this issue. We list two on pages 419 and 420.

People who are grieving usually get a lot of support at first, but it can taper off quickly. It's important for you to let your friend know that you're still there. One way to do this is to organize a support team. Team members take turns checking up on the person, telephoning her, sending her cards, inviting her to dinner. How long should you keep doing this? Hospice programs provide grief support for up to twelve months. Try to maintain your own commitment for as long as it takes—until you're sure that your friend no longer needs it.

"Don't be afraid to talk about the loved one," says therapist Carol Landt. "As people talk, so can they heal. And when your friend wants to talk," says Landt, "listen! You might want to remind your friend how well they cared for their loved one, or acknowledge how difficult it was for them. Encourage people who are grieving to be kind to themselves, to care for themselves."[5]

We agree with Carol. If there's one point we'd like to make, it's this: Be kind to the person who is grieving—even (especially) when that person is you.

Just as you need not face cancer alone, so you need not face death alone. And in facing death, as in facing cancer, what you do can make a difference—whether you are the dying patient or the patient's loved ones.

> *"Don't be afraid to talk about the loved one. As people talk, so can they heal. And when your friend wants to talk, listen!"*
>
> –Carol Landt

In order of their first appearance, the patients who contributed to this appendix are: Arnold Schraer, Marcie Wienecke, John Chapman, and Charles Fuhrman. The family members who contributed to this appendix are: Kris Richardson, James Carse, Lois Ryder, and Carol Landt.

Recommended Reading

Ahronheim, Judith, and Doron Weber. *Final Passages: Positive Choices for the Dying and Their Loved Ones.* **New York: Simon & Schuster, 1992.**

This guidebook for dying patients and their families tells what to expect from modern medical technology; offers advice for dealing with your doctor; and discusses pain control, clinical depression, and the issues surrounding life support, suicide, and euthanasia. It shows you how to take advantage of the options that will enable you to live life fully until the end. Dr. Ahronheim is a physician and an associate professor at Mt. Sinai Hospital in New York City; Doron Weber writes on health care issues. Both authors are affiliated with the Society for the Right to Die.

Doore, Gary, ed. *What Survives? Contemporary Explorations of Life after Death.* **Los Angeles: Jeremy P. Tarcher, 1990.**

This collection of essays by psychologists, scientists, and religious scholars examines the belief in life after death in a variety of different cultures. It discusses altered states of consciousness, mysticism, and shamanistic practices from the perspective of modern scientific thought. Doore concludes that survival cannot be either proven or disproven, and presents a strong case for believing in it anyway.

Kramer, Kenneth. *The Sacred Art of Dying: How World Religions Understand Death.* **New York: Paulist Press, 1988.**

A professor of religious studies explains what Christians, Jews, Hindus, Buddhists, and Muslims believe about death and describes how they prepare themselves to die. There are chapters on Chinese and Native American beliefs and on the beliefs of ancient civilizations as well. Each chapter includes journal exercises that will help you to explore your own attitudes toward death.

Kübler-Ross, Elisabeth. *On Death and Dying*. New York: Macmillan Publishing Co., 1969.

This landmark book describes in detail the five stages that dying patients go through and explains how best to help the patient during each of these stages. The author also discusses the emotional effects that the patient's death may have on the family. Although it was written for professionals, this book is easy to read; it will be helpful to anyone who wants to understand, and learn from, the dying patient. Dr. Kübler-Ross is a physician, a psychiatrist, and a world-famous authority on death.

—————————————. *On Children and Death*. New York: Macmillan Publishing Co., Collier, 1985.

How dying children think about death, and how to talk, and live, with the dying child. This book is based on stories told by the parents themselves and on Kübler-Ross's own extensive experience in working with dying children. The tone is somewhat inspirational; there is a long chapter on spiritual issues. The bibliography is exceptionally good.

LeShan, Eda. *Learning to Say Goodbye: When a Parent Dies*. New York: Macmillan Publishing Co., 1976.

Speaking directly to the child, Eda LeShan talks about how it feels when a parent dies. She describes in terms that a child can understand the stages that he or she will go through in recovering from grief. This book is written for older children, but young children might like to have parts of it read to them. The whole family can benefit from this simple, clear, compassionate little book. LeShan is an educator and family counselor who writes for children and about them.

Morse, Melvin. *Closer to the Light: Learning from the Near-Death Experiences of Children*. New York: Ballantine Books, Ivy Books, 1990.

This book offers a glimpse of what it may be like to die; it suggests that death may be a peaceful, joyous experience. It is based on hundreds of interviews that the author conducted with children who had once been declared clinically dead. Dr. Morse examines the near-death experience in light of contemporary neuroscience; he believes that it is possible that some part of the mind may live on after death. This book is very easy to read; it includes an extensive bibliography of books and articles on the near-death experience. Dr. Morse is a pediatrician and a pioneer in near-death research.

Rando, Therese A. *Grief, Dying, and Death: Clinical Interventions for Caregivers.* **Champaign, IL: Research Press Co., 1984.**

Written for health care professionals, this book offers detailed suggestions on working with dying patients and grieving family members. It is well organized and clearly written in a somewhat dry but fairly readable style. It includes a chapter on funerals and funerary rituals and one on the caregiver's personal concerns. There is a long list of scientific references. The author is a clinical psychologist who specializes in issues of loss, grief, and terminal illness.

Schaefer, Dan, and Christine Lyons. *How Do We Tell the Children? A Parents' Guide to Helping Children Understand and Cope When Someone Dies.* **New York: Newmarket Press, 1986.**

The authors explain how children of different ages view death. They list the questions children are likely to ask and suggest how to answer them in ways that are sensitive, accurate, and appropriate. Children's grief reactions are discussed in detail. There is a quick reference section that parents can turn to for answers when they haven't time to read the whole book. Dan Schaefer has been a funeral director for twenty-five years; he has worked directly with thousands of grieving children and their parents. Christine Lyons is a journalist who specializes in children's issues.

Schiff, Harriet Sarnoff. *The Bereaved Parent.* **New York: Penguin USA, Viking, 1978.**

Parents who must deal with the death of a child will find solid information, understanding, and support in this guidebook, written by a woman whose own son died at the age of ten. She discusses practical decisions as well as emotional reactions and explains how the death may affect your marriage and your other children. This book is compassionate, easy to read, and full of concrete advice from someone who has been there.

Stoddard, Sandol. *The Hospice Movement: A Better Way of Caring for the Dying.* **New York: Random House, Vintage, 1992.**

Written for the general reader, this book describes in detail how hospices are managed and what services they provide. It also gives the history of the hospice movement. The writing is anecdotal and frequently poetic. The author is a professional writer and a hospice volunteer.

Tatelbaum, Judy. *The Courage to Grieve: Creative Living, Recovery, and Growth through Grief.* **New York: HarperCollins Publishers, 1984.**

A self-help book about surviving grief, written by a Gestalt therapist. It explains how to deal with the fear of death and describes the various phases of grief, recovery, and resolution. The author provides self-help exercises and offers advice on working with a therapist. Readers who need help understanding, or working through, their grieving will find this book full of valuable suggestions.

You can order books on death and grieving through Compassion Book Service (1-704-675-9670) and Centering Corporation (1-402-553-1200). Call to request their current catalogues.

Financial, Legal, Insurance, and Employment

If you have cancer now or if you are recovering from cancer, you are probably facing a great many practical problems. These may include legal or financial problems, problems with insurance, or even problems with employment. In this appendix we give you the basic information that you will need to deal with these problems and we tell you where you can learn more.

Money Problems

Having cancer can be very expensive. Here are some ways to ease the strain on your pocketbook.

How to Get Financial Aid

If you need help paying your bills, many agencies offer financial aid. To get in touch with the ones that are most suitable for you, start by calling the National Cancer Institute (NCI) Cancer Information Service (1-800-4-CANCER). If you have leukemia, you might also want to get in touch with the Leukemia Society of America, Inc. (1-212-573-8484). This organization may provide financial aid directly under certain conditions.

You may qualify for state financial aid. If your cancer is work related, you may be eligible for worker's compensation. If your cancer is not work related but it has left you disabled, you may qualify for state unemployment-disability benefits. The laws that govern both of these programs vary from state to state. To learn more about the laws in your state, contact the Department of Labor, listed in the white pages under State Government.

You may also qualify for federal support. Social Security offers two forms of support for people who are disabled. You may be eligible for disability insurance benefits if you have paid enough into Social Security and if you have been disabled for five consecutive months. You may be eligible for Supplemental Security Income (SSI) if your income falls below the federal poverty level, provided you are sixty-five or older *or* blind *or* disabled. It is not necessary to have paid into Social Security in order to qualify for SSI.

Social Security also offers retirement benefits to workers who have paid into the system, whether they are disabled or not. To receive partial benefits, you must be at least sixty-five. Survivors of workers who qualify for Social Security retirement benefits may be eligible for spouses', survivors', or dependents' benefits.

To learn whether you are eligible for any of these programs, contact the Social Security Administration office nearest you. It will be listed in the white pages of your telephone directory under U.S. Government, Department of Health and Human Services.

Your union or your employer may also pay disability benefits. Contact one or both of them to find out. To be eligible, you will usually have to have belonged to the union, or have worked for the employer, for at least five years.

No matter what kind of disability benefits you file for, file as soon as you verify that you are eligible. It can take weeks to process your claim.

There are also many organizations that will provide you with services, such as transportation, or equipment, such as wheelchairs, at no cost. To find out more about these organizations, call 1-800-4-CANCER. You might also contact the social services department of your hospital and religious and community service organizations in your area. If you qualify for public assistance, contact your local public assistance office. If you belong to a labor union, talk to your union representative. Some pharmaceutical companies offer free drugs to patients who cannot afford to buy them.[1]

APPENDIX 2

Taxes

Keep a record of all of your medical expenses. You can deduct part of these expenses from your income for federal tax purposes. As of tax year 1992, you could take a medical deduction for expenses that exceeded 7.5 percent of your adjusted gross income. Deductible expenses include the cost of prescription drugs, doctors' fees, and hospital expenses. They also include health insurance premiums, the cost of home nursing care, and travel costs to get medical care. For more on medical deductions, see IRS publication 502; call 1-800-TAX FORM to get a copy.

Financial Counseling

If you are having trouble paying your bills, you may want to get financial counseling. A counselor can help you to budget your income and work with your creditors. To locate a financial counselor, look in the yellow pages under Consumer Credit Counseling Services. A for-profit service will charge a fee, so look for a nonprofit service. If none is listed, contact the National Foundation for Consumer Credit, Inc., at 1-301-589-5600. This organization will put you in touch with a nonprofit credit counseling service in your area.

Legal Problems

You need to know the legal issues that concern you as a patient. The first of these is the issue of informed consent.

Informed Consent

For more on getting this information from your doctor, see Chapter 4.

You must sign an informed consent form before you can undergo certain procedures. This form states that you agree to be treated and that you have been told

- What is going to be done and why
- The probable consequences
- The risks of having the procedure and of not having it
- The medically acceptable alternatives

Make sure that you have been given—and that you understand—this information before you sign the form. And remember that you can cross out any line of the form that you do not agree to. Remember too that signing the form simply gives the doctor permission to treat you. It does not absolve the doctor if he or she is negligent.

An informed consent is not necessary in the case of a life-threatening emergency. It is not necessary if your doctor discovers in the course of performing one surgery that another surgery must be done. It is not necessary if you waive your right to an informed consent. But otherwise, when the procedure is one that requires your informed consent, the doctor cannot legally treat you until he or she has obtained that consent.

Children under eighteen do not usually have the right to informed consent, but their parents exercise this right on their behalf.

Your Medical Records

You also have legal rights with respect to your medical records. Exactly what rights you have here will depend on the laws in your state. To find out how to gain access to your hospital records, check first with the medical records department of the hospital itself. If this doesn't give you the information you need, check with the state office of the American Medical Association to learn exactly what your rights are and how to exercise them. To learn how to gain access to your physician's records, check first with his or her office. If you need more information, check with the State Board of Medical Examiners (sometimes called the State Licensing Board), listed in the white pages under State Government.

Your Rights as a Patient

In 1973 the American Hospital Association adopted a guideline for hospital policy that is known as the Patient's Bill of Rights. Here is a summary of the rights to which

APPENDIX 2

you as a patient are entitled, regardless of sex, age, race, creed, or ability to pay:

- The right to be treated courteously and with respect
- The right to know your physician's name, address, and specialty
- The right to obtain information about your treatment, including alternatives; to obtain information about your rights as a patient; and to review your medical records
- The right to privacy
- The right to refuse treatment
- The right to examine your hospital bill and to have it explained to you.
- The right to know the hospital rules that apply to you
- The right to refuse to participate in experimental treatment

In some states these rights also apply to the person whom you designate as your advocate.

Only a few states have actually legislated the Patient's Bill of Rights, and various states have revised it in one way or another. But in most hospitals you will find posted some version of the Patient's Bill of Rights, and most hospitals make at least some attempt to implement it. If you want to learn more about your rights as a patient, or if you suspect that your rights are not being respected, talk to the patient ombudsman. It is this staff member's job to act as your advocate. If you still aren't satisfied, you may want to complain (in writing) to the medical director of the hospital (sometimes called the hospital chief of staff).

Finally, you should know that it is illegal for the hospital to refuse to discharge you until you have paid your bill. If you have questions about the bill, don't pay it or sign an agreement to pay it until those questions have been answered. Ask for a fully itemized bill and examine each item carefully. If there are major discrepancies between what you think you owe and what the hospital says you owe, consult an attorney or ask your insurance company to step in.

Power of Attorney

Most people's lives are full of paperwork–bills to pay, taxes to pay, checks to deposit. When you are ill, the paperwork piles up quickly; if allowed to pile up, it can soon become unmanageable. If you will be unable to manage your own affairs for some time, you may want to prevent this from happening by appointing another person to manage them for you. This is called granting that person *power of attorney*. The person whom you appoint can make legal and financial decisions on your behalf; in some states, he or she can make medical decisions on your behalf as well. The power of attorney lasts until you revoke it or until you become incapacitated.

A *durable power of attorney* extends the terms of the power of attorney. It must be made while you are mentally competent, but once made, it lasts until you die or until you revoke it. A durable power of attorney, then, lets you designate someone to manage your financial affairs if you become permanently incapacitated. In many states you can also use a durable power of attorney to designate someone to manage your health care.

In some states it is also possible to draw up a *springing durable power of attorney*. This differs from the durable power of attorney in two ways: it takes effect only when you become incapacitated and it ends when you become competent again.

State laws vary when it comes to drawing up any version of the power of attorney. Consult a lawyer who is familiar with the legal requirements in your state.

Trusts and Wills

Establishing a trust is a complex procedure. It is generally worthwhile only for people who have a large estate and who want a bank or other dependable trustee to manage that estate for them during their lifetime (a living trust) or for their heirs, if the latter are children

APPENDIX 2

or are otherwise inexperienced at managing money.

No matter how large or small your estate, it is always wise to make sure that you have a will. It is especially wise, of course, if you are facing a terminal prognosis. Note that once the will is drawn up you can change it at any time; this is called adding a *codicil* to the will. Computer software is available for drawing up simple wills, but in general we strongly recommend that you consult an attorney. He or she will help you to draw up a valid will– one that will ensure that your wishes are followed concerning the disposition of your estate.

Living Wills

If you are facing a terminal prognosis, you may want to draw up a Living Will. This document lets you specify, while you are still mentally competent, exactly how much you want done to prolong your life once it is clear that you will not recover. If you do not wish to be kept alive by artificial means or by "heroic measures," think seriously about drawing up a Living Will. The Living Will is legally valid in most, but not all, states; however, simply express-ing your wishes on paper will encourage your physicians to follow them (and may make them liable for damages if they do not).

If you decide to draw up a Living Will, be sure to discuss the issues involved with your doctor. Each of the people who participate in your care should have a copy. To be valid, a Living Will must be signed and dated in the presence of two adult witnesses who are not family members or other interested parties. For more on Living Wills, contact Choice in Dying (formerly Concern for Dying/Society for the Right to Die) at 1-212-366-5540.

In addition to the legal and financial problems summa-rized in this section, cancer patients face legal problems that are related to employment and financial problems that are related to insurance. We discuss these special problems in the next two sections.

Insurance

For most cancer patients, *insurance problems* means problems with medical insurance. In this section we summarize what you will need to know.

Private Medical Insurance

You can buy private medical insurance as an individual or as a member of a group. Most people carry group insurance provided by their employers. Group plans are also available through associations such as AARP and religious or professional organizations. If you are not eligible for group insurance, it is also possible to buy individual coverage directly from insurers such as Blue Cross/Blue Shield. If you are shopping for individual insurance, be sure to buy it from a licensed independent broker. Look in the yellow pages under Insurance for the names of licensed brokers in your area. We shall have more to say presently about choosing a policy.

Public Medical Insurance

If you meet the requirements, you may be eligible for public medical insurance. If you are over sixty-five or are otherwise eligible for Social Security, you are also eligible for Medicare. The rules that govern what Medicare covers and how to apply for benefits are complicated and they change frequently. To learn more about Medicare, consult *Your Medicare Handbook*, available at the nearest Social Security Administration office. Look in the white pages under U.S. Government, Department of Health and Human Services.

If your income is limited, you may be eligible for Medicaid. Medicaid is provided by the states, so rules on eligibility vary, but in general you are eligible if you get Supplemental Security Income or if you qualify for "medically needy" status. To learn more about Medicaid, contact your State Department of Public Welfare or State

Department of Social Services, listed in the white pages under State Government.

If you are a veteran, you will be eligible for service-related health care benefits. Cancer is not usually service related, but if you have reason to believe that yours is (if you were exposed to Agent Orange, for example), you may want to investigate this possibility. Even if your cancer is not service related, you may be eligible for certain benefits, especially if your income is limited. Contact the Department of Veterans' Affairs, listed in the white pages under U.S. Government. Or consult the booklet *Federal Benefits for Veterans and Dependents,* available from the Superintendent of Documents, U.S. Government Printing Office, Washington, DC 20402.

Special Problems for Cancer Patients

If you had medical insurance before you were diagnosed, you will probably not lose your coverage after your diagnosis (although your rates may go up). However, once you have been diagnosed with cancer, it is difficult to obtain private insurance. The company may refuse to insure you altogether, or it may charge very high premiums or deny certain benefits based on your medical history. The problem is especially acute for patients who are insured by their employer and who change jobs after they have been diagnosed. As a rule, the coverage on your new job will not cover preexisting conditions until you have been free of treatment for six months to a year. And it is considered insurance fraud if you don't disclose preexisting conditions. A few plans will cover you immediately, even for a preexisting condition, but you will pay a very high premium for the privilege of joining such a plan.

All of this helps to explain why one out of four cancer survivors cannot get adequate medical insurance.[2]

Although there is no law that guarantees cancer patients the right to medical insurance, there are two laws that can help you to keep the insurance that covered you on your old job. The Comprehensive Omnibus Budget

Reconciliation Act (COBRA) mandates that employers of over twenty employees offer continued coverage to employees and their dependents who have lost coverage through individual circumstances. This means that if your hours are reduced or if you quit or are terminated for any reason other than gross misconduct, you will still be covered (although you will have to pay your own premiums). The coverage must be continued for up to eighteen months after termination of employment. Spouses and dependents are covered for up to thirty-six months.

The Employer Retirement and Income Security Act (ERISA) mandates that an employer may not discriminate against an employee for the purpose of denying benefits. This means, for example, that your employer cannot fire you when he learns you have cancer in order to keep you from collecting benefits under an employee benefit plan. To learn more about COBRA and ERISA, contact the Pension and Welfare Benefits Administration of the U.S. Department of Labor, Room N-5658, 200 Constitution Avenue NW, Washington, DC 20210.

Many states have high-risk pools for state residents who are otherwise uninsurable. Coverage usually goes into effect after a six-month waiting period. As of this writing, high-risk pools are available in California, Colorado, Connecticut, Florida, Georgia, Illinois, Indiana, Iowa, Louisiana, Maine, Minnesota, Missouri, Montana, Nebraska, New Mexico, North Dakota, Oregon, Rhode Island, South Carolina, Tennessee, Texas, Utah, Washington, Wisconsin, and Wyoming. If you live in one of these states, contact the State Department of Insurance to learn more about the program. (And if you do not live in one of these states, call anyway and ask whether your state is planning to set up a high-risk pool.)

Finally, some health maintenance organizations (HMOs) and private insurance companies will insure you regardless of your medical history on a so-called open-enrollment plan. There is usually a waiting period of three months to one year before these plans will pay benefits on preex-

APPENDIX 2

isting conditions. Some open-enrollment plans are offered year-round; others are offered for a brief period once a year. Blue Cross/Blue Shield periodically offers open enrollment in several states. To find out more about their programs, look in the yellow pages under Insurance for the names of Blue Cross/Blue Shield agents in your area.

Choosing the Best Policy

If you are difficult to insure, you may have to settle for any policy you can get. But whenever possible, it pays to shop for insurance. In general it is preferable to get group insurance; it costs less and it offers more benefits. This is an important point to consider when you are changing jobs. If you have to choose between two new jobs, it may pay you to take the one that pays less but offers the better insurance plan. Note too that the larger the company, the less likely it is that its group insurance plan will exclude you based on your medical history. If you leave some companies, you can convert your coverage under the company group policy to individual coverage. This coverage usually lasts about a year.

In any case, don't give up one plan until you are covered by another. And if you are buying individual insurance, shop around. Compare the policies that different companies offer. Make sure that the one you choose is guaranteed renewable. Choose the one that has the shortest waiting period relevant to your preexisting condition. Make sure that the policy will pay for at least 80 percent of the cost of covered services (an exception is often made for inpatient psychiatric care). Make sure that the policy will pay at least $250,000 for catastrophic illness coverage. Be careful not to buy duplicate coverage—that is, don't buy a special cancer insurance policy, for example, when you can get the same coverage on a comprehensive policy. —And if possible, buy your insurance while you're still healthy.

Whether you are shopping for insurance or reviewing your existing coverage, it's important to read the policy carefully. Find out *exactly* what it covers. Get a *current* copy of the plan booklet from your carrier and find out

- The amount of the deductible (for example, $2,000)
- The maximum amount over the deductible that you will be expected to pay. (For example, you may be expected to pay 20 percent of expenses over $2,000 up to $10,000. In this example, you would pay a deductible of $2,000 plus 20 percent of $8,000 or $1,600. Your total out-of-pocket expenses would be $3,600, and the insurance company would pay all expenses over $10,000.)
- What percentage of the hospital and nonhospital charges the policy will pay
- The amount of maximum lifetime coverage
- How much mental health coverage the policy provides
- What the policy stipulates concerning second opinions
- What things are not covered
- How to file a claim. The policy will specify that claims must be filed within a certain period of time.

If you have questions, ask your insurance broker to answer them. If you still have questions, talk to the company's claims representative or contact the American Council on Life Insurance at 1-800-423-8000.

Once you have an insurance policy, don't risk letting it lapse. Keep it in force by paying your premiums promptly. Note that if you have a disability policy, the premiums may be waived under certain conditions. Check the fine print. The waiver of premium does not usually apply to hospitalization or major medical policies.

Filing a Claim

You should file claims for any expenses that are covered by your insurance. This is one reason why it's important to know what your policy covers. Some people don't file claims even when they know they are covered simply because they can't face the paperwork. If this sounds like you, get a friend or family member to help you, or ask someone from your church or temple to help. You can also ask a social worker or an American Cancer Society (ACS) volunteer. If all else fails, there are medical claims companies that will provide this service for a fee. To find one, look in the yellow pages under Insurance Claim Processing Services.

What should you do if your claim is rejected? The first thing to do is to check to make sure that you filled it out correctly. Next check to make sure that your hospital or your physician provided the company with the information it needed to process the claim. If everything seems to be in order and you believe that the company has made a mistake, talk to your insurance broker (or to your company's benefits people, if you are insured through your employer). If this doesn't bring results, contact the insurance company directly. Ask first to speak to the claims representative and then to the claims supervisor. Next send a letter to the company's corporate offices. If you still aren't satisfied, contact your State Department of Insurance. If all else fails, you can file a complaint in small-claims court or consult an attorney who specializes in insurance law.

Whenever you deal with your insurance company, whether you're filing a complaint or simply filing a claim, be sure to keep a record of all your correspondence. This includes claim forms, payment vouchers, notifications, bills, and letters to and from the company. Make notes of any telephone calls, including the date of the call and the names of the people you talked to. This is a good way to keep everything straight and to keep track of the money that you are owed. It will be essential if you should ever be involved in a dispute with your insurance company.

Life Insurance

If you are a cancer patient, you will probably have trouble buying life insurance. Whether or not you are able to obtain it will depend on the type of cancer you have, on when it was diagnosed, and on your prognosis. (No company will issue life insurance to a patient whom it believes to be terminal.) You may, however, wish to apply for life insurance if you have young children, or a spouse or parent who depends on you for support. You can improve your chances if you go with the large companies (because they grade carefully for type and stage of tumor); if you can get insured through a group plan (because companies that write insurance for large groups don't evaluate the health of individual members); or if you apply for a graded policy (which will pay full benefits only after a three-year waiting period). In buying life insurance, as in buying medical insurance, shop around. Get estimates from several different companies, and work with an independent broker, who can help you to get the best possible deal.

Employment

One out of four people who have had cancer face employment problems. They may not be hired at all. They may be demoted or denied benefits. They may even be dismissed outright. The prejudice against cancer survivors stems from a variety of myths—the myth that cancer is contagious, the myth that cancer survivors cannot work hard, the myth that they are facing imminent death. In fact, however, employees who have had cancer are just as productive as any other employees, and their absentee records are comparable.[3]

Your Legal Rights

The law protects your rights as a cancer survivor. The Federal Rehabilitation Act of 1973 outlaws discrimination based on handicap; it applies to any employer who receives federal assistance. In 1988 a federal court ruled that this act protected healthy cancer survivors from job discrimination. Employers covered by the Federal Rehabilitation Act include federal, state, and local governments; most schools and universities; and any institution that receives grants from the government. To be eligible for protection under the act, you must be currently healthy, however, and you must be qualified to "perform the basic functions of the job."

You may also be protected by the Americans with Disabilities Act (ADA). This law protects more cancer survivors than the Rehabilitation Act, because it covers private employers who do not receive federal funds. As of this writing, ADA applies only to private employers who have at least twenty-five employees; in mid-1994, however, that minimum will be reduced to fifteen.

Under both the Federal Rehabilitation Act and the ADA it is illegal for an employer to require you to disclose your medical history until after he or she has agreed to hire you. It is also illegal for an employer to require you to take a physical examination designed to screen out any disability, including cancer.

If you are not covered by either the Rehabilitation Act or the ADA, you may still be protected by state law. Every state protects handicapped employees from job discrimination. However, only a few states expressly prohibit discrimination against people who have had cancer. To learn what the law is in your state, contact the nearest office of the ACS or telephone the National Coalition for Cancer Survivors at 1-301-650-8868.

If your rights under the Rehabilitation Act are violated, you can file a private lawsuit against your employer or you can file a complaint with the federal agency that provides your employer with funds. If you don't know the name of this agency, you can find out by contacting the Civil Rights Division of the United States Department of Justice at 1-202-514-4718. If your rights under the ADA are violated, you can file a complaint with the Equal Employment Opportunities Commission. For information, phone the local office of the EEOC, listed in the white pages under U.S. Government.

To learn more about your rights as an employee with cancer, see the ACS booklet *Cancer: Your Job, Insurance, and the Law.* To obtain a copy of this booklet, contact the nearest office of the ACS or telephone 1-800-ACS-2345.

Dealing with Your Employer

Before you resort to legal means, it is wise to try dealing with your employer directly. If you are experiencing job discrimination, here are some things to try.

First, let your employer know (politely) that you know your rights. Make it clear that you prefer to work things out amicably if possible. If necessary, ask your employer to adjust to your needs. Suggest several different ways in which this could be done. (If you need help coming up with suggestions, contact the Job Accommodation Network at 1-800-526-7234.) Seriously consider any changes that your employer offers to make.

It helps to provide your employer with accurate information. Explain that cancer patients are dependable employees. (The ACS can supply you with statistics.) Provide information on your own condition. Ask your doctor to back you up by explaining exactly how your condition will affect your ability to work. Fortify your attempts with articles from medical journals. Ask your social worker, your oncology nurse, and the staff at your local ACS office to phone your employer and offer to answer any questions that he or she may have.

Try to get your fellow workers to support you. Point out that if the company discriminates against disabled workers, it could discriminate against them too someday.

Finally, learn what the deadline is for filing a complaint. These deadlines are specified under your state's antidiscrimination laws. That way if worst comes to worst and your employer refuses to recognize your rights, you won't have missed your chance to take legal action.

APPENDIX 2

Vocational Rehabilitation

If your cancer interferes with your ability to work, perhaps your state vocational rehabilitation agency can help. This agency provides disabled employees with counseling and guidance, rehabilitation evaluation, and placement services. It can also suggest how your employer might make "reasonable accommodations" to meet your needs. Reasonable accommodations might include modifying your work hours or your duties, redesigning facilities or equipment in order to make them easier for you to use, or even retraining you to do a different job. To locate your state rehabilitation agency, look in the white pages under State Government. It may be listed under Rehabilitation, Public Welfare, Labor, Human Resources, Human Services, or Education. This agency is required to provide you with the services that you are entitled to under federal law. If your state rehabilitation agency is not providing you with the services to which you believe you are entitled, contact the U.S. Department of Education, Office of Special Education Programs and Rehabilitation Service Administration at 1-202-205-5507.

Dealing with Your Coworkers

Why are some people uncomfortable around cancer patients? See page 174 and page 270.

You may have problems dealing with your coworkers. As we explained in Chapter 6 and Chapter 7, some people are uncomfortable around cancer patients. In those chapters we offer general suggestions for dealing with this problem. In addition, the NCI suggests that you take the following steps:[4]

- Decide before you go back to work whether you want to discuss your cancer with your coworkers. This is a personal decision, so do what feels right to you.

- Keep in touch with your coworkers during your treatment and recovery. Let them know what is happening and how you are coming along. The more they know, the less uncomfortable they will be with the idea that you are a cancer patient. This can prevent a lot of problems when you come back to work.

- When you have educated your employer about cancer, ask your employer to educate your coworkers. See whether your company (or your union) will sponsor an educational program, perhaps with a speaker from the ACS, an oncologist, or representatives from cancer support groups, followed by a question-and-answer session.

- Form a workplace support group for cancer survivors.
- Consider sharing your own experiences with coworkers who have just learned that they have cancer.
- If, after all this, your coworkers' attitudes still interfere with your ability to do your job, and if you can't resolve the situation yourself, don't hesitate to ask management to step in. It is in your employer's interest, as well as your own, to resolve any problems that interfere with your work.

Applying for a New Job

State and federal antidiscrimination laws cover hiring practices as well as other forms of employment discrimination. But when you apply for a new job, there are things that you can do to protect yourself from being discriminated against in the first place.

- Be realistic about your abilities. Don't apply for jobs that call for skills you don't have; but *don't underestimate your own abilities, either.* It's important to assess your skills as accurately as you can and then look for a job that uses those skills to the fullest.
- Organize your resume by skills rather than by dates of employment. That way you don't make it obvious that there were periods when you were unemployed.
- Don't lie on your employment application. On the other hand, don't say that you're a cancer survivor unless you are asked. You are not legally obligated to say that you have had cancer unless it has a direct effect on your ability to do the job.

APPENDIX 2

- Seek employment from organizations that receive federal assistance. These employers are specifically prohibited from discriminating against cancer patients under the Federal Rehabilitation Act, as we have just explained.
- You may want to consult a job counselor. He or she can help you to avoid the pitfalls and show you how to present yourself to best advantage.
- List the questions that you think an employer might ask and practice answering those questions. That way you will go into your interview relaxed, confident, and well prepared.

Recommended Reading

Clifford, Denis, and Mary Randolph. *Who Will Handle Your Finances If You Can't?* **Berkeley, CA: Nolo Press, 1992.**

The authors answer all of your questions about the durable power of attorney for financial management and provide the information and the forms you need to draw up this document for yourself. The book includes a short chapter on the respective advantages of hiring a lawyer or doing your own legal research. Denis Clifford and Mary Randolph are both attorneys. Nolo Press offers an update service to keep readers informed about changes in the law that may affect their books.

Colen, B. D. *The Essential Guide to a Living Will: How to Protect Your Right to Refuse Medical Treatment.* **New York: Prentice Hall Press, 1991.**

This book explains in detail how to prepare a Living Will–and why it is necessary to have one. It describes the technologies that are currently used to keep dying patients alive and discusses legal and ethical factors that influence the decision to cut off life support. It explains what issues you will need to consider, and what actions you can take, to increase the likelihood that your wishes in this matter will be followed. The book includes Living Will forms for the forty-one states that have Living Will laws. Short, clearly written, and very readable. B. D. Colen is a Pulitzer Prize-winning reporter who specializes in medical issues.

Larschan, Edward J. *The Diagnosis Is Cancer.* **Palo Alto, CA: Bull Publishing, 1986.**

This book contains excellent advice on dealing with legal, financial, and insurance issues. We describe it further in the Recommended Reading for Chapter 1.

APPENDIX 2

National Coalition for Cancer Survivorship. *Charting the Journey: An Almanac of Practical Resources for Cancer Survivors.* **Edited by Fitzhugh Mullan, Barbara Hoffman, and the Editors of Consumer Reports Books. Mount Vernon, NY: Consumers Union, 1990.**

An invaluable resource book for cancer patients and their families. Chapter 6: "Taking Care of Business" is full of specific, detailed information about employment, insurance, and financial issues. This book includes thirty pages of cancer survivorship resources and an excellent bibliography. Most of the authors are cancer survivors, as well as professionals in their respective fields.

Resources

National Cancer Institute-Designated Comprehensive Cancer Centers

University of Alabama at Birmingham Comprehensive Cancer Center
1824 Sixth Avenue S
Birmingham, AL 35294
1-205-934-5077

University of Arizona Cancer Center
1501 N Campbell Avenue
Tucson, AZ 85724
1-602-626-6372

Jonsson Comprehensive Cancer Center
University of California at Los Angeles
10833 LeConte Avenue
Los Angeles, CA 90024
1-310-825-5268

The Kenneth T. Norris, Jr. Comprehensive Cancer Center
University of Southern California
1441 Eastlake Avenue
Los Angeles, CA 90033
1-213-226-2370

Yale University Comprehensive Cancer Center
PO Box 3333, LEPH-139
New Haven, CT 06510
1-203-785-6338

Lombardi Cancer Research Center
Georgetown University Medical Center
3800 Reservoir Road NW
Washington, DC 20007
1-202-687-2192

Sylvester Comprehensive Cancer Center
University of Miami Medical School
1475 NW 12th Avenue
Miami, FL 33136
1-305-545-1000

The Johns Hopkins Oncology Center
600 N Wolfe Street
Baltimore, MD 21205
1-410-955-8638

Dana-Farber Cancer Institute
44 Binney Street
Boston, MA 02115
1-617-632-3000

University of Michigan
Comprehensive Cancer Center
101 Simpson Drive
Ann Arbor, MI 48109
1-313-936-9583

Meyer L. Prentis Comprehensive
Cancer Center of Metropolitan
Detroit
110 E Warren Avenue
Detroit, MI 48201
1-313-745-4329

Mayo Comprehensive
Cancer Center
200 First Street SW
Rochester, MN 55905
1-507-284-3413

Norris Cotton Cancer Center
Dartmouth-Hitchcock Medical Center
1 Medical Center Drive
Lebanon, NH 03756
1-603-650-5527

Roswell Park Cancer Institute
Elm and Carlton Streets
Buffalo, NY 14263
1-800-767-9355

Columbia University
Comprehensive Cancer Center
College of Physicians and Surgeons
630 W 168th Street
New York, NY 10032
1-212-305-6905

Kaplan Cancer Center
New York University Medical Center
462 First Avenue
New York, NY 10016
1-212-263-6485

Memorial Sloan-Kettering
Cancer Center
1275 York Avenue
New York, NY 10021
1-800-525-2225

UNC Lineberger Comprehensive
Cancer Center
University of North Carolina School
of Medicine
Chapel Hill, NC 27599
1-919-966-3036

Duke Comprehensive Cancer Center
PO Box 3814
Durham, NC 27710
1-919-684-5810

Cancer Center of Wake Forest
University at the Bowman Gray
School of Medicine
Medical Center Blvd.
Winston-Salem, NC 27157
1-919-748-4354

James Cancer Hospital and
Research Institute
410 W 10th Avenue
Columbus, OH 43210
1-614-293-8619

Fox Chase Cancer Center
7701 Burholme Avenue
Philadelphia, PA 19111
1-215-728-2570

University of Pennsylvania
Cancer Center
Penn Tower Hotel, 6th floor
3400 Spruce Street
Philadelphia, PA 19104
1-215-662-6364

Pittsburgh Cancer Institute
200 Meyran Avenue
Pittsburgh, PA 15213
1-800-537-4063

The University of Texas M.D. Anderson Cancer Center
1515 Holcombe Blvd.
Houston, TX 77030
1-713-792-3245

Vermont Cancer Center
University of Vermont
1 S Prospect Street
Burlington, VT 05401
1-802-656-4414

Fred Hutchinson Cancer Research Center
1124 Columbia Street
Seattle, WA 98104
1-206-667-5000

Wisconsin Clinical Cancer Center
University of Wisconsin
600 Highland Avenue
Madison, WI 53792
1-608-263-8600

Hospitals with Multidisciplinary Second-Opinion Clinics

St. Vincent Cancer Center
Little Rock, AR
1-501-660-3900

Arizona Cancer Center
Tucson, AZ
1-602-626-2900

City of Hope National Medical Center
Los Angeles, CA
1-800-423-7119
1-800-535-1390 (in California)

University of California at San Diego Cancer Center
San Diego, CA
1-619-543-3456

Regional Cancer Foundation
San Francisco, CA
1-415-775-9956

University of Colorado Cancer Center
Denver, CO
1-303-372-1550

Yale University School of Medicine
Department of Medical Oncology
New Haven, CT
1-203-785-6222

Cedars Medical Center
Miami, FL
1-305-325-5691

DeKalb Medical Center
Atlanta-Decatur, GA
1-404-501-5559

University of Iowa Cancer Center
Iowa City, IA
1-319-356-3584

Loyola University Medical Center
Chicago, IL
1-708-216-3336

Northwestern University
Chicago, IL
1-312-908-5284

Meyer L. Prentis Comprehensive
Cancer Center of Metropolitan
Detroit
Detroit, MI
1-313-993-0335

Dartmouth-Hitchcock
Medical Center
Hanover, NH
1-603-650-5527

Regional Cancer Center Lourdes
Binghamton, NY
1-607-798-5431

Montefiore Medical Center
Bronx, NY
1-212-920-4826

Roswell Park Memorial Institute
Buffalo, NY
1-800-685-6825

Memorial Sloan-Kettering
Cancer Center
New York, NY
1-800-525-2225

Mount Sinai Cancer Center
New York, NY
1-212-241-6361

University of Rochester
Cancer Center
Rochester, NY
1-716-275-4911

Ireland Cancer Center
Cleveland, OH
1-216-844-5432

Arthur G. James Cancer Hospital
and Research Institute
Columbus, OH
1-614-293-8890

Fox Chase Cancer Center
Philadelphia, PA
1-215-728-2986
1-800-728-2680

University of Pennsylvania
Cancer Center
Philadelphia, PA
1-800-777-8176

Pittsburgh Cancer Institute
Pittsburgh, PA
1-800-537-4063

Roger Williams Cancer Center
Providence, RI
1-401-456-2072

Thompson Cancer Survival Center
Knoxville, TN
1-615-541-1757

St. Jude Children's Research
Hospital
Memphis, TN
1-901-522-0301

UTMB Cancer Center
Galveston, TX
1-409-772-1164

University of Wisconsin
Cancer Center
Madison, WI
1-608-263-8600

Information, Services, and Support for Cancer Patients

Air Life Line
1716 X Street
Sacramento, CA 95818
1-916-446-0995
1-800-446-1231
Provides air transportation for patients

American Brain Tumor Association
3725 N Talman Avenue
Chicago, IL 60618
1-312-286-5571
1-800-886-2282
Provides information on brain tumor research and treatments

American Cancer Society (ACS)
1599 Clifton Road NE
Atlanta, GA 30329
1-404-320-3333
1-800-ACS-2345 (hotline)

American Medical Support Flight Team (Angel Flight)
3237 Donald Douglas Loop S
Santa Monica, CA 90405
1-310-390-2958
1-310-456-2035 (24-hour hotline)
Provides air transportation for patients

American Red Cross
431 18th Street NW
Washington, DC 20006
1-202-737-8300

Better Together Club
PO Box 4277
Syossct, NY 11791
1-800-422-8811
Provides information and referrals for ostomy patients

Cancer Guidance Hotline
1323 Forbes Avenue, Suite 200
Pittsburg, PA 15239
1-412-261-2211
Provides information and support for patients and families

Cancer Support Network
802 E Jetterson
Bloomington, IL 61701
1-309-829-2273
Provides support groups, lending library, wig bank

Candlelighters Foundation
7910 Woodmont Avenue, Suite 460
Bethesda, MD 20814
1-301-657-8401 (Maryland)
1-800-366-2223
Provides information and support for parents of children with cancer

CanSurmount
(contact a local ACS office)
An ACS program that provides information and support for cancer survivors, family members, and health professionals

Center for Attitudinal Healing
19 Main Street
Tiburon, CA 94920
1-415-435-5022
Provides support for patients with life-threatening illnesses

APPENDIX 3

447

Center for Medical Consumers
237 Thompson Street
New York, NY 10012
1-212-674-7105
Provides information, referrals to
national health organizations, and a
medical consumers' public library

**Children's Oncology Camps
of America**
2309 W Whiteoaks Drive, Suite B
Springfield, IL 62704
1-217-793-3949
Publishes an annual directory of
children's oncology camps

Choice in Dying
200 Varick Street
New York, NY 10014
1-212-366-5540
Provides Living Will forms,
information, and advice

**Consumer Health Information
Research Institute**
3521 Broadway
Kansas City, MO 64111
1-800-821-6671
Provides information about alternative
treatments

DES Action USA
Long Island Jewish Medical Center
New Hyde Park, NY 11040
1-516-775-3450
2845 24th Street
San Francisco, CA 94110
1-415-826-5060
Provides information about diethyl-
stilbestrol (DES)

Encore
YWCA of the United States
726 Broadway, 5th floor
New York, NY 10003
1-212-614-2827
Provides support and rehabilitation for
postmastectomy patients

Food and Drug Administration
Office of Consumer Affairs HFE-88
Room 16-63
5600 Fishers Lane
Rockville, MD 20857
1-301-443-3170
Provides information on federal
regulation of drugs

I Can Cope
(contact a local ACS office)
An ACS program that provides
information on treatment for cancer
patients and family members

**International Association of
Laryngectomees**
(contact a local ACS office)
An ACS program that provides
information and services for
laryngectomy patients

International Pain Foundation
909 NE 43rd Street, Suite 306
Seattle, WA 98105
1-206-547-2157
Provides information about
pain control

Let's Face It
PO Box 711
Concord, MA 01742
1-508-371-3186
Provides information and support for
patients with facial disfigurements

Leukemia Society of America, Inc.
600 Third Avenue
New York, NY 10016
1-212-573-8484
1-800-955-4572 (information hotline)
Provides information, referrals,
support, and financial aid for patients
with leukemia, Hodgkin's disease, and
lymphoma

Look Good...Feel Better
1-800-558-5005
(contact a local ACS office)
An ACS program that teaches makeup
techniques to women patients

**Make-a-Wish Foundation of
America**
1624 E Meadowbrook
Phoenix, AZ 85016
1-602-248-9474
Grants wishes to children with life-
threatening illnesses

Man to Man
910 Contento Street
Sarasota, FL 34242
1-813-349-1719
1-813-355-4987
Provides information and support for
patients with prostate cancer

**National Alliance of Breast Cancer
Organizations (NABCO)**
1180 Avenue of the Americas,
2nd floor
New York, NY 10036
1-212-719-0154
Provides information for patients with
breast cancer; prefers written inquiries

**National Bone Marrow Donor
Program**
3433 Broadway Street NE, Suite 400
Minneapolis, MN 55413
1-800-654-1247 (hotline and donors)
1-800-526-7809 (general business and
recipients)

**National Cancer Care
Foundation/Cancer Care, Inc.**
1180 Avenue of the Americas,
2nd floor
New York, NY 10036
1-212-221-3300
Provides information on nonmedical
resources, support, financial aid

National Cancer Institute (NCI)
Cancer Information Service
1-800-4-CANCER
Provides information and publications
on all aspects of cancer; provides
physicians and patients with access
to Physician Data Query (PDQ)

APPENDIX 3

National Coalition for Cancer Survivorship
1010 Wayne Avenue, 5th floor
Silver Spring, MD 20910
1-301-650-8868
Provides information on services and materials for patients; publishes the *Cancer Survivors Almanac of Resources*

National Council against Health Fraud
Resource Center
3521 Broadway
Kansas City, MO 64111
1-800-821-6671
Provides information on questionable health practices and health organizations

National Health Information Center
PO Box 1133
Washington, DC 20013
1-301-565-4167 (Maryland)
1-800-336-4797
Provides referrals to organizations that provide information about cancer and other health issues, including insurance

National Hospice Organization
1901 N Moore Street, Suite 901
Arlington, VA 22209
1-800-658-8898
Provides information, referrals, and support

National Institute of Neurological Disorders and Strokes
Building 31, Room 8A06
National Institutes of Health
Bethesda, MD 20892
1-301-496-5751
1-800-352-9424
Provides information on brain tumors

National Leukemia Association, Inc.
585 Stewart Avenue, Suite 536
Garden City, NY 11530
1-516-222-1944
Provides information and financial aid for patients with leukemia

National Lymphedema Network
2211 Post Street, Suite 404
San Francisco, CA 94115
1-800-541-3259
Provides information and support for patients with lymphedema

National Women's Health Network
1325 G Street NW
Washington, DC 20005
1-202-347-1140
Provides information on women's cancers and other issues related to women's health

Ostomy Rehabilitation Program
(contact a local ACS office)
An ACS program that provides information and services for ostomy patients

Prostate Health Program of New York
785 Park Avenue
New York, NY 10021
1-212-988-8888

Reach to Recovery Program
(contact a local ACS office)
An ACS program that provides information and services for patients with breast cancer

Ronald McDonald Houses
McDonald's Campus Office Building
Crock Drive
Oak Brook, IL 60521
1-708-575-7418
Provides inexpensive lodging near cancer treatment centers for children with cancer and their families

Share
19 W 44th Street, Suite 415
New York, NY 10036
1-212-382-2111
Provides support for patients with breast cancer

Skin Cancer Foundation
PO Box 561
New York, NY 10156
1-212-725-5176
Provides information and support for patients with skin cancer

Sunshine Foundation
2001 Bridge Street
Philadelphia, PA 19124
1-215-335-2622
1-800-767-1976
Grants wishes to children with chronic or terminal illnesses

Sunshine Kids
2902 Ferndale Place
Houston, TX 77098
1-713-524-1264
Provides activities for children with cancer

United Cancer Council, Inc.
1803 N Meridian Street
Indianapolis, IN 46202
1-317-923-6490
Provides services, medications, and prostheses

United Ostomy Association, Inc.
36 Executive Park, Suite 120
Irvine, CA 92714
1-714-660-8624
1-800-826-0826
Provides information and support for ostomy patients

Us-Too, the American Foundation for Urologic Disease
300 W Pratt Street, Suite 401
Baltimore, MD 21201
1-800-828-7866
Provides support for patients with prostate cancer

Visiting Nurse Associations of America
3801 E Florida Avenue, Suite 900
Denver, CO 80210
1-800-426-2547
Provides skilled nurses, therapists, home care aides

APPENDIX 3

Vital Options
4419 Coldwater Canyon Avenue,
Suite A-C
Studio City, CA 91604
1-818-508-5657
Provides information and support
for young adults with cancer

Wellness Community National Headquarters
2200 Colorado Avenue
Santa Monica, CA 90404
1-310-453-2300
Provides support; helps patients
to improve their quality
of life

Y-Me Breast Cancer Support Program, Inc.
18220 Harwood Avenue
Homewood, IL 60430
1-708-799-8228 (24-hour hotline)
1-800-221-2141
Provides information and support;
wig and prosthesis bank for patients
with breast cancer

Newsletters and Magazines

For Cancer Patients

Cancer Communication
Patient Advocates for Advanced
Cancer Treatment (PAACT)
1143 Parmelee NW
Grand Rapids, MI 49504
1-616-453-1477
1-616-453-1351 (information
available on Voicemail)

Medical options and advances in the
treatment of prostate cancer

Candlelighters
7910 Woodmont Ave., Suite 460
Bethesda, MD 20814
1-301-657-8401 (Maryland)
1-800-366-2223
Free quarterly devoted to information
on childhood cancer

Coping
2019 N Carothers
Franklin, TN 37064
1-615-790-2400
This quarterly carries articles on
subjects of interest to cancer patients
and new developments in cancer
treatment and research.

Living through Cancer
323 Eighth Street SW
Albuquerque, NM 87102
1-505-242-3263
Personal stories, poetry, book reviews,
articles, and resource lists by and for
cancer patients and their families

Nabco News
2280 Avenue of the Americas
New York, NY 10036
1-212-719-0154
The quarterly publication of the
National Alliance of Breast Cancer
Organizations. Members receive the
newsletter, the NABCO resource list,
and special mailings.

NCCS Networker
1010 Wayne Avenue
Silver Spring, MD 20910
1-301-650-8868
The quarterly newsletter of the
National Coalition for Cancer
Survivorship

SEARCH
National Brain Tumor Foundation
323 Geary Street, Suite 510
San Francisco, CA 94102
1-415-296-0404
1-800-934-CURE
Research data and practical
information for people with brain
tumors

Surviving!
Stanford University Medical Center
Patient Research Center,
Room H0103
Division of Radiation Oncology
300 Pasteur Drive
Stanford, CA 94305
1-415-723-7881
This patient newsletter provides infor-
mation on Hodgkin's disease, plus
stories, essays, and artwork by
Hodgkin's survivors.

Y-Me Hotline
18220 Harwood Avenue
Homewood, IL 60430
1-708-799-8338
1-708-799-8228 (24-hour hotline)
1-800-221-2141
A newsletter for women who are
coping with breast cancer

General Interest

*American Health: Fitness of
Body and Mind*
28 W 23rd Street
New York, NY 10010
1-800-365-5005
This magazine carries carefully
researched articles on all aspects
of health.

Harvard Health Letter
Harvard Medical School Health
Publication Group
164 Longwood Avenue
Boston, MA 02115
Many libraries carry this newsletter;
it is also available by subscription.

Health
PO Box 56863
Boulder, CO 80322
1-800-274-2522
A clearly written, reliable magazine;
deals with prevention, fitness, and
disease

Mayo Clinic Health Letter
200 First Street SW
Rochester, MN 55905

Medical Abstracts Newsletter
PO Box 2170
Teaneck, NJ 07666
Abstracts (summaries) of the research
studies that are published in profes-
sional journals

APPENDIX 3

Nutrition Action Health Letter
1875 Connecticut Avenue NW,
Suite 300
Washington, DC 20009
Published by the Center for Science
in the Public Interest

*Tufts University Diet and
Nutrition Letter*
53 Park Place
New York, NY 10007
1-800-274-7581

*University of California at Berkeley
Wellness Letter*
PO Box 420148
Palm Coast, FL 32142

Information on Board Certification and Accreditation

American Board of Medical Specialties
1007 Church Street, Suite 404
Evanston, IL 60201
1-708-491-9091
1-800-776-2378 (to verify a
physician's certification)
Maintains a national list of board-
certified physicians in all specialties;
publishes the *ABMS Compendium of
Certified Medical Specialists*, available
in public and medical libraries

American College of Radiology
1891 Preston White Drive
Reston, VA 22091
1-703-648-8900

Provides a list of accredited mammography facilities; monitors equipment
and staff qualifications

American College of Surgeons
Office of Public Information
55 E Erie Street
Chicago, IL 60611
1-312-664-4050
Provides a list of board-certified
surgeons in all specialties; prefers
written inquiries

College of American Pathologists
325 Waukegan Road
Northfield, IL 60093
1-800-323-4040 (to verify accreditation of a laboratory)
Maintains a national list of accredited
hospital and nonhospital laboratories

Community Health Accreditation Program, Inc.
350 Hudson Street
New York, NY 10014
1-800-669-9656
Provides a list of accredited home care
organizations

Joint Commission on Accreditation of Health Care Organizations (JCAHO)
1 Renaissance Blvd.
Oak Brook Terrace, IL 60181
1-708-916-5800 (to verify
accreditation of a hospital)
Maintains a national list of
accredited hospitals

Notes

Chapter 1:
The Verdict Is Cancer

1. Samuel D. Spivack, MD, interview with Alpha Institute, San Francisco, CA, September 21, 1988.

2. Andrew Moyce, MD, interview with Alpha Institute, Oakland, CA, January 30, 1989.

3. Spivack.

4. Spivack, interview with Alpha Institute, San Francisco, CA, July 27, 1988.

5. John Laszlo, *Understanding Cancer* (New York: Harper & Row Publishers, 1987), 206.

Chapter 2:
Understanding Cancer

1. Paula Carroll, *Life Wish* (Alameda, CA: Medical Consumers Publishing Co., 1986).

2. On the role of oncogenes in carcinogenesis, see Morag Park and George F. Vande Woude, "Principles of Molecular Cell Biology of Cancer: Oncogenes," in *Cancer: Principles and Practice of Oncology*, 3d ed., ed. Vincent T. DeVita, Jr., Samuel Hellman, and Steven A. Rosenberg (Philadelphia: J.B. Lippincott Co., 1989), 1145-66; W. Davis Merritt et al., "Oncogene Amplification in Squamous Cell Carcinoma of the Head and Neck," *Archives of Otolaryngology: Head and Neck Surgery* 116 (December 1990): 1394-98; Rena S. Wong and Edward Passaro, Jr., "Growth Factors, Oncogenes and the Autocrine Hypothesis," *Surgery, Gynecology and Obstetrics* 168 (May 1989): 469-70. See also Robert A. Weinberg, "Finding the Anti-Oncogene," *Scientific American* (September 1988): 44-51. On the role of viruses in carcinogenesis, see L. Austin Doyle, "Viral Carcinogenesis," in *Comprehensive*

Textbook of Oncology, 2d ed., vol. 1, ed. A.R. Moosa, S.C. Schimpf, and M.C. Robson (Baltimore, MD: Williams & Wilkins, 1991), 45-51; Johng S. Rhim, "Viruses, Oncogenes, and Cancer," *Cancer Detection and Prevention* 11 (1988): 139-49; Fred Rappe et al., "Properties of Viruses Associated with Human Cancer," in *American Cancer Society Textbook of Clinical Oncology,* ed. Arthur I. Holleb, Diane J. Fink, and Gerald P. Murphy (Atlanta, GA: American Cancer Society, 1991), 133-47.

3. For a general discussion of the ways in which cancer kills, see John Laszlo, *Understanding Cancer* (New York: Harper & Row Publishers, 1987), 70-71.

4. Dennis J. Templeton and Robert A. Weinberg, "Principles of Cancer Biology," in Holleb, Fink, and Murphy, 681.

5. National Cancer Institute, Cancer Information Service, telephone conversation with Alpha Institute, July 14, 1992.

6. American Cancer Society, *Cancer Facts and Figures: 1992* (Atlanta, GA: American Cancer Society, 1991), 9.

7. Ibid., 8, 18.

8. On the role of carcinogens in the development of cancer, see John H. Weisburger and Clara L. Horn, "The Causes of Cancer," in Holleb, Fink, and Murphy, 80-98; Thomas J. Slaga, "Mechanisms of Chemical Carcinogenesis," in Moosa, Schimpf, and Robson, 31-44; Henry C. Pitot and Yvonne P. Dragan, "Facts and Theories Concerning the Mechanisms of Carcinogenesis," *FASEB Journal* 5 (June 1991): 2280-86.

9. On the role of the immune system in combating cancer, see Ronald B. Herberman, "Principles of Tumor Immunology," in Holleb, Fink, and Murphy, 69-79; Philip D. Greenberg, "Mechanisms

of Tumor Immunology," in *Basic and Clinical Immunology,* 7th ed., ed. Daniel P. Stites and Abba I. Terr, (Norwalk, CT: Appleton & Lange, 1991), 580-87. There is some controversy regarding the role of the immune system in combating cancer. For other viewpoints, see W. John Martin, "Tumor Immunology Overview," in Moosa, Schimpf, and Robson, 101-103; Carmelita G. Frondoza, "Current Views on Immune Surveillance," in Moosa, Schimpf, and Robson, 104-107; John L. Ziegler, "Cancer in the Immunocompromised Host," in Stites and Terr, 588-98. On the failure of immunological controls, see also G. Klein, "Tumor Immunology: A General Appraisal," in *Scientific Foundations of Oncology,* ed. T. Symington and R.L. Carter (London: William Heinemann Medical Books, 1976), 497-504.

10. On the relationship between aging and immune function, see William O. Weigle, "Effects of Aging on the Immune System," *Hospital Practice* (December 15, 1989): 112-19; Richard A. Miller, "Aging and Immune Function," *International Review of Cytology* 124 (1991): 187-215. See also Paul R. Kaesberg and William B. Ershler, "The Importance of Immunesenescence in the Incidence and Malignant Properties of Cancer in Hosts of Advanced Age," *Journal of Gerontology* 44, no. 6 (1989): 63-66; Richard A. Miller, "Gerontology as Oncology: Research on Aging as the Key to the Understanding of Cancer," *Cancer* 68 (1991): 2496-2501. For another viewpoint, see Henry C. Pitot, "Aging and Cancer: Some General Thoughts," *Journal of Gerontology* 44, no. 6 (1989): 5-9; Douglas Dix, "The Role of Aging in Cancer Incidence: An Epidemiological Study," *Journal of Gerontology* 44, no. 6 (1989): 10-18; Richard G. Cutler and Imre Semsei, "Development, Cancer, and Aging: Possible Common Mechanisms of Action and Regulation," *Journal of Gerontology* 44, no. 6 (1989): 25-34.

11. David M. Prescott and Abraham S. Flexner, *Cancer, the Misguided Cell* (Sunderland, MA: Sinauer Associates, 1986), 234. For a dissident view, see Dix.

12. On the role of viruses in causing cancer, see Fred Rapp, "Properties of Viruses Associated with Human Cancer," in Holleb, Fink, and Murphy,

133-52; Elaine Blume, "1971-1991: Virus Cancer Research Pays Rich Dividends," *Journal of the National Cancer Institute* 83, no. 21 (November 6, 1991): 1528-31. See also James K. Roche and Christopher P. Crum, "Local Immunity and Uterine Cervix: Implications for Cancer-Associated Viruses," *Cancer Immunology and Immunotherapy* 33 (1991): 203-209.

13. Geoffrey M. Cooper, "Elements of Human Cancer" (Boston: Jones & Bartlett Publishers, 1992), 77.

14. Jay R. Harris et al., "Cancer of the Breast," in *Cancer: Principles and Practice of Oncology,* 2d ed., ed. Vincent T. DeVita, Jr., Samuel Hellman, and Steven A. Rosenberg (Philadelphia: J.B. Lippincott Co., 1985), 1119. See also Graham A. Coldlitz et al., "Family History, Age, and Risk of Breast Cancer: Prospective Data from the Nurses' Health Study," *Journal of the American Medical Association* 270, no. 3 (July 21, 1993): 338-43.

15. Mary-Claire King, "Genetic Analysis of Cancer in Families," *Cancer Surveys* 9, no. 3 (1990): 419.

16. On the role of heredity in the development of cancer, see Henry T. Lynch, ed., *Cancer Genetics* (Springfield, IL: Charles C. Thomas Publisher, 1976).

17. "Gains against Cancer since 1930 Are Overstated, Congress Is Told," *New York Times,* April 16, 1987, A1.

18. American Cancer Society, 1.

19. Lewis Thomas, "Getting at the Roots of a Deep Puzzle," *Discover* (March 1986): 65-66.

20. Michael Lerner with R. Naomi Remen, "Varieties of Integral Cancer Therapies," *Advances* 2, no. 3 (Summer 1985): 27.

Chapter 3:
Getting the Best Care

1. Sheldon Greenfield, Sherrie Kaplan, and John E. Ware, Jr., "Expanding Patient Involvement in Care," *Annals of Internal Medicine* 102 (1985): 520-28; Judith Rodin and Ellen J. Langer,

"Long-Term Effects of a Control-Relevant Intervention with the Institutionalized Aged," *Journal of Personality and Social Psychology* 35, no. 12 (1977): 897-902. See also documentation for the discussion of control in Chapter 8.

2. Theresa Koetters, RNMS, interview with Alpha Institute, San Francisco, CA, June 13, 1992. All quotations from Theresa Koetters in Chapter 3 are taken from this interview.

3. Samuel D. Spivack, MD, interview with Alpha Institute, San Francisco, CA, January 12, 1989. All quotations from Dr. Spivack in Chapter 3 are taken from this interview.

4. Andrew Moyce, MD, interview with Alpha Institute, Oakland, CA, January 30, 1989. All quotations from Dr. Moyce in Chapter 3 are taken from this interview.

5. Annette Bloch and Richard Bloch, *Fighting Cancer* (Kansas City, MO: Cancer Connection, 1985), 21.

Chapter 4:
Standard Treatments

1. John Laszlo, *Understanding Cancer* (New York: Harper & Row Publishers, 1987), 29.

2. *Journal of the National Cancer Institute* (July 6, 1988): 620.

3. Ian Burn, "Progress in Surgical Oncology," in *Cancer Research and Treatment Today: Results, Trends and Frontiers,* ed. K. Lapis and S. Eckhardt (Budapest: Akademiai Kiado, 1987), 112.

4. Samuel D. Spivack, MD, interview with Alpha Institute, San Francisco, CA, September 21, 1988.

5. Julien M. Goodman, MD, interview with Alpha Institute, Alameda, CA, April 27, 1990.

6. James W. Forsythe, MD, interview with Alpha Institute, Reno, NV, August 23, 1990.

7. Adapted from Carlos A. Pellegrini, "What Happens in Surgery," in *Everyone's Guide to Cancer Therapy,* ed. Malin Dollinger, Ernest H. Rosenbaum, and Greg Cable (Kansas City, MO:

Andrews & McMeel, 1991), 41-42.

8. Karin Selbach, RN, interview with Alpha Institute, Oakland, CA, February 23, 1992.

9. Andrew Moyce, MD, interview with Alpha Institute, Oakland, CA, February 10, 1990.

10. Adapted from National Institutes of Health, *Chemotherapy and You: A Guide to Self-Help during Treatment,* Publication no. 91-1136, revised June 1990, 36-37.

11. See, for example, Abraham Mittelman, "Life-Threatening Toxicity of Cancer Therapy," *Critical Care Clinics* (January 1989): 1-9; Bruce D. Minsky et al., "Combined Modality Therapy of Rectal Cancer: Decreased Acute Toxicity with the Preoperative Approach," *Journal of Clinical Oncology* 10, no. 8 (August 1992): 1218-24; Pieter Sonneveld et al., "Modulation of Multidrug-Resistant Multiple Myeloma by Cyclosporin, *Lancet* 340 (1992): 255-59; Eliahu Gez et al., "Methylprednisolone as Antiemetic Treatment in Breast-Cancer Patients Receiving Cyclophosphamide, Methotrexate, and 5-Fluorouracil: A Prospective, Crossover, Randomized Blind Study Comparing Two Different Dose Schedules," *Cancer Chemotherapy and Pharmacology* 30 (1992): 229-32.

12. Laszlo, 153-58.

13. See Michael P. Carey and Thomas G. Burish, "Etiology and Treatment of the Psychological Side Effects Associated with Cancer Chemotherapy: A Critical Review and Discussion," *Psychological Bulletin* 104, no. 3 (1988): 307-25.

14. Theresa Koetters, RNMS, interview with Alpha Institute, San Francisco, CA, April 27, 1990.

15. On the risks and side effects of chemotherapy, see National Institutes of Health, 15-28; Paul E. Rosenthal et al., "Complications of Cancer and Cancer Treatment," in *Cancer Manual,* 8th ed., ed. Robert T. Osteen et al. (Boston: American Cancer Society, Massachusetts Division, 1990), 433-49.

16. National Institutes of Health, *Radiation Therapy and You: A Guide to Self-Help during*

Treatment, Publication no. 92-2227, revised October 1990, 3.

17. For a more complete discussion on the internal and external methods, see ibid., 9-20. See also Frank R. Hendrickson and H. Rodney Withers, "Principles of Radiation Oncology," in *American Cancer Society Textbook of Clinical Oncology,* ed. Arthur I. Holleb, Diane J. Fink, and Gerald P. Murphy (Atlanta, GA: American Cancer Society, 1991), 35-46.

18. On the risks and side effects of radiation therapy, see National Institutes of Health, *Radiation Therapy,* 21-37; Paul E. Rosenthal et al., "Complications of Cancer and Cancer Treatment," in Osteen et al., 425-33. See also J. Denekamp and A. Rojas, "Cell Kinetics and Radiation Pathology," *Experientia* (January 15, 1988): 33-41; J.M. Vaeth and J.L. Meyer, eds., *Radiation Tolerance of Normal Tissues* (Basel: Karger, 1988).

19. James Menafee, "The Stanford Zone," *Surviving!* Department of Therapeutic Radiation, Stanford University Medical Center (October 1987): 11.

20. On hormonal therapy, see Nelson A. Burstein, Christopher Longcope, and Herbert H. Wotiz, "Overall Principles of Cancer Management: Hormonal Therapy," in Osteen et al., 109-14; B.J. Kennedy, "Principles of Endocrine Therapy," in *Cancer Medicine,* 2d ed., ed. James F. Holland and Emil Frei III (Philadelphia: Lei & Febigeer, 1982), 945-46. See also Jay R. Harris et al., "Cancer of the Breast," in *Cancer: Principles and Practice of Oncology,* 3d ed., ed. Vincent T. DeVita, Jr., Samuel Hellman, and Steven A. Rosenberg (Philadelphia: J.B. Lippincott Co., 1989), 1248-52; John T. Hamm and Joseph C. Allegra, "New Hormonal Approaches to the Treatment of Breast Cancer," *Critical Reviews in Oncology/Hematology* 11 (1991): 29-41.

21. On the risks and side effects of hormonal therapy, see Hamm and Allegra, 30; Peter Henriksson, "Estrogen in Patients with Prostatic Cancer: An Assessment of the Risks and Benefits," *Drug Safety* 6, no. 1 (1991): 47-53; V.C. Jordan, "The Role of Tamoxifen in the Treatment and Prevention of Breast Cancer," *Current Problems in Cancer* 16, no. 3 (May-June 1992): 129-76;

Richard R. Love, "Tamoxifen Therapy in Primary Breast Cancer: Biology, Efficacy, and Side Effects," *Journal of Clinical Oncology* 7, no. 6 (June 1989): 809-12; Donna Glover and John H. Glick, "Oncologic Emergencies," in Holleb, Fink, and Murphy, 519.

22. For a detailed discussion of the way in which clinical trials are designed, see Seth M. Steinberg and Margaret N. Wesley, "Clinical Trials: Design and Evaluation," in *Comprehensive Textbook of Oncology,* 2d ed., vol. 1, ed. A.R. Moosa, S.C. Schimpf, and M.C. Robson (Baltimore, MD: Williams & Wilkins, 1991), 415-25.

23. Adapted from National Institutes of Health, *What Are Clinical Trials All About?* Publication no. 90-2706, 8-9.

24. On the pros and cons of participating in clinical trials, see Michael B. Bracken, "Clinical Trials and the Acceptance of Uncertainty," *British Medical Journal* (May 2, 1987): 1111-12; Richard D. Geber and Aron Goldhirsch, "Can a Clinical Trial Be the Treatment of Choice for Patients with Cancer" *Journal of the National Cancer Institute* (August 17, 1988): 886-87; "Recruiting Patients for Clinical Trials," *Journal of the National Cancer Institute* (July 6, 1988): 619-20.

25. On private research programs, see William Boly, "Cancer, Inc.," *Hippocrates* (January-February 1989): 38-48.

26. Blake Cady and Robert Quinlan, "Overall Principles of Cancer Management: Surgery," in Osteen et al., 84; "New High-Tech Cure Uses Light to Conquer Cancer," *Men's Health Newsletter* (May 1991): 3-5. See also Barbara W. Henderson, "Photodynamic Therapy: Coming of Age," *Photo-Dermatology* (October 1988): 200-211.

27. William J. Slichenmyer and Daniel D. Von Hoff, "New Natural Products in Cancer Chemotherapy," *Journal of Clinical Pharmacology* 30 (1990): 770-88. For more on new anticancer drugs, see Charles M. Haskell, "Investigational Chemotherapeutic Agents," in *Cancer Treatment,* 3d ed., ed. Charles M. Haskell (Philadelphia: W.B. Saunders Co., 1990), 941-45.

28. H. Rodney Withers, "Biological Basis of Radiation Therapy for Cancer," *Lancet* 339 (January 18, 1992): 158.

29. Jeffrey S. Tobias, "Clinical Practice of Radiotherapy," *Lancet* 339 (January 18, 1992): 159-63. On recent advances in radiation therapy, see Ralph R. Dobelbower, Jr. et al., "Radiation Therapy in Cancer Management: New Frontiers," in Moosa, Schimpf, and Robson, 502-22.

30. Hamm and Allegra, 37.

31. Warren E. Leary, "Drug to Be Tested as Cancer Preventer," *New York Times,* April 30, 1992.

32. For a more complete discussion of immunotherapy, written for the lay reader, see Raphael Catane and Malcolm S. Mitchell, "What Happens in Biological Therapy," in Dollinger, Rosenbaum, and Cable, 62-69. See also Timothy J. Eberlein et al., "Overall Principles of Cancer Management: Biologic Response Modifiers," in Osteen et al., 115-24.

33. Bob Rust, "Monoclonals: The Body's Cruise Missiles," *Coping* 2 (1990): 42-43.

34. K.A. Fackelmann, "New Anticancer Strategy Targets Gene," *Science News* 141 (June 6, 1992): 372.

35. Michael R. Cooper and M. Robert Cooper, "Principles of Medical Oncology," in Holleb, Fink, and Murphy, 65.

36. Steven A. Rosenberg, "Adoptive Immunotherapy for Cancer," *Scientific American* (May 1990): 62-69. See also Steven A. Rosenberg et al., "Use of Tumor-Infiltrating Lymphocytes and Interleukin-2 in the Immunotherapy of Patients with Metastatic Melanoma," in *New England Journal of Medicine* (December 22, 1988): 1676-80; Eva Lotzova and Ronald B. Herberman, eds., *Interleukin-2 and Killer Cells in Cancer* (Boca Raton, FL: CRC Press, 1990); John F. DiPersio and David W. Golde, "Hematopoietic Growth Factors," in Haskell, 931-40.

37. National Cancer Institute, "Biological Therapies: Newest Form of Cancer Treatment," *Cancer Facts* (December 1988): 9-10; Eberlein et al., 121-22. See also DiPersio and Golde.

38. National Cancer Institute, "Gene Therapy Vaccine Trial," *Cancer Facts* (October 1991), 1-3.

39. Charles D. Bankhead, "Optimal Hyperthermia Temp Cited," *Medical World News* (February 12, 1990): 29. On hyperthermia, see also F. Kristian Storm, "Hyperthermia," in Haskell, 915-18.

40. The study suggested that ultrasound may promote the absorption of doxorubicin by the tumor. See John Urbon et al., "Retrospective Analysis of Hyperthermia for Use in the Palliative Treatment of Cancer: A Multi-Modality Evaluation," *International Journal of Radiation Oncology* 18, no. 1 (January 1990): 155-63.

41. Laszlo, 241.

Chapter 5: Alternative Treatments

1. These categories are based on similar ones developed by Michael Lerner, a nationally recognized expert on alternative cancer treatments. Michael Lerner is president of Commonweal, a health service and research center in Bolinas, California, and founder of the Commonweal Cancer Help Program, a residential psychoeducational program for cancer patients. He is a lecturer in the Division of Family and Community Medicine, University of California, San Francisco, School of Medicine, and a primary consultant to a study of unconventional cancer therapies by the Office of Technology Assessment of the United States Congress. A periodically updated collection of works in progress and papers by Lerner and his colleagues is published by Commonweal under the title *Varieties of Integral Cancer Therapy.*

2. "Unproven Methods of Cancer Management: Laetrile," *CA: A Cancer Journal for Clinicians* (May-June 1991): 187. In a study of laetrile conducted by the National Cancer Institute, "no substantive benefit was observed in terms of cure, improvement, or stabilization of cancer, improve-ment of symptoms related to cancer, or extension of lifespan. The hazards of [laetrile] were evidenced in several patients by symptoms of cyanide toxicity or by blood cyanide levels approaching the lethal range." Charles G. Moertel

et al., "A Clinical Trial of Mygdalin (Laetrile) in the Treatment of Human Cancer," *New England Journal of Medicine* 306, no. 4 (1982): 201.

3. Because it has not been approved by the FDA, laetrile cannot legally be transported across state lines or brought from another country into the United States. Beginning in 1977, an exception was made if the laetrile was for the personal use of a patient whose physician had signed an affidavit stating that he or she was terminally ill. This exception was overturned in 1987. It is also illegal to use laetrile *within* a state that has no explicit law allowing such use. As of this writing, twenty states do have such laws. It is therefore legal to use laetrile in those states *provided* that the laetrile *is legally manufactured, distributed, and administered within the state*. To the best of our knowledge, however, there is no state where these conditions are currently being met.

4. James W. Forsythe, MD, interview with Alpha Institute, Reno, NV, August 23, 1990. All quotations from Dr. Forsythe in Chapter 5 are taken from this interview.

5. The American Cancer Society has published nonclinical studies of selected alternative therapies. These studies are based on a review of existing literature in the field. See "Unproven Methods of Cancer Management: Livingston-Wheeler Therapy," *CA: A Cancer Journal for Clinicians* (March-April 1990): 103-8; "Unproven Methods of Cancer Management: Gerson Method," *CA: A Cancer Journal for Clinicians* (July-August 1990): 252-56.

6. U.S. Food and Drug Administration, *Laetrile: The Commissioner's Report,* HEW Publication no. 77-3056, July 29, 1977. See also Gerald E. Markel and James Peterson, *Politics, Science, and Cancer: The Laetrile Phenomenon* (Boulder, CO: Westview Press, 1980), 51; and note 2 above.

7. Andrew Moyce, MD, memorandum to Alpha Institute, August 13, 1990.

8. American Cancer Society, *Cancer Facts and Figures: 1992* (Atlanta, GA: American Cancer Society, 1991), 13, 14, 8.

9. New York Botanical Garden, telephone conversation with Alpha Institute, September 23, 1992.

10. Peter Barry Chowka, "Cancer 1988," *East/West Journal* (December 1987): 52.

11. Michael Lerner, "A Report on Complementary Cancer Therapies," *Advances* 2, no. 1 (Winter 1985): 34.

12. Douglas Brodie, MD, interview with Alpha Institute, Incline Village, NV, August 8, 1990.

13. Barrie R. Cassileth, "Contemporary Unorthodox Treatments in Cancer: A Study of Patients, Treatments, and Practitioners," *Annals of Internal Medicine* 7 (1984): 105-12.

14. Michael Lerner has encountered similar complaints. See Michael Lerner, "Exceptional Cancer Patients as an Emerging Force in Cancer Therapy and Care" (Paper delivered at the World Health Organization Conference, Bad Honnef, Germany, June 1987), in Varieties of Integral Cancer Therapy, 10th ed., ed. Michael Lerner (Bolinas, CA: Commonweal, 1990), unpaginated.

Chapter 6:
Coping: Meeting the Challenges

1. Andrew W. Kneier, memorandum to Alpha Institute, July 21, 1992. Andrew Kneier is affiliated with the UCSF Cancer Center at Mt. Zion Hospital, in San Francisco. We are indebted to him for many of the ideas that we present in the first part of this chapter.

2. Ricki Dienst, interview with Alpha Institute, Berkeley, CA, August 20, 1992. All quotations from Ricki Dienst in Chapter 6 are taken from this interview.

3. Massimo Biondi and Giorgio D. Kotzalidis, "Human Psychoneuroimmunology Today," *Journal of Clinical Laboratory Analysis* 4 (1990): 24.

4. Hal Stone and Sidra Stone, *Embracing Your Inner Critic* (New York: HarperCollins Publishers, HarperSan Francisco, In press).

5. Ibid.

6. For a good general discussion of psychoneuroimmunology, see G.F. Solomon, "Psychoneuroimmunology: Interactions between Central Nervous System and Immune System," *Journal of Neuroscience Research* 18 (1987): 1-9.

7. Ronald Glaser et al., "Stress Depresses Interferon Production by Leukocytes Concomitant with a Decrease in Natural Killer Cell Activity," *Behavioral Neuroscience* 100, no. 5 (1986): 675-78.

8. Biondi and Kotzalidis, 24.

9. Ibid., 23.

10. Lawrence S. Sklar and Hymie Anisman, "Stress and Cancer," *Psychological Bulletin* 89, no. 3 (May 1981): 369-406; Ann O'Leary, "Stress, Emotion, and Human Immune Function," *Psychological Bulletin* 108, no. 3 (November 1990): 372-73; Amanda J. Ramirez et al., "Stress and Relapse of Breast Cancer," *British Medical Journal* 298 (February 4, 1989): 291-95; Jeremy Wood, O.J.A. Gilmore, and R.J. Pope, "Stress and Relapse of Breast Cancer," *British Medical Journal* 298 (April 8, 1989) 962-63.

11. Sklar and Anisman, 395; O'Leary; Ramirez et al. See also W.H. Redd and P.B. Jacobsen, "Emotions and Cancer: New Perspectives on an Old Question," *Cancer* 62 (1988): 1871-79; S. Ben-Eliyahu et al., "Stress Increases Metastatic Spread of a Mammary Tumor in Rats: Evidence for Mediation by the Immune System," *Brain, Behavior, and Immunity* 5 (1991): 193-205; Joanne Weinberg and Joanne T. Emerman, "Effects of Psychosocial Stressors on Mouse Mammary Tumor Growth," *Brain, Behavior, and Immunity* 3 (1989): 234-46.

12. David Speigel et al., "Effect of Psychosocial Treatment on Survival of Patients with Metastatic Breast Cancer," *Lancet* 2 (1989): 888-91.

13. Janice K. Kiecolt-Glaser et al., "Modulation of Cellular Immunity in Medical Students," *Journal of Behavioral Medicine* 9, no. 1 (1986): 5-21.

14. Norman Cousins, *Anatomy of an Illness* (New York: W.W. Morton & Co., 1979), 39.

15. Rosemary Cogan et al., "Effects of Laughter and Relaxation on Discomfort Thresholds," *Journal of Behavioral Medicine* 10, no. 2 (1987):

139-44; Lee S. Berk et al., "Neurendocrine and Stress Hormone Changes during Mirthful Laughter," *American Journal of the Medical Sciences* 298, no. 6 (December 1989): 390-96. See also L.S. Berk et al., "Eustress of Mirthful Laughter Modifies Natural Killer Cell Activity," *Clinical Research* 37, no. 1 (1989): 115A.

16. American Cancer Society, *Cancer Facts and Figures: 1992* (Atlanta, GA: American Cancer Society, 1991), 1, 13.

17. Arthur T. Skarin et al., "Lymphoma," in *Cancer Manual*, 8th ed., ed. Robert T. Osteen et al. (Boston: American Cancer Society, Massachusetts Division, 1990), 336.

18. Martin E.P. Seligman, *Learned Optimism* (New York: Alfred A. Knopf, 1991); David D. Burns, *The Feeling Good Handbook: Using the New Mood Therapy in Everyday Life* (New York: William Morrow & Co., 1989).

19. Nancy Heck, RPT, memorandum to Alpha Institute, August 20, 1992. All quotations from Nancy Heck in Chapter 6 are taken from this memorandum.

20. On the relationship between social support and healing, see Dean Ornish, "Lifestyle Changes of the Rich and Famous," Chap. 4 in *Dr. Dean Ornish's Program for Reversing Heart Disease* (New York: Random House, 1990), 85-93. This chapter cites numerous studies that suggest a connection between the two factors. Some of these studies had cancer patients as their subjects; others examined the effect of social support on immune function or on cardiac disease.

21. Paul Brenner, MD, telephone interview with Alpha Institute, San Francisco, CA, September 9, 1992. All quotations from Dr. Brenner in Chapter 6 are taken from this interview.

22. Karin Selbach, RN, interview with Alpha Institute, Oakland, CA, February 23, 1992. On support groups, see also Shelley E. Taylor et al., "Social Support, Support Groups, and the Cancer Patient," *Journal of Consulting and Clinical Psychology* 54, no. 5 (October 1986): 608-15.

23. Robert Fuhr, interview with Alpha Institute, Menlo Park, CA, February 18, 1992.

24. On the benefits of counseling for cancer patients, see S. Greer, "Can Psychological Therapy Improve the Quality of Life of Patients with Cancer?" *British Journal of Cancer* 59, no. 2 (February 1989): 149-51.

25. Douglas Brodie, MD, interview with Alpha Institute, Incline Village, NV, August 8, 1990.

26. Robert Fried, "Integrating Music in Breathing Training and Relaxation: I. Background, Rationale, and Relevant Elements," *Biofeedback and Self-Regulation* 15, no. 2 (1990): 161-69. See also Mark S. Rider et al., "The Effect of Music, Imagery, and Relaxation on Adrenal Corticosteroids and the Re-enactment of Circadian Rhythms," *Journal of Music Therapy* 22, no. 1 (1985): 46-58.

27. See, for example, Alan Beck and Aaron Katcher, *Between Pets and People: The Importance of Animal Companionship* (New York: Putnam Publishing, 1983); Phil Arkow, ed., for the Latham Foundation, *The Loving Bond: Companion Animals in the Helping Professions* (Saratoga, CA: R & E Publishers, 1987).

28. Herbert Benson, *The Relaxation Response* (New York: William Morrow & Company, 1975), 18.

29. For an interesting discussion of the history of meditation in a religious context, see Herbert Benson, John F. Beary, and Mark P. Carol, "The Relaxation Response," *Psychiatry* 37 (February 1974): 38-40.

30. Herbert Benson, *Your Maximum Mind* (New York: Avon Books, 1989), 200-202.

31. Ibid., 202.

32. Benson, *Relaxation Response,* 65ff.

33. For a good discussion of the uses of imagery in healing, written for the lay reader, see Mike Samuels and Nancy Samuels, *The Well Adult* (New York: Summit, 1988), 64-70.

34. Lily Kravcisin, interview with Alpha Institute, Woodside, CA, January 8, 1990.

35. Carol Landt, memorandum to Alpha Institute, May 20, 1992.

36. William H. Redd and Michael Andrykowski, "Behavioral Intervention in Cancer Treatment: Controlling Aversion Reactions to Chemotherapy," *Journal of Consulting and Clinical Psychology* 50, no. 6 (December 1982): 1018-29; Michael P. Carey and Thomas G. Burish, "Etiology and Treatment of the Psychological Side Effects Associated with Cancer Chemotherapy: A Critical Review and Discussion," *Psychological Bulletin* 104, no. 3 (November 1988): 307-25; Jeanne Lyles et al., "Efficacy of Relaxation Training and Guided Imagery in Reducing the Aversiveness of Cancer Chemotherapy," *Journal of Consulting and Clinical Psychology* 50, no. 4 (August 1982): 509-24.

37. Carey and Burish.

38. Deborah Blumenthal, "Massage Goes Main," *American Health* (October 1991): 70.

39. Karry M. Miller and Patsy A. Perry, "Relaxation Technique and Postoperative Pain in Patients Undergoing Cardiac Surgery," *Heart and Lung* 19 (1990): 136-46; Karry M. Miller, "Deep Breathing Relaxation: A Pain Management Technique," *AORN Journal* 45, no. 2 (February 1987): 484-88. See also Geraldine G. Flaherty and Joyce J. Fitzpatrick, "Relaxation Technique to Increase Comfort Level in Postoperative Patients: A Preliminary Study," *Nursing Research* 27, no. 6 (1978): 352-55. For an interesting discussion of the use of breathing to decrease physical and emotional pain, see Joan Borysenko, *Minding the Body, Mending the Mind* (Reading, MA: Addison-Wesley Publishing Co., 1987), 83-87.

40. On the uses of breathing training to control anxiety, see P. Grossman, J.C.G. de Swart, and P.B. Defares, "A Controlled Study of a Breathing Therapy for Treatment of Hyperventilation Syndrome," *Journal of Psychosomatic Research* 29, no. 1 (1985): 49-58; George A. Hibbert and Michael Chan, "Respiratory Control: Its Contribution to the Treatment of Panic Attacks," *British Journal of Psychiatry* 154 (1989): 232-26.

Chapter 7:
For Family and Friends

We are indebted to Andrew W. Kneier and Robert Fuhr for many of the ideas that we present in this chapter.

1. For a general discussion of these issues, see Nancy F. Woods, Frances Marcus Lewis, and Edythe S. Ellison, "Living with Cancer: Family Experiences," *Cancer Nursing* 12, no. 1 (1989): 28-33.

2. Annette Pont-Gwire, memorandum to Alpha Institute, October 19, 1992. All quotations from Annette Pont-Gwire in Chapter 7 are taken from this memorandum.

3. Carol Landt, memorandum to Alpha Institute, May 20, 1992. All quotations from Carol Landt in Chapter 7 are taken from this memorandum.

4. Andrew W. Kneier, memorandum to Alpha Institute, September 16, 1992. All quotations from Andrew W. Kneier in Chapter 7 are taken from this memorandum.

5. Robert Fuhr, memorandum to Alpha Institute, October 4, 1992. All quotations from Robert Fuhr in Chapter 7 are taken from this memorandum.

6. Lily Kravcisin, interview with Alpha Institute, Woodside, CA, February 7, 1990.

7. For a discussion of the ways in which children cope, see L. Michele Issel, Mary Ersek, and Frances Marcus Lewis, "How Children Cope with Mother's Breast Cancer," *Oncology Nursing Forum* 17, no. 3 (Supplement, 1990): 5-13.

8. Dian Marino, "White Flowers and a Grizzly Bear: Living with Cancer," *New Internationalist* (August 1989): 8-9.

Chapter 8:
...and Living

1. Shannon Ruff Dirksen, "Perceived Well-Being in Malignant Melanoma Survivors," *Oncology Nursing Forum* 16, no. 3 (1989): 353-58; Alastair J. Cunningham, Gina A. Lockwood, and John A. Cunningham, "A Relationship between Perceived Self-Efficacy and Quality of Life in Cancer Patients," *Patient Education and Counseling* 17 (1991): 71-78. See also J. Bloom, "Social Support, Accommodation to Stress, and Adjustment to Breast Cancer," *Social Service and Medicine* 16, no. 14 (1982): 1329-38.

2. Frances Marcus Lewis, "Experienced Personal Control and Quality of Life in Late-Stage Cancer Patients," *Nursing Research* 31, no. 2 (March-April 1982): 113-19.

3. Cunningham, Lockwood, and Cunningham, 75-76; Lewis, 116.

4. Lewis, 116.

5. Cunningham, Lockwood, and Cunningham, 76.

6. Ibid.

7. Melvin Seeman and Teresa E. Seeman, "Health Behavior and Personal Autonomy: A Longitudinal Study of the Sense of Control in Illness," *Journal of Health and Social Behavior* 24 (June 1983): 144-60.

8. Sue A. Wiedenfeld et al., "Impact of Perceived Self-Efficacy in Coping with Stressors on Components of the Immune System," *Journal of Personality and Social Psychology* 59, no. 5 (1990): 1082-94.

9. William J. Knaus, *Do It Now: How to Stop Procrastinating* (New York: Prentice-Hall, 1979).

10. George Somogyi, interview with Alpha Institute, Alameda, CA, December 9, 1991.

11. Joy L. Johnson and Janice M. Morse, "Regaining Control: The Process of Adjustment after Myocardial Infarction," *Heart and Lung* 19 (1990): 133.

12. Lynn P. Rehm, "Mood, Pleasant Events, and Unpleasant Events: Two Pilot Studies," *Journal of Consulting and Clinical Psychology* 46, no. 5 (1978): 855.

13. Ibid., 854-59; Arthur A. Stone, "Event Content in a Daily Survey Is Differentially Associated with Concurrent Mood," *Journal of Personality and Social Psychology* 52, no. 1 (1987): 56-58.

14. Stone, 57.

15. Paul Rohde et al., "Dimensionality of Coping and Its Relation to Depression," *Journal of Personality and Social Psychology* 58, no. 3 (1990): 505.

16. Arthur A. Stone et al., "Evidence That Secretory IgA Antibody Is Associated with Daily Mood," *Journal of Personality and Social Psychology* 52, no. 5 (1987): 988-93.

17. Clark W. Heath, Jr., "Cancer Prevention," in *American Cancer Society Textbook of Clinical Oncology,* ed. Arthur I. Holleb, Diane J. Fink, and Gerald P. Murphy (Atlanta, GA: American Cancer Society, 1991), 101; Lawrence E. Lamb, "Understanding Cancer," *Health Letter,* special report 123 (November 1991): 1.

18. Heath, 101.

19. B.E. Henderson, R.K. Ross, and M.C. Pike, "Toward the Primary Prevention of Cancer," *Science* 254 (November 22, 1991): 1137. The authors define the causes of cancer as "categories of human environmental exposure for which epidemiologic evidence alone is sufficiently consistent and strong" to categorize them as such.

20. The Work Study Group on Diet, Nutrition, and Cancer: Sidney Weinhouse et al., "American Cancer Society Guidelines on Diet, Nutrition, and Cancer," *CA: A Cancer Journal for Clinicians* 41, no. 6 (November-December 1991): 335.

21. Ibid., 337.

22. Bruce Ames, "Be Most Wary of Nature's Own Pesticides," *Consumer's Research* (May 1989): 14.

23. Work Study Group, 335-36.

24. Ibid., 336. See also Bernard E. Statland, "Nutrition and Cancer," *Clinical Chemistry* 38, no. 8 (1992): 1587-94.

25. G. Block, "Epidemiologic Evidence Regarding Vitamin C and Cancer," *American Journal of Clinical Nutrition* 54, supp. 6 (December 1991): 1310S-14S. See also J.F Dorgan and A. Schatzkin, "Antioxidant Micronutrients in Cancer Prevention," *Hematology/Oncology Clinics of North America* 5, no. 1 (February 1991): 43-68.

26. Statland, 1592.

27. See, for example, Henry D. Janowitz, *Your Gut Feeling: A Complete Guide to Living Better with Intestinal Problems* (New York: Oxford University Press, 1987).

28. K.K. Carroll, M. Lipkin, and J.H. Weisburger, "Diet's Key Role in Preventing Cancer," *Patient Care* (May 15, 1989): 54.

29. Ritva R. Butrum, Carolyn K. Clifford, and Elaine Lanza, "NCI Dietary Guidelines: Rationale," *American Journal of Clinical Nutrition* 48 (1988): 889.

30. Carroll, Lipkin, and Weisburger, 54-74.

31. Henderson, Ross, and Pike, 1131-38.

32. E. Danforth, Jr., "Diet and Obesity," *American Journal of Clinical Nutrition* 41 (1985): 1132-45; Statland, 1592-93.

33. "Changing U.S. Consumption Trends," *Nutrition Research Newsletter* (October 1989): 116.

34. "Figures: Twelve Tips for Trimming Fat Back to the Magical 30 Percent of Calories," *In Health* (November-December 1990): 73.

35. Work Study Group, 336.

36. Jerome L. Knittle and David P. Katz, "Weight Control," in *The Mount Sinai School of Medicine Complete Book of Nutrition,* ed. Victor Herbert and Genell J. Subak-Sharpe (New York: St. Martin's Press, 1990), 283.

37. W. Virgil Brown, "Fats and Cholesterol," in Herbert and Subak-Sharpe, 61.

38. Nancy A. Bennett, MS, RD, interview with Alpha Institute, San Francisco, CA, September 16, 1992. All quotations from Nancy A. Bennett in Chapter 8 are taken from this interview.

39. On the beneficial effects of aerobic exercise, see K.H. Cooper, *The Aerobics Program for Total Well-Being* (New York: M. Evans & Co., 1982), 112-16.

40. Cooper, 111; Carolyn D. Berdanier and Michael K. McIntosh, "Weight Loss–Weight Regain: A Vicious Cycle," *Nutrition Today* (September-October 1991): 10.

41. Steven N. Blair et al., "Physical Fitness and All Cause Mortality, A Prospective Study of Healthy Men and Women," *Journal of the American Medical Association* 262, no. 17 (November 3, 1989: 2395-2401.

42. H.W. Kohl, Ronald E. LaPorte, and Steven N. Blair, "Physical Activity and Cancer: An Epidemiological Perspective," *Sports Medicine* 6 (1988): 222-37.

43. John E. Vena et al., "Lifetime Occupational Exercise and Colon Cancer," *American Journal of Epidemiology* 122, no. 3 (September 1985): 357-65.

44. R.E. Frisch et al., "Lower Prevalence of Breast Cancer and Cancers of the Reproductive System among Former College Athletes Compared to Non-Athletes," *British Journal of Cancer* 52 (1985): 885-91.

45. Blair et al., 2398.

46. Kurt Elward and Eric B. Larson, "Benefits of Exercise for Older Adults: A Review of Existing Evidence and Current Recommendations for the General Population," *Clinics in Geriatric Medicine* 8, no. 1 (February 1992): 35-46; Per-Olof Astrand, "Physical Activity and Fitness," *American Journal of Clinical Nutrition* 55 (1992): 1231S-36S; Judith M. Riffee, "Osteoporosis: Prevention and Management," *American Pharmacy* NS32, no. 8 (August 1992): 68-69.

47. James A. Blumenthal et al., "Cardiovascular and Behavioral Effects of Aerobic Exercise Training in Healthy Older Men and Women," *Journal of Gerontology* 44, no. 5 (1989): M 147-57. See also Posner et al., "Low to Moderate Intensity Endurance Training in Healthy Older Adults: Physiological Responses after Four Months," *Journal of the American Geriatrics Society* 40, no. 1 (January 1992): 1-7; Elward and Larson, 42; Astrand, 1233S.

48. M. Brown and J.O. Holloszy,"Effects of a Low Intensity Exercise Program on Selected Physical Performance Characteristics of Sixty- to Seventy-one-Year Olds," *Aging* 3, no. 2 (1991): 129-39.

49. For more on setting up an exercise program, see Cooper 123-36.

50. Lynn Fitzgerald, "Exercise and the Immune System," *Immunology Today* 9, no. 11 (1988): 337-39; Heyward L. Nash, "Can Exercise Make Us Immune to Disease?" *The Physician and Sportsmedicine* 14, no. 3 (March 1986): 250-53.

51. Bess H. Marcus et al., "Usefulness of Physical Exercise for Maintaining Smoking Cessation in Women," *American Journal of Cardiology* 68 (August 1, 1991): 406-7. See also C.B. Taylor et al., "Smoking Cessation after Acute Myocardial Infarction: The Effects of Exercise Training," *Addictive Behaviors* 13 (1988): 331-34.

52. Nancy L. Keim, Teresa F. Barbieri, and Amy Z. Belko, "The Effect of Exercise on Energy Intake and Body Composition in Overweight Women," *International Journal of Obesity* 14 (1990): 335-46. See also R. Woo, J.S. Garrow, and F.X. Pi-Sunyer, "Effect of Exercise on Spontaneous Calorie Intake in Obesity," *American Journal of Clinical Nutrition* 36 (1982): 470-77.

53. David C. Nieman, Jeann M. Onasch, and Jerry W. Lee, "The Effects of Moderate Exercise Training on Nutrient Intake in Mildly Obese Women," *Journal of the American Dietetic Association* 90 (1990): 1557-62.

54. Daniel B. Carr et al., "Physical Conditioning Facilitates the Exercise-Induced Secretion of Beta-Endorphin and Beta-Lipotropin in Women," *New England Journal of Medicine* (September 3, 1981): 560-62.

55. David Sinyor et al., "Aerobic Fitness Level and Reactivity to Psychosocial Stress: Physiological, Biochemical, and Subjective Measures," *Psychosomatic Medicine* 45, no. 3 (June 1983): 205-17.

56. Lisa McCann and David S. Holmes, "Influence of Aerobic Exercise on Depression," *Journal of Personality and Social Psychology* 46, no. 5 (1984): 1142-47. See also John H. Greist et al., "Running as Treatment for Depression," *Comprehensive Psychiatry* 20, no. 1 (1979): 41-53.

57. Greist et al., 48-49.

58. Edward McAuley, Kerry S. Courneya, and Janice Lettunich, "Effects of Acute and Long-Term Exercise on Self-Efficacy Responses in Sedentary, Middle-Aged Males and Females," *Gerontologist* 31, no. 4 (1991): 534-42.

59. Lawrence Garfinkel, "Overweight and Cancer," Annals of Internal Medicine 103, no. 6 (December 1985): 1034-36.

60. Edward A. Lew and Lawrence Garfinkel, "Variations in Mortality by Weight among 750,000 Men and Women," *Journal of Chronic Disease* 32 (1979): 569.

61. Berdanier and McIntosh, 12.

62. Editors of the *University of California at Berkeley Wellness Letter, The Wellness Encyclopedia* (Boston: Houghton Mifflin, 1991), 33.

63. Ibid., 32-34.

64. Robert Fuhr, interview with Alpha Institute, Alameda, CA, June 6, 1992, and subsequent correspondence. All quotations from Robert Fuhr in Chapter 8 are taken from these sources.

65. "Facts about Cigarette Smoking," brochure published by the American Lung Association, 0171, 1990.

66. American Cancer Society, *Cancer Facts and Figures: 1992* (Atlanta, GA: American Cancer Society, 1991), 18.

67. Ibid.

68. Ibid., 9, 18.

69. Ibid., 18.

70. Ibid., 19.

71. Studies cited in Charles B. Sherman, "Health Effects of Cigarette Smoking," *Clinics in Chest Medicine* 12, no. 4 (December 1991): 643-58.

72. Jonathan E. Fielding, "Smoking: Health Effects and Control," *New England Journal of Medicine* 313, no. 8 (August 22, 1985): 491.

73. American Cancer Society, 19.

74. Ibid.

75. Cited in Fielding, 495. See also Anne L. Wright et al., "Relationship of Parental Smoking to Wheezing and Nonwheezing Lower Respiratory Tract Illness in Infancy," *Journal of Pediatrics* 118 (February 1991): 207-14; Louis I. Landau, "Smoking and Childhood Asthma," *Medical Journal of Australia* 154 (June 3, 1991): 715-16.

76. American Cancer Society, 19.

77. American Thoracic Society, "Health Effects of Smoking on Children," *American Review of Respiratory Disease* 132, no. 5 (November 1985): 1137-38.

78. Donald P. Kadunce et al., "Cigarette Smoking: Risk Factor for Premature Facial Wrinkling," *Annals of Internal Medicine* 114, no. 10 (May 15, 1991): 840-44.

79. M. Condra et al., "Prevalence and Significance of Tobacco Smoking in Impotence," *Urology* 27, no. 6 (June 1986): 495-98. See also S. Glina et al., "Impact of Cigarette Smoking on Papaverine-Induced Erection," *Journal of Urology* 140, no. 3 (September 1988): 523-24.

80. "Facts about Cigarette Smoking."

81. Carolyn Gloeckner, "Where There's Smoke, There's Disease," *Current Health* (November 2, 1990): 14-15.

82. U.S. Department of Health and Human Services, Public Health Service, Centers for Disease Control, *The Health Benefits of Smoking Cessation: A Report of the Surgeon General*, 1990, DHHS Publication no. (CDC) 90-8419.

83. Jerome L. Schwartz, "Methods for Smoking Cessation," *Clinics in Chest Medicine* 12, no. 4 (December 1991): 739.

84. "Public Health Focus: Effectiveness of Smoking Control Strategies–United States," *Journal of the American Medical Association* 268, no. 13 (October 7, 1992): 1645.

85. Liro S. Covey and Alexander Glassman, "New Approaches to Smoking Cessation," *Physician Assistant* (November 1991): 70.

86. "Nicotine Patches," *Medical Letter on Drugs and Therapeutics* 34, no. 868 (April 17, 1992): 38. See also Transdermal Nicotine Study Group,

"Transdermal Nicotine for Smoking Cessation," *Journal of the American Medical Association* 226, no. 22 (December 11, 1991): 3133-38.

87. Covey and Glassman, 74.

88. "Smoking Cessation: The Best Ways to Kick the Deadliest, Most Expensive Addiction," *Public Citizen Health Research Group Health Letter* 4, no. 10 (October 1988): 6. See also Schwartz, 744-46.

89. "Facts about Cigarette Smoking."

90. International Agency for Research on Cancer, "Alcohol Drinking," *IARC Monograph on the Evaluation of the Carcinogenic Risk to Humans* 44 (1988): 255.

91. S.Y. Choi and H. Kahyo, "Effect of Cigarette Smoking and Alcohol Consumption in the Aetiology of Cancer of the Oral Cavity, Pharynx, and Larynx," *International Journal of Epidemiology* 4 (December 20, 1991): 878-85.

92. William J. Blot et al., "Smoking and Drinking in Relation to Oral and Pharyngeal Cancer," *Cancer Research* 48 (June 1, 1988): 3282-87.

93. Regina G. Ziegler, "Alcohol-Nutrient Interactions in Cancer Etiology," *Cancer* 58 (1986): 1942-48.

94. Marsha Hudnall, "Alcohol Poses Many Health Risks, Few Benefits," *Environmental Nutrition* 12 (July 1989): 1-3.

95. See Bassam Moushmoush and Pierre Abi-Mansour, "Alcohol and the Heart: The Long-Term Effects of Alcohol on the Cardiovascular System," *Archives of Internal Medicine* (January 1991): 36-43. See also Emanuel Rubin, "How Alcohol Damages the Body," *Alcohol Health and Research World* 13 (Fall 1989): 322-28.

96. Rubin.

97. U.S. Department of Health and Human Services, Public Health Service, *Morbidity and Mortality Weekly Reports* 39, no. 49 (December 14, 1990).

98. State of California Department of Health Services, "Alcohol-Related Mortality, California 1990," *A Data Summary* (February 1991).

99. Michael J. Lewis, "Alcohol: Mechanisms of Addiction and Reinforcement," *Advances in Alcohol and Substance Abuse* 9, no. 1-2 (1990): 48.

100. For a detailed description of the neurological processes involved, see Michael E. Charness, "Alcohol and the Brain," *Alcohol Health and Research World* 14 (Spring 1990): 85-90.

101. "Ways to Detox Your Home: Safe Houses," *American Health* (March 1992): 88, 90; American Cancer Society, 17, 19, 20; Robert Berkow, ed., *The Merck Manual of Diagnosis and Therapy,* 16th ed. (Rahway, NJ: Merck & Co., 1992), 2644-45; "The Pollutants That Matter Most: Lead, Radon, Nitrate," *Consumer Reports* (January 1990): 31.

102. "Ways to Detox."

103. American Cancer Society, 17, 13.

104. Alexandra Greeley, "No Tan Is a Safe Tan: Depletion of the Ozone Layer Impairs Protective Screen against Cancer," *Nutrition Health Review* (Summer 1991): 14-16; "Sunlight, DNA, and Skin Cancer," *Lancet* 1 (June 1989): 1362-63.

105. John Stephen Taylor, "Immune Suppression Caused by Sun Exposure," *NCI Weekly* (September 4, 1989): 4-6.

106. Quoted in Greeley, 16.

107. Quoted in "The Rising Risk of Skin Cancer," *University of California at Berkeley Wellness Letter* 7, no. 10 (July 1991): 2.

108. For more on this subject, see Raphael Warren et al., "Age, Sunlight, and Facial Skin: A Histologic and Quantitative Study," *Journal of the American Academy of Dermatology* (November 1991): 751-61.

109. Antony W. Sedgwick et al., "Follow-up of Stress-Management Courses," *Medical Journal of Australia* 150 (May 1, 1989): 485-89.

110. Dean Ornish et al., "Effects of Stress Management Training and Dietary Changes in Treating Ischemic Heart Disease," *Journal of the American Medical Association* 249, no. 1 (January 7, 1983): 57.

111. Maurizio Fava et al., "Psychological and Behavioral Benefits of a Stress/Type A Behavior Reduction Program for Healthy Middle-Aged Army Officers," *Psychosomatics* 32, no. 3 (Summer 1991): 341.

112. American Cancer Society, 10.

113. American Cancer Society, 1. We define the term "cured" on page 33.

114. Tim Friend, "The Overlooked Disease," *Men's Health* (February 1992): 31.

115. American Cancer Society, 10.

116. In one national survey, fewer than half of the men who had *ever* had a physical said that it included a rectal exam. "Prostate Cancer: Some Good News Men Can Live With," brochure published by the National Cancer Institute, copyright 1989 by the Prostate Cancer Education Council.

117. Diane J. Fink, *Guidelines for the Career-Related Checkup* (Atlanta, GA: American Cancer Society, 1991), 20-21.

118. Ibid., 18-19, 29, 15.

Appendix 1:
The Dying Patient

1. James P. Carse, telephone interview with Alpha Institute, June 8, 1992. All quotations from James P. Carse in Appendix 1 are taken from this interview.

2. Elisabeth Kübler-Ross, *On Death and Dying* (New York: Macmillan Publishing Co., 1969), 104.

3. Robert Fuhr, memorandum to Alpha Institute, October 23, 1992. All quotations from Robert Fuhr in Appendix 1 are taken from this memorandum.

4. Kübler-Ross, 156.

5. Carol Landt, memorandum to Alpha Institute, December 14, 1992.

Appendix 2:
Financial, Legal, Insurance, and Employment

Much of the material in this appendix is adapted from Barbara J. Hoffman, "Taking Care of Business: Employment, Insurance, and Money Matters," in National Coalition for Cancer Survivorship, *Charting the Journey: An Almanac of Practical Resources for Cancer Survivors,* ed. Fitzhugh Mullan, Barbara Hoffman, and the Editors of Consumer Reports Books (Mount Vernon, NY: Consumer's Union, 1990), 97-142.

1. The names of these companies are listed in Appendix A: "Cancer Survivorship Resources," in Mullan, Hoffman, and Consumer Reports Books, 192-93.

2. Ibid., 118.

3. National Institutes of Health, *Facing Forward: A Guide for Cancer Survivors,* Publication no. 90-2424, July 1990, 37.

4. Ibid., 36-37.

Index

B